Powerful Cancer-Fighting Foods

Exposing Medical Myths and Deceptions

Pauline White

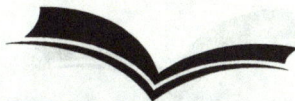

TEACH Services, Inc.
PUBLISHING
www.TEACHServices.com • (800) 367-1844

Copyright © 2022 Pauline White
Copyright © 2022 TEACH Services, Inc.
ISBN-13: 978-1-4796-0839-3- (Paperback)
ISBN-13: 978-1-4796-0840-9 (ePub)
Library of Congress Control Number: 2022912018

All Bible references are taken from the 1611 King James Version of the Bible. Public domain.

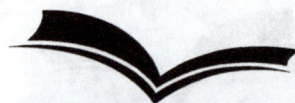

Published by

TEACH Services, Inc.
P U B L I S H I N G
www.TEACHServices.com • (800) 367-1844

Dedication

This book is dedicated to the memory of my late father. I have been encouraged by others to keep pressing forward with the research, writing and publishing of this life-enhancing and life-saving information, and I hope that it will be a blessing to many.

I wish you abundant health.

Pauline White.

Table of Contents

Introduction

This book is written and punctuated in British English.

The scriptures that are quoted herein are in red and from the 1611 King James Bible. They are generally spiritual reflections of the provided health information.

My original intention was to write small health nuggets for a whole-food, plant-based recipe and cooking DVD. I have been diligently working toward this goal for some years. However, as time passed, the nuggets grew into articles, which eventually became longer as time went on, and I was inspired to develop them into this book. I wrote this book to provide hope and encouragement, and to give others confidence in natural God-given plants that have been in existence for thousands of years and utilized for their life-giving properties, which have proven their effectiveness. This book is full of knowledge-based information that will benefit many lives. Most people have been affected in some way by cancer or other health issues that the medical establishment has deemed incurable by their methods. Drugs are not *health-care* but *sick-care*, and nature has been wisely designed so that healthful medicine is within reach in natural plant-foods. The most powerful healing substances in the world are masquerading as foods. Therefore, enjoying a healthy diet is not only health-care but also a form of self-respect. These natural plant-foods cannot be patented by drug companies, but are nevertheless very powerful, naturally detoxifying, and not harmful.

An article from the European Molecular Biology Organization (EMBO) provided through the National Center for Biotechnology Information (NCBI) discusses what disease *IS* and *IS NOT*:

> At first sight, the answer to "What is a disease?" is straightforward. Most of us feel we have an intuitive grasp of the idea, reaching mentally to images of memories of colds, cancer or tuberculosis. But a look through any medical dictionary soon shows that articulating a satisfactory definition of disease is surprisingly difficult. And it is not much help defining disease as the opposite of health, given that definitions of health are equally tricky.[1]

The most important medicine of all is educating people on how not to want unnatural medicine. A healthy diet and lifestyle can change the mind, body, mood, and attitude. According to studies, lifestyle choices determine health and

---

1 Jackie Leach Scully, "What is a disease?" EMBO reports, July 2004, https://1ref.us/1ne (accessed February 28, 2021).

not genes. Are you sick and tired of being sick and tired? Do you need help to overcome an addiction? Do you find yourself stressed and unable to cope with an illness? Do you want to feel full of life and energy? If so, read on and learn how to do this and so much more, because what you do not know can kill you and what you think you know can harm you. With God's natural plant-foods, you can heal yourself from the inside, out, without becoming harmed from the outside, in. I would like to encourage you to take responsibility for your own health and cancer-proof your life because good health should be your natural state and you can become your own best doctor, as sound knowledge and healthy, whole, unprocessed food is the safest and most powerful form of therapy. Good health is a right and not a privilege, so enjoy and get *vegucated* without being medicated as true education is far superior to drug medication, because those who have health have hope and real wealth, so invest in yourself.

"Be of good courage, and He shall strengthen your heart all ye that hope in the LORD" (Psalm 31:24).

Chapter 1

My Story

"THE ABILITY OF YOUR BODY TO HEAL IS MUCH GREATER THAN ANYONE HAS ALLOWED YOU TO BELIEVE."

On March 14th, 1983, my dearly beloved dad, Herbert W. P. White, died at the age of sixty-seven. This major event made an overwhelming impact on me and completely turned the direction of my life towards searching for the reasons why he died the way that he did. In the early 1970s he was diagnosed with bladder cancer and was given an overabundance of drugs, surgery, X-rays, radiation, and chemotherapy (which has never been a *therapy*), which caused him tremendous suffering and made him much worse. After undergoing a great many of these extremely painful protocols with no relief in sight, the former bladder cancer metastasized into bone cancer following the removal of his bladder. In mid-February 1983, an oncologist informed him that he had only four weeks to live and that there were no natural cures to help him at all.

I vividly recall the day when my mum and I went to visit my dad in hospital just before he died. He was laid out on a stretcher and trembling violently from excruciating pain. I immediately asked a staff nurse what was happening to him. She coldly informed me that they were using him for experiments. The next time we saw him he was breathing his last. He died exactly four weeks after he was told that he has only four weeks to live, and I have been on a quest for more knowledge on this and many other health subjects ever since. He was a Captain in the Queen's Own Royal West Kent Regiment and fought with the Eighth Army. He was a significantly decorated war hero and received a citation from King George V1 of the UK together with his Military Cross medal for bravery. He was also my hero. He survived a gunshot wound to his head during the World War II battle of Monte Cassino, and as a consequence suffered much pain from his head wound as well as vivid nightmares and post-traumatic stress disorder for many years afterwards until he died. He survived the gunshot wound of the enemy, but unfortunately not the poisonous treatments that came from the same source as the holocaust, which was the biggest battle of his entire life.

"He healeth the broken in heart, and bindeth up their wounds" (Psalm 147:3).

Both of my grandmothers were professional cooks in London, and my maternal grandmother also assisted her neighbours with natural health remedies, so these epigenetic traits have likely been passed on to me. When I was a young child, I often became very ill. Our local doctor was a regular visitor to our household of six, as it seemed we were a sickly bunch. But even after many bottles of different coloured, unpleasant-tasting concoctions were unceremoniously dispatched down my throat, I did not improve. It was following my second operation when I was five years old, and while I was still sick in hospital, that I was held fast by several hospital staff while they forced smallpox poison into my arm by multiple skin punctures, which was very painful. At a young age, I consumed a fair amount of sugar and other unhealthy substances and was often vaccinated at school.

Not long after my dad died, I started to research about health. I also attended numerous courses which I thought would help me to learn about good health, but I later discovered that they had questionable principles which were not rooted and grounded in the truth. When I read some information that nitrogen mustard (an active component of World War I mustard gas) was used in chemotherapy I could hardly believe it, so I asked two medical doctors with whom I was completing a course, and they informed me that mustard gas and its derivative, nitrogen mustard, was indeed used in chemotherapy. I was horrified as that was what they had used on my dad that made his suffering so much worse. I have always loved to cook and be creative, and before I started to learn about good health I was consuming a lot of animal products, tea, coffee, chocolate, sugar, and other injurious substances, which I decided to forgo when I discovered that there was a better way to live, and started to put into practice what I had learnt about a healthy whole plant-food diet.

I have learnt much about cancer and other health issues over many years through diligent research and study, and have discovered that it is the simple and inexpensive God-given natural remedies that can reverse not only cancer but also many other health issues. Drugs never cure disease, but just change its form and location. I also became a Seventh-day Adventist Christian eight years after my dad died, and now I also follow what the Bible says about healthy living and feel so much better for it and have much more energy.

There is hope for those who have cancer or other health issues if they are willing to follow the natural ways of a healthy diet and lifestyle. A well-informed person who chooses to take care of themselves is a powerful form of activism. Choosing natural healthy foods should be the healthy way to live, and making and consuming healthy, delicious, and satisfying recipes can easily become a way of life. Unfortunately, it is often the case that people consume junk foods and processed foods. Most people want to save time and money, but when they buy these products they are really doing neither in the long term, because when they become sick it generally costs them a lot more time and money and can even take their life prematurely, thereby losing precious time on this earth to bless others.

"The LORD bless thee, and keep thee: The LORD make His face to shine upon thee, and be gracious unto thee: The LORD lift up His countenance upon thee, and give thee peace" (Numbers 6:24–26).

Chapter 2

General Health Information

"SYMPTOMS ARE NOT DANGEROUS ENEMIES TO BE DESTROYED BUT FRIENDLY MESSENGERS WHO ENCOURAGE US TO TAKE MORE CARE OF OUR PRECIOUS GOD GIVEN BODIES."

Cancer Is Not a Disease but a Survival Mechanism

The body can remain healthy well into advanced age if it is given the opportunity to do so by maintaining a healthy diet and lifestyle. Cancer is not a disease but is part of an innately complex, intelligently-designed, healing and survival mechanism of the body, as no scientific proof exists to show that cancer is a disease.[2] Genes do not accidentally malfunction but can be the result of a traumatic past event, prolonged and intense stress, the death of a loved one, deep-seated frustration, worries, guilt, resentment, shame, and poor self-image. Unresolved emotional conflicts, accompanied by prolonged emotional stress, are able to compromise, suppress, and even shut down the immune system, thereby preventing healing and rendering the body susceptible to all types of illnesses. Childhood stress, including unborn and premature infants, can disrupt early brain development, compromise the function of the immune and nervous systems, and later impact adult health issues such as depression, heart disease, cancer, and other chronic health issues. Cancer can also be a spiritual result of unforgiveness. Those that are sick should first realize that their only hope is to surrender to Jesus Christ, who is the only true healer, as nature is the servant of God, who heals and restores.

"Let the people praise thee, O God; let all the people praise thee"
(Psalm 67:3).

---

[2] Jackie Leach Scully, "What is a disease?" EMBO reports, July 2004, https://1ref.us/1ne (accessed February 28, 2021).

It is a recognized fact that everyone has millions of cancer cells in their body at all times during their life. Even though the body makes millions of cancer cells daily, under severe temporary stress, some individuals produce more cancer cells than usual, which cluster together as tumours, and which disappear after a healing response when the impact of the stress has subsided. The body produces cancer cells continually, thereby keeping the immune system activated. Cancer cells can signal the immune system to allow them to grow, which results in larger tumours, as killing cancer cells with conventional methods can jeopardize the body's survival. These cancer cells keep toxic, deadly, carcinogenic substances and caustic metabolic waste matter away from vital organs as well as the blood and lymph. A tumour is comprised of this waste matter, which is surrounded by a membrane to protect the rest of the body. To remove the necessity for cancer initiation, the body should be cleansed of waste products and toxins. Without any scientific facts whatsoever, doctors and cancer researchers have falsely assumed that cancer results from cell mutations, which then have a life of their own. However, uncontrolled random cancer cell division does not occur. Cancer does not need to be treated with conventional methodologies which stem from unproven ideas that it will grow, spread, and kill its host if they do not conform to the establishment practices, which do great harm to the body. However, a healthy diet and lifestyle can prevent cancer from developing, assist the immune system, and deliver anti-cancer nutrients to the body which can also reverse health issues.

Those that are sick should first realize that their only hope is to surrender to Jesus Christ, who is the only true healer, as nature is the servant of God, who heals and restores.

It is untrue that healthy food cannot affect the progression and spread of cancer. Utilizing anti-cancer foods to prevent cancer can be clearly explained using current scientific research. There are many more natural, spontaneous remissions of cancer than there are from medical establishment diagnosed and treated cancers, and there is a growing undeniable weight of evidence that cancers can regress, stop, and disappear on their own. When the body has been abused it can restore balance if nature is given the opportunity to do so. Almost all cancers dissipate by themselves without any intervention from *big pharma*. However, if a tumour is located in a position that is blocking vital bodily functions, then surgical intervention may help in the interim if absolutely necessary. Cancer is not the killer that most people assume it to be, as up to 95% of all tumours that occur heal themselves when the causal factors are removed, as a cancer cell does not have the ability to kill anything. Nor has a cancerous tumour the ability of continuous destruction, or is a malicious process to overtake healthy cells, disrupt vital body functions, and annihilate the body. Self-destruction is not the purpose of any cell unless it has deteriorated and needs to be replaced, as health is optimal cell functioning. Cancer cells, as well as all other cells, do not exist to destroy the body. It is the wasting away of the body's cell tissue by the continued deprivation of life forces and nutrients together with a toxic overload that eventually leads to a demise of the body and is the predominant cause of cancerous tumours.

> *"And said, If thou wilt diligently hearken to the voice of the LORD thy God, and wilt do that which is right in His sight, and wilt give ear to His commandments, and keep all His statutes, I will put none of these diseases upon thee, which I have brought upon the Egyptians: for I am the Lord that healeth thee"*
> *(Exodus 15:26).*

A symptom is not a disease but is an expression of the body showing that it is actively engaged in cleansing itself, as cancer is a healing process. The entire body supports the growth of cancer when it is in its best interest to do so, and when healing is complete and the cancer no longer serves a purpose, it regresses or changes into a harmless, dormant state. A tumour does not cause itself, but there are root causes behind it which need to be dealt with to facilitate healing. Not recognizing that cancer is a healing mechanism can be fatal, and often is. When the body has been poisoned, burned, or cut, the body may need to grow another tumour to complete its healing process.

> *"Our help is in the name of the LORD, who made heaven and earth"*
> *(Psalm 124:8).*

Cancer cells are immature cells that function differently than normal cells and often have an abnormal shape. Unlike normal cells, they can be larger or smaller in size, have a larger nucleus, which contains more DNA, and often have an abnormal number of chromosomes. Cancer cells do not communicate as normal cells do, but ignore signals from normal cells, reproduce rapidly, and evade the immune system. Normal cells stay in the area of the body where they belong, but cancer cells lack adhesion molecules that cause stickiness and can travel to other regions of the body via the bloodstream. By definition, a cancer cell is a normal healthy cell that has undergone genetic mutation, which, as a survival mechanism, is responding to its environment. Cancers are not only caused by cell mutations, as they require more than mutations to progress, they also require the co-operation, participation, and support of the surrounding cells and the entire body organism. The healing mechanism of cancer is not only coordinated by the entire organism to correct an underlying imbalance but as the body has its own innate wisdom, it halts or regresses the growth of a tumour when it is deemed necessary to do so and not otherwise.

Cancer healing does not come at the expense of destroying other vital, indispensable body parts and is attainable only when the causes of excessive cancer cell growth have been dealt with, while the body is being adequately supported through its healing process. If the body is afflicted with any of the root causes of cancer, the body may quickly die unless it grows cancer cells. It can take many years for tumours to form unless the body is exposed to large quantities of carcinogens, which may subsequently require an aggressively rapid cancerous growth to deal with it. Cancer is a healing attempt by the body and for the body, and stopping this healing effort with destructive methods can destroy the body, but supporting it in its healing efforts can save it. Cancer is the final and most desperate healing survival mechanism that the body has at its disposal when all other measures have failed.

"For God sent not His Son into the world to condemn the world;
but that the world through Him might be saved"
(John 3:17).

When cancer cells can no longer import oxygen for their energy supply, as normal cells do, then their only remaining option is to import sugar for their energy. Normal cells create thirty-six ATP (adenosine triphosphate) of energy for every molecule of glucose. However, when they convert to cancer cells, they only create two ATP of energy for every molecule of glucose. Glucose is the primary fuel of cancer cells, and when cancer cells absorb glucose this generates large amounts of lactic acid, which creates a lower pH. This lactic acid by-product of cancer cells must be metabolised by the liver, which quickly converts the lactic acid to glucagon. Glucagon is a peptide hormone that is formed in the pancreas and raises the concentration of glucose in the blood by promoting glycogenolysis, which is the breakdown of glycogen to glucose, thereby

> ### Glucose is the primary fuel of cancer cells.

causing a vicious circle. Cancer cells are unable to import a fuel source for energy, and as a survival mechanism, they must convert and import more sugar in an oxygen-deprived environment. This survival mechanism is a final attempt of the body to heal itself, as cancer is initiated when the detoxification and primary waste removal mechanisms of the body have been rendered inefficient. Cancer is a healing mechanism which the body may choose from its arsenal to re-establish allostasis (stability through change). According to medical research, under mental and physical duress, the powerful DNA anti-cancer hormone, interleukin-II, decreases. It only increases again after the stress has dissipated, as low secretions of interleukin-II increase cancer incidences. Emotional stress can not only shut down the immune system and cause illness, but also prevent the body from healing. Medical evidence shows that people can die from a massive heart attack during severe stress without having any previous heart condition. Cancer develops over many years as a result of the combined effects of daily lifestyle choices together with environmental pollutants. Therefore, to heal the body, the cause needs to be removed.

"I will praise thee; for I am fearfully and wonderfully made: marvellous are thy works; and that my soul knoweth right well" (Psalm 139:14).

In the early nineteenth century, it was perceived that inflammation was linked to cancer, and epidemiological studies have revealed that chronic inflammation causes different forms of cancer. Every cancer cell has inflammation, which is a critical component of tumour progression. Symptoms of inflammation and oxidative stress are common denominators in diseases, with every symptom emanating from a shortage of cellular bio-energy. Cells surrounded by inflammation cannot survive because oxygen and nutrients cannot enter these cells and toxins cannot escape. As well as originating from sites of inflammation, cancers can also arise from areas of infections and chronic irritation. Researchers have discovered that exposure to DNA-damaging chemicals, after the formation of inflammation, boosts mutations even further, thereby increasing the risk of cancer. Findings suggest that chronic inflammation potentially results in increased DNA damage and proliferation that can co-operate together to increase the risk of cancer formation. It is an illness that causes cancer as cancer does not cause an illness.

"Whether therefore ye eat, or drink, or whatever ye do, do all to the glory of God" (1 Corinthians 10:31).

Unfortunately, the unscientific, unproven, and ungodly false theory of evolution, which became popularized by Charles Darwin in the nineteenth century, drives the hypothesis that the evolution of healthy cells into cancerous cells is a process very similar to the assumed terminology of natural selection. This idea is misleading, as a fundamental presumption of evolution is that random mutations are usually harmful, resulting in instantaneous cell death. However, rather than dying, as normal cells do when faced with random mutations, cancer cells exhibit the exact opposite response. Tumours are capable of building their own blood supply (angiogenesis) and they also express highly organized behaviours which are deemed impossible to induce through mutations alone. They protect themselves by silencing cancer-suppression genes and activating tumour-promoting genes. They secrete corrosive enzymes which enable them to move freely throughout the body. They can also change their metabolism, thus enabling them to survive in a highly acidic environment with low oxygen, while ingeniously removing their own surface-receptor proteins to avoid detection by white blood cells.

"Blessed is the man that walketh not in the counsel of the ungodly, nor standeth in the way of sinners, nor sitteth in the seat of the scornful" (Psalm 1:1).

Matter by itself cannot give rise to information and a code. All human life begins when a sperm and an egg (gametes) fuse together at fertilization to form a single diploid zygote or microscopic one-cell embryo. How does just one cell know the steps to build a body with many trillions of cells of hundreds of different kinds? The body is complex beyond comprehension and is encoded with an instruction manual on how to build and operate every part of its incredible self. DNA contains information, and the scientific laws of information show that there must be an intelligent source, as it is impossible for this to happen by chance over millions of years of random mutations and natural selection. DNA is not as complicated as cells, each of which is a miniature city which works together as one unit. To assume that everything we see around us evolved from nothing, a similar scenario could be a whirlwind sweeping through and junkyard and assembling a jumbo jet.

"For nothing is secret, that shall not be made manifest; neither any thing hid, that shall not be known and come abroad" (Luke 8:17).

ANIMAL PRODUCTS

A healthy, whole plant-food diet, containing a variety of fruits, vegetables, legumes, grains, nuts, and seeds is what the body is designed to eat. Taste bud cells undergo a continual turnover throughout life, with their average lifespan estimated at approximately ten days. This means that those partaking of unhealthy diets can transition to a varied, healthy whole plant-food diet in a relatively short period of time without feeling deprived, as new taste bud cells adapt to new tastes. Healthy, whole plant-food diets do have a profound effect on the metabolism, and the least energy-efficient plant-food is about ten times more efficient than the most efficient meat product. Most whole plants are high-protein foods, and all whole plant-foods contain protein. For example, 25% of wheat protein is in the bran and germ of whole wheat. In addition to protein, there is an enormous variety of nutrients in all plants. The human body only needs about 0.75 grams of protein for every kilo (approximately 2.2 pounds) of body weight, and there will not be a deficiency of protein if enough calories are consumed. A protein deficiency is almost exclusively seen in those suffering from a calorie and nutrient deficiency. In fact, consuming too much protein can cause cancer, and even at advanced stages of the disease, reducing its intake can turn cancer off.

> *There is nothing humane about the barbaric and torturous slaughter of these animals.*

The word protein comes from the Greek word *proteos*, meaning primary place. Proteins are made up of amino acids which join together to form long chains. Proteins perform the majority of their work in the cells and are also used for growth and maintenance. The body's protein needs are dependent upon health and activity levels. Some proteins are hormones, which are chemical messengers that aid communication between tissues, cells, and organs. Proteins are made and secreted by endocrine glands or tissues and then transported in the blood to their selected organs or tissues where they bind to protein receptors on cell surfaces. Some proteins are fibrous and provide cells and tissues with rigidity. They also play a vital role in regulating the concentrations of acids and bases in the blood and other bodily fluids. Protein plays many roles in the body. It helps to repair and build the body's tissues, allows metabolic reactions to occur, and coordinates bodily functions. In addition to providing the body with a structural framework, proteins also maintain the correct pH and fluid balance.

It is a medically and scientifically established fact that protein obtained from plant foods is far superior to protein obtained from flesh foods. Therefore, the consumption of animal products cannot be justified on a nutritional basis. The flavour of meat is partly due to the presence of uric acid, a purine which is a poisonous, toxic waste. If this is not quickly and thoroughly removed from the blood by the kidneys, it will be deposited in the tissues and give rise to health problems including gout and gallbladder and kidney stones. All animal products are stimulants by nature and act similar to drugs. Animal blood contains haemoglobin, albumin, and gamma globulin, and all of these chemicals activate opioid receptors, which are linked to food addictions, reward, and pain control.

One of the primary reasons that animal products are difficult for humans to digest is that the human body does not secrete the enzyme uricase, as meat-eating animals do. Protein fermentation is detrimental to the body. It mainly occurs in the lower end of the colon and results in the production of potentially toxic metabolites. Animal proteins tend to have more sulphur-containing amino acids such as methionine, which can convert into hydrogen sulphide in the colon. Hydrogen sulphide gas can contribute to the development of inflammatory bowel disease, which seldom occurs amongst whole plant-food eaters. The toxic effects of hydrogen sulphide appear to be a result of blocking the ability of the cells lining the colon from utilizing butyrate, which is a substance that beneficial bacteria make from consumed starch and fibre. Many are reluctant to follow a healthful, whole plant-food diet because they are concerned about what they assume are incomplete proteins from plant sources. This huge misconception is one of the oldest myths related to whole plant-food diets and was disproved long ago. It was popularized by Frances Moore Lappé in her 1971 book called *Diet for a Small Planet*. She later retracted her unproven myth. The medical evidence is overwhelming, clear, and consistent that those consuming healthy whole plant-food diets are far less likely to be overcome by debilitating and major life-threatening diseases because they have superior immune systems and more energy, as true wealth comes from the ground. Delicious, satiating, and nourishing anti-inflammatory recipes for every occasion can be made from the vast array of God-given healthy, whole plant-foods.

"It shall be a perpetual statute for your generations throughout all your dwellings, that ye eat neither fat nor blood" (Leviticus 3:17).

Raising animals for food (including land for grazing and growing feed crops) now uses approximately 30% of the earth's land-mass, and nearly 40% of the world's grain is fed to livestock. Raising livestock is directly associated with a topsoil loss of about 85%, which lowers crop productivity by about 70%. A healthy whole plant-food diet makes small demands on the soil as compared to a meat-based diet. For every kilo of animal flesh that is produced, livestock are fed over seven kilos of grain. It also takes an enormous amount of water to grow crops for animals to eat. One acre of land can produce about 9,000 kilos of potatoes, but only about seventy-five kilos of meat. One milking cow can drink up to 450 litres of water per day, and it takes about 670 litres of water to produce one litre of milk. About 4,400 litres of water are required to produce one kilo of boneless beef, and this includes irrigation of pastureland for grazing, drinking water, irrigation of crops fed to the cattle, as well as for the processing of the meat. Whereas, it only takes about 250 litres of water to produce one kilo of wheat. Livestock can also be fed very unhealthy cheap materials including unwanted animal parts such as skin, hair, feathers, hooves, blood, or even diseased animals, including pets, road kills, manure and other animal waste (including arsenic-laden chicken manure, as arsenic is fed to chickens), sugar-laden candies, plastics, drugs, chemicals, and other unsavoury substances. All cattle leftover parts are rendered and fed to poultry and pigs, which are in turn rendered and fed back to the cattle, and this is legal. These livestock produce about twenty times as much waste as humans do, and this washes into waterways and causes increased ammonia, bacteria, phosphates, and nitrates, whilst also decreasing the oxygen content, which kills animal and plant life. Meat contains about fifteen times more pesticides than plant-foods, and pesticides become more concentrated as they move up the food chain and are more easily retained in fatty tissues. Consuming a healthy, whole plant-food diet uses less energy, land, and water than any other diet.

"See, I have set before thee this day life and good, and death and evil" (Deuteronomy 30:15).

Genetically modified feed is fed to animals, and the unhealthy properties of that feed, together with noxious pesticides, are transferred to the consumer, who then becomes more prone to contracting various health issues. Antibiotics are used in abundance to keep animals alive in horrific living conditions that would otherwise kill them, as there is horrendous cruelty in the animal industry. Meat consumption produces disease-causing inflammation, contains no fibre, putrefies in the gut for about three days where it removes more water from the system, and causes cancer and other health issues. Meat-eaters are also nine times more likely to be obese than plant-eaters. Chicken and fish are even more toxic than other meats, and a very large percentage of food poisoning is caused by consuming contaminated animals. Meat is red when it is sold, even if it is spoiled, because to retain its red colour it needs to be treated with carbon monoxide (a toxic gas), otherwise the oxidation from air exposure would gradually change the meat into an unappetizing brownish-grey colour within just a few days. A very large study showed that eating meat increases the likelihood of dying from all diseases by 20%. Other studies showed significant reductions in cancer risks amongst those who avoid meat, which is not only devoid of fibre but also other nutrients which have a protective effect. According to the World Health Organization, processed meats are classified as Class 1A carcinogens for humans, which is the same carcinogenic classification as alcohol, cigarettes, arsenic, and asbestos, and are the leading causes of human cancers. It is known that bowel cancer occurs mainly in countries that are the largest meat producers and consumers in the world. In the middle of the last century, the bacterium Streptococcus bovis was isolated from the colon of a large proportion of bowel cancer sufferers. This bacterium exists in the intestines of both dairy and beef cattle and is transmitted to the human intestine through the consumption of meat products while having the effect of being an insidious long-term carcinogen.

"But flesh with the life thereof, which is the blood thereof, shall ye not eat" (Genesis 9:4).

Cows are generally intelligent, gentle animals who possess good memories and interact in socially complex ways. These gentle giants have some similar human traits and mourn over the deaths of, and even separation from, those that they love, even shedding tears over their losses. Cows raised for the beef industry are often kept in intensive, artificially lit factory farms for their entire lives without ever grazing outside or having space to move around. They are often brutally treated and are generally fed on a highly unnatural genetically modified corn and soy diet, which they would never eat if they were given the choice to roam free in green pastures. This causes them almost constant digestive pain which can lead to metabolic diseases. Cows that are fed corn produce a lot more E. coli in their gut and this can contaminate their meat when slaughtered. E. coli can be deadly. Even cows that are grass-fed usually spend some time inside, often in crowded, manure-filled feedlots. As a result of this many animals develop respiratory ailments due to the choking ammonia and other chemicals in the air produced by their manure. Putrefactive bacteria are colon or manure germs that all meats are infected with during the process of slaughtering, and the average meat-eater is quite oblivious to the fact that they are ingesting a mass of swarming micro-organisms identical with those of manure. The number of these manure germs increases with the length of time that the meat is kept in storage. While the animal is alive the putrefactive bacteria in the colon are prevented from entering the rest of the body by the osmotic process of the colon. However, during the slaughtering process, the animal's tissues become thoroughly infected with these filthy manure germs, which rapidly penetrate through their colon walls and into their flesh within just a few hours after slaughter. Ammonia and bleach are used to try to disinfect the contaminated meats. Millions of drugged and diseased animals are consumed every year along with their adrenaline and considerable amounts of the poisonous end products of cell metabolism, which result from their slaughter. Endotoxins are inside the bacteria on meat and cannot be neutralized by very high temperatures. The presence of endotoxins in the blood, known as endotoxemia, can trigger problematic immune responses in animals. They also stimulate the human immune system to produce systemic inflammation, which makes holes in the intestinal tract, leading to a plethora of diseases. There are absolutely no safe animal products.

"He causeth the grass to grow for the cattle, and herb for the service of man: that He may bring forth food out of the earth" (Psalm 104:14).

It is a myth that dairy products are healthy and build strong bones. The consumption of dairy products causes chronic inflammation and excess mucus and is not the innocuous substance that many have been led to believe. It drives common health issues such as cancer, diabetes, and dementia, and dairy has been linked to a higher risk of cancers and contains pesticides and synthetic hormone contaminants. When introduced into the human body these synthetic hormones can affect normal hormonal functioning and, coupled with the dairy products in which they are contained, can also cause infertility as dairy clogs the amazing finely-tuned human machinery. Drinking one glass of dairy milk per day raises the risk of dying from all causes by 15% and one to two glasses increases the risk to 21%. Drinking three or more glasses of dairy milk per day increases mortality risk by 93%.[3] Women who drink three or more glasses of dairy milk per day also have a 60% increased risk of developing a hip fracture. Humans barely absorb the calcium in dairy milk, especially if it is pasteurized. It also causes osteoporosis, which is scurvy of the bones, as it increases calcium loss from the bones. Many scientific studies have shown a large number of detrimental health effects that are directly linked to dairy consumption, including parasites, constipation, and an increase in bone fracture risks by 50%. Dairy products do not decrease the risk of bone fractures but sufficient vitamin D can prevent fractures. Dairy products also increase the body's level of insulin-like growth factor 1 (IGF), formerly called somatomedin, a known cancer promoter. Dairy products contain the fat - arachidonic acid (an Omega-6 unsaturated fatty-acid) which, when consumed on a regular basis, sabotages DHA. As with all animal protein, dairy acidifies the pH of the body, initiating a biological correction.

Calcium is an excellent acid neutralizer, and the biggest storage of calcium in the body is in the bones. The calcium, which the bones need to stay strong, is utilized to neutralize the acidifying effect of dairy products, and calcium is pulled from the bones, leaving a calcium deficit, which is excreted by the body via the urine. After about thirty years of age bone loss is normal. The Nurses' Health Study discovered that calcium supplements weaken the bones. They also provide no benefits for reducing fracture risks. A large ten-year calcium supplement study showed that consuming calcium supplements can cause damage to the vascular system, which includes the heart and brain. Another recent study, which was the first of its kind, revealed that even low doses of calcium supplements are linked to brain lesions. Consuming calcium supplements that contain substances that are unnatural to the body, such as chalk (a form of limestone), bone meal, and the shells of eggs and oysters, is unhealthy. Women are often advised to take calcium supplements, but since their bones are naturally less dense when they are older, these unnecessary supplements can do more harm than good as they cause the bones to become not only more brittle but also more prone to breaking. High bone density is associated with higher endogenous estrogen levels, which are associated with a higher risk of breast cancer. Women in the highest hip bone mineral density category are 62% more likely to develop breast cancer than women in the lowest bone mineral density category. Calcification of arteries and brain structures can also occur due to unnatural calcium being deposited in soft tissues. The body is designed

---

[3] Karl Michaëlsson, et al, "Milk intake and risk of mortality and fractures in women and men," *BMJ* 2014; 349: g6015, https://1ref.us/1nh (accessed February 28, 2021).

to obtain calcium from food, as bone is a living tissue which requires many nutrients to be healthy and not just calcium. There is also a much higher breast cancer risk for those with the highest bone density. According to a study, excessive inflammation is linked to severe and rapid bone loss as too much swelling destroys bones. Conversely, weight-bearing exercises help to build bone strength. Approximately 65% of the world's population cannot properly digest dairy products and are lactose intolerant. The RNA-binding protein tristetraprolin controls inflammation. Any food or lifestyle that is acidic will acidify the blood and thin the bones, and all drugs, including calcium supplements, acidify the body.

Statistics show that countries with the lowest consumption of dairy products also have the lowest incidences of fractures in their populations. Surprisingly, the lowly chia seed contains five times more calcium than dairy milk as well as healthy high-antioxidant Omega-3 fatty acids, and chia seeds can be quickly and easily made into a healthy, whole plant-food milk. Omega-3 fatty acids are an integral part of cell membranes throughout the body and also affect the functioning of these membranes' cell receptors. They also help to protect against glaucoma. Dairy milk protein is comprised of approximately 86% casein, which is a significantly potent tumour-causing chemical carcinogen and the most relevant food-based carcinogen in existence. Research has shown that all dairy products contain casomorphin peptides, which are protein fragments that are derived from the digestion of casein. Casomorphins have an opioid-like addictive factor that can trigger dopamine receptors in the brain, thereby triggering an addictive element. Opioid receptors are linked to addiction, reward, and pain control. The substance with a morphine effect in dairy milk is identical in biochemical, chemical, immunological, and pharmacological properties to authentic morphine. This is the reason why some individuals find it difficult to relinquish unhealthy dairy cheeses, as they are particularly concentrated and potent with high levels of opiates.[4] These opiates are not only found in cow's milk, but human milk also at concentrations of 200–500 nanograms per litre for both cow's and human milk. Dairy cheese contains the most condensed form of casein; it contains an abundance of casomorphins which make it more addictive than other dairy products. This very acidic, unhealthy substance remains in the stomach for many hours as the stomach has difficulty dealing with it and finally

---

[4] E. Hazum, et al, "Morphine in cow and human milk: could dietary morphine constitute a ligand for specific morphine (mu) receptors?" *Science*, August 28, 1981, PubMed, https://1ref.us/1ni (accessed February 28, 2021).

ejects it through the pyloric sphincter valve at the base of the stomach. Food opiates cause food addictions which have a hard-wired organic component that contains powerful narcotic properties and are associated with the presence of psychoactive chemicals that bind to opioid receptors in the nervous system. God designed cow's milk to be addictive to a baby calf so that it will grow quickly and thrive and human milk to a baby human so that it will also grow and thrive. The greatest source of Alzheimer's disease is brain-toxic, sodium aluminium phosphate (aluminium), which is contained in cheeses and is the most common substance used in its manufacture. It is utilized as an emulsifying agent when producing all processed cheeses. An emulsification process surrounds the fat in the cheese with this aluminium substance, which gives the cheese a smooth, soft meltable texture and is typically 3% sodium aluminium phosphate. Aluminium is widely used by the food processing industry and is also contained in drugs and cosmetics.

Animal products are popular because they are addictive stimulants. Many people love their pets and would never think of killing them for food, but they happily eat the meat of other animals. Many do not realize the horrors that exist in the brutal animal industry. If they saw for themselves the terrible cruelty, then they would have a better understanding of the barbaric practices that happen behind the scenes. People could then see how terribly these animals suffer just to please their taste buds.

Cows quite often have a very painful inflammatory condition of their mammary glands called mastitis, and the pus from these conditions can get into their milk, due to normal dairy practices. Millions of dairy cows are frequently specially bred and routinely drugged to produce unnatural quantities of milk due to artificial hormones, antibiotics, and steroids, and after about four to five years of constant exhaustive calving and milk production, they are routinely slaughtered for their meat. Nearly all male calves and approximately three-quarters of female calves are slaughtered within a few days of their misery filled lives. These beautiful, helpless little calves are taken away from their mothers within a few hours of birth so that their mothers can be constantly milked. These mothers spend days frantically crying out for their hapless little calves after they are taken away, as they form strong bonds with their calves, who often do not even receive any basic care while they await a terrifying and painful slaughter. The calves are not even considered noteworthy by dairy farmers but are regarded as just a surplus by-product of the dairy industry. They are sold for veal, as their flesh is light pink because they have mostly been starved. There is nothing humane about the barbaric and torturous slaughter of these animals.

"Have mercy upon me, O LORD; for I am weak: O LORD, heal me; for my bones are vexed" (Psalm 6:2).

Chickens are inquisitive, sensitive, intelligent, social creatures, who, in nature, have social hierarchies and care for their young. Chickens can normally live for more than ten years in natural surroundings, but when they are raised for eggs and meat in factory farms, they have a horrendous existence. They are generally debeaked, which is a barbaric and agonizing practice which leads to the death of many birds. Debeaking is also standard practice for many organic, free-range farms. Egg production begins to decrease when laying hens are about two years old and then they are mercilessly slaughtered.

Both chickens and their eggs are the source of a myriad of diseases. Next to chickens, eggs are the second largest cause of Salmonella poisoning. Eggs are not a health food, as many people think. Salmonella bacterial infection can cause serious health complications and has been found to contaminate a fair percentage of raw chicken meat. Salmonella can infect the ovaries of healthy-looking chickens, thereby contaminating the eggs inside the chicken before the shells are even formed.

Campylobacteriosis is an infectious disease which is caused by bacteria of the genus Campylobacter. Its major source is considered to be due to the consumption of contaminated chicken meat. Egg industry hens have been genetically manipulated to lay 200–350 eggs per year, while hens that have not been genetically manipulated normally lay about a dozen eggs per year for reproductive purposes. If a hen's natural brooding process of protecting and nesting with her eggs is interfered with by their being constantly removed, her body instinctively responds by producing more eggs. Developing chicks require large amounts of nutrients, especially calcium to form the shells, for which a hen must mobilize about 10% of the calcium that is stored in her bones. For yearly egg production, a hen will utilize a quantity of calcium that is far greater than her entire skeleton by thirty-fold or more. This is the main reason why egg production hens are commonly afflicted with weak and broken bones, as their sick bodies lose more calcium than they can assimilate from their food to enable them to continuously produce more eggshells.

It takes about three kilos of grain, in the form of chicken feed, to produce one kilo of eggs, and about 200 litres of water is needed to grow the grain to produce one average-sized egg. Many millions of these cruelly treated defense-less animals are killed annually for their meat and eggs, and their viruses can also contribute to human cancers. It is estimated that there are nearly 400 trillion harmless viruses in the human body. This is collectively known as the human virome. Only infected viruses can be harmful. When male chicks are just one day old they are usually thrown alive into a macerator (high-speed grinder) because they are unprofitable for the egg industry. Adult birds are also ground up alive. The females raised for their flesh have a much more horrifying and atrocious existence, as most of them spend their pain-filled lives crammed into small battery cages with other hens in multi-layered tiers in filthy, huge, win-dowless, ammonia-filled warehouses with artificially manipulated lighting that is designed to induce the birds to eat often. They are hardly able to move around as the use of growth-promoting drugs ensure large, fast-growing birds while the cage wire cripples their feet, rubs off their feathers and grazes their skin. These drugs and the condition of the birds also affect the health outcome of those that consume them. Chickens have now been gene-edited in order to create flu-resis-tant birds. Some chickens and turkeys have been specially bred to be top-heavy and cannot even stand on their feet. They are drugged to grow so quickly that their lungs, hearts, and limbs often cannot keep up. Most chicken farms are so dirty that the meat has to be washed with chlorine before being sold for human consumption.

Consuming chicken flesh is not a healthier option than red meat. The bar-baric conditions of their existence necessarily create a product riddled with ill-ness. It is standard practice to starve hens in order to shock their bodies into a rapid egg-laying cycle for bigger profits. Hens are also adversely afflicted by fatty liver disease due to their liver cells working constantly to produce the pro-tein and fat required for egg yolks. Hens become very weakened due to these conditions, and when they are exhausted and unable to lay any more eggs they are referred to as *egg-bound*. Eggs exit the hen's body from the same place as her urine and faecal matter do. They succumb to many infections, one of which is from broken eggs that become stuck inside their oviduct. They also succumb to prolapses and ovarian cancer from their rapidly ageing hyperactive reproductive systems. These are common causes and conditions leading to premature death for these hapless creatures. When the time arrives for them to be mercilessly and torturously slaughtered, they are hung upside down in shackles, which further injures their often broken legs. Their throats are then cut open by machines and they are usually not even stunned before this process. They are then immersed in

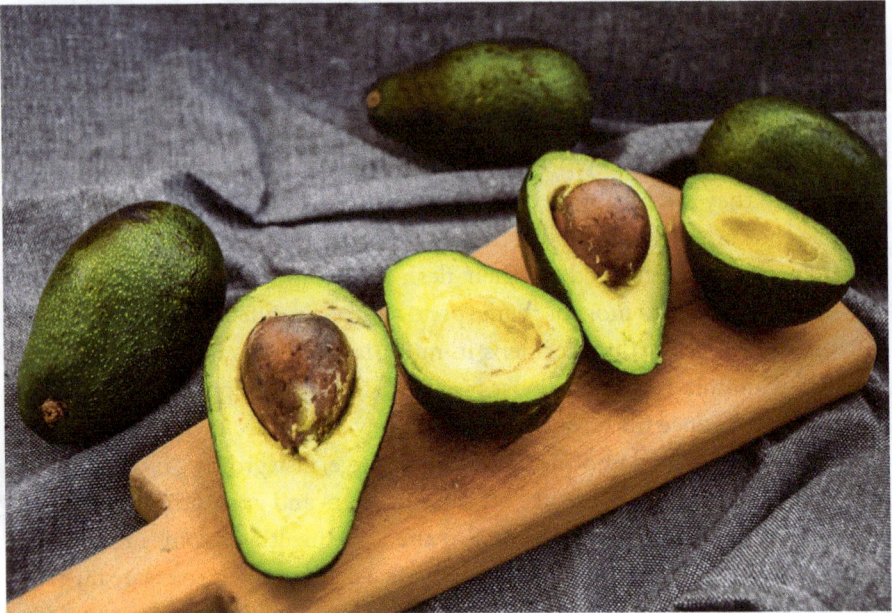

scalding-hot water for feather removal and are often conscious throughout the entire process. Following these barbaric processes eviscerating machines are used to remove their internal organs and salmonella cross-contamination is spread by this method. Dead diseased birds are then turned into animal feed for livestock.

Recent studies show that the consumption of eggs, chicken, and turkey causes inflammation, which is a precursor to cancer, diabetes, heart disease, and more. Having high levels of the cardiotoxicant trimethylamine-N-oxide (TMAO) in the bloodstream is associated with a significantly higher risk of having a stroke or a heart attack. The choline in eggs can be changed into TMAO by gut bacteria and is then absorbed back into the body system, but levels of TMAO increase with higher egg consumption. TMAO is not produced if there are no TMAO producing bacteria present in the gut. If a whole plant-food gut eco-system is established then the gut does not produce TMAO, and the avoidance of animal products also reduces the risk of cancer, stroke, and heart attack. Conversely, beautiful green egg-shaped avocados are alkalizing, extremely nutritious, versatile and can be consumed regularly as part of a whole plant-food diet.

"Which leaveth her eggs in the earth, and warmeth them in the dust" (Job 39:14).

Ducks and geese are intelligent, social, and curious animals who enjoy being in flocks with other birds. They thrive in their natural habitat, where they waddle around investigating their surroundings and forage for insects and grubs in ponds and vegetation. Every year millions of geese and ducks are intensively farmed for their flesh. They, too, suffer enormously at the hands of the cruel meat industry and are crammed into tiny, filthy cages in torturous, cramped conditions in windowless warehouses, which are totally devoid of anything remotely similar to their natural habitat. Day-old females, who do not gain weight as fast as the males, are thrown alive into a grinder. The more unfortunate male birds endure a still more horrific ordeal by being force-fed for the production of the agony-causing substance, pâté de foie gras, which is a taste of death. Foie gras is French for *fat liver*. These dying, vomit-tainted, distressed creatures are riddled with painful sores, abscesses, and eye injuries while also suffering in agony from broken wings and legs, and are slaughtered before reaching maturity. To force the bird's livers to become unnaturally fatty, workers grab geese and ducks by their necks and shove metal pipes down their throats in a barbaric process known as *gavage*. They then pump huge amounts of grain through the pipes into their stomachs, which they do several times a day. Millions die from this process alone. This disgusting torture continues until the unfortunate animals' livers swell to up to ten times their normal size, pressing against other organs, including their lungs, causing them to constantly pant. At slaughter, these hapless birds are hung upside down, have their throats cut and are left to bleed to death. Consuming their flesh or eggs is acidifying to the human system and causes inflammation which leads to many diseased states.

"Who teacheth us more than the beasts of the earth, and maketh us wiser than the fowls of heaven?" (Job 35:11).

Sheep have incredibly unique personalities and are exceptionally intelligent creatures with a whole host of endearing and adorable qualities. Although sheep are flock animals, they have the ability to act independently of one another and show amazing natural behaviours. They are intuitive animals that in nature look after their even more adorable offspring. Unfortunately, lambs are killed for their inflammatory disease-causing meat, and male lambs may be slaughtered when they are only ten weeks old. Many millions of lambs die from malnutrition, disease, or exposure within days of their birth. During their short lives, they are forced to undergo painful mutilations, such as having their tails cut off and being castrated without painkillers. Sheep left out on the hillsides hardly fare any better and are often shamefully neglected and suffer from painful infections, flystrike, lameness, and parasites, such as ticks. Flystrike, also known as myiasis, is caused by maggots feeding on an animal's flesh, as flies are drawn to lay their eggs in moist and dirty fur. Flystrike is not only painful but can also be deadly if not quickly treated. In the winter thousands of animals freeze to death in icy conditions. Others are sent to terrifying deaths after traumatic journeys in overcrowded trucks to livestock markets, or even worse, they are crammed onto ships to be transported on grim voyages that can last for many days or weeks, to overseas slaughterhouses.

"I am the good shepherd: the good shepherd giveth his life for the sheep" (John 10:11).

Pigs are intelligent, loyal, and friendly animals who naturally live in small family groups and enjoy exploring their surroundings, foraging for food, playing, and building nests for their offspring. They are normally lean, unless overfed by humans, and are misunderstood in many ways. They also like to wallow in mud to cool down. Pigs are naturally smarter than other domesticated animals and their ability to solve problems is well documented. Animal experts consider them to be more trainable than dogs. They are also reliable truffle hunters with a keen sense of smell which enables them to locate the pricey fungi. Pigs are one of the only large mammals to exist in every part of the world. Unfortunately, they carry many viruses and toxins. They are also teaming with multiple parasites such as trichinae, flukes, worms, and tapeworms, which, when consumed, can lodge in the human brain, spinal cord, and gut. Pork tapeworms literally hatch in the human stomach and can grow to a length of ten meters whilst feeding off ingested nutrients. Pig flesh also has the ability to transfer the parasitic disease trichinosis to humans. Trichinosis is a parasitic disease caused by roundworms. During the initial infection, an invasion of the intestines can cause vomiting, abdominal pain, and diarrhea. Some of these parasites, along with their eggs and cysts, are not even killed by cooking, and some parasite species are also freeze resistant. Parasite infections are often mistaken for the symptoms of other health conditions including pneumonia, severe malnutrition, food poisoning, diarrhoea, epileptic seizures, abdominal pain, vomiting, fever, weight loss, hormone deficiency, sleep problems, rashes,

> *Symptoms do not usually appear until long after a parasitic infection has taken hold of the body.*

and general weakness; however, symptoms do not usually appear until long after a parasitic infection has taken hold of the body.

Pigs are scavengers and will eat just about anything, including rotting dead carcasses and manure. Consequently, they retain very high, potent levels of toxins in their own fatty tissues because the transit time of what they consume is very short. Unlike other mammals, pigs do not sweat, and therefore they cannot sweat out toxins. Because of this, their flesh is extremely toxic and produces many life-threatening inflammatory, diseased conditions in those that consume them.

The preservative sodium nitrite is cancer-causing and is used to keep the flesh of dead animals a pink colour. It is contained in bacon, prosciutto, pastrami, pepperoni, ham, sausages, corned beef, salami, hot dogs, and other processed meat products. A high intake of cured meat is directly associated with the aggravation of asthma symptoms, as the nitrites are responsible for oxidative stress related to lung damage, lung cancer, asthma, and chronic obstructive pulmonary disease (COPD). Cured meat is considered to be any type of meat that has been preserved and flavoured by adding a combination of nitrates, nitrites, refined sugar, and unhealthy white processed salt.

"And the swine, because it divideth the hoof, yet cheweth not the cud, it is unclean unto you: ye shall not eat of their flesh, nor touch their dead carcase" (Deuteronomy 14:8).

Pigs suffer horrendously when they are imprisoned in factory farms, as they have no chance there to carry out their natural behaviours. They are crammed into barren concrete pens and may never even breathe fresh air or see the sun. Being naturally intelligent, the boredom and stress of being in extremely confined spaces can drive the pigs to engage in aggressive behaviour, such as tail-biting. Farmers routinely cut off their tails and grind down their sensitive teeth, often without painkillers. Female pigs endure chronic pain after having rings forced through their noses, while male piglets may be castrated without anaesthetics, which is a barbaric procedure that is still legal in many countries. Sows in factory farms are repeatedly forced to become pregnant. Before they give birth, they are often confined to gestation crates that are so small that they cannot even turn around, lie down comfortably, or fulfil their strong natural urge to build a nest. Each litter of piglets are torn away from their mother when they are just a few weeks old. These are then sent to fattening pens before being sent to the slaughterhouse. There the cruelty continues, and the animals are hoisted upside down by their back legs and their throats are cut, often without having been effectively stunned.

God did not design pigs to be eaten or their carcases touched. He designed them to clean up the planet, which is why the Bible says that unclean animals, such as pigs, should not be touched or eaten.

"Thou shalt not eat any abominable thing"
(Deuteronomy 14:3).

There is a common misunderstanding that if you are a vegetarian then you can eat fish as it is not really *meat*. as the British Vegetarian Society classes a vegetarian as a person who does not eat meat or fish and sometimes other animal products. There are sub-categories of being a vegetarian, but eating fish is not one of them. According to research, fish are sentient, intelligent, sensitive, and social creatures with good memories. They live in complex social communities and learn from and recognise others. Records indicate that, for every pound of fish that is caught and utilized, up to five pounds of unintended marine species are also caught. These include many hundreds of thousands of dolphins, seals, whales, and turtles, which are caught and then discarded every year after suffering cruel deaths in commercial fishing nets.

Every year millions of tons of plastic end up in the oceans. Microplastics (smaller than five millimetres) pose the greatest threat to marine life and are so small that they are easily ingested by marine creatures. Many of these creatures, which contain microplastics, are consumed by humans, as evidenced by gut samples supplied by volunteers from around the world. The seafood industry is dangerously underregulated and is an enormous cause of food poisoning, which can result in extreme discomfort, kidney, and nervous system damage—and even death. Consuming fish is not a healthier option than eating meat. Many bodies of water are polluted with animal and human waste, which carries dangerous bacteria. Fish flesh is very acidic and causes many inflammatory diseases, such as cancer and heart disease. Fish also contain parasites, which can penetrate the skin of humans who touch their flesh. Fish absorb toxic chemicals contained in the surrounding water, such as methylmercury, arsenic, dioxins, lead, cadmium, radioactive strontium 90, chromium, and PCBs (polychlorinated biphenyls are man-made industrial chemicals). These toxic, inflammatory agents not only cause cancers and kidney damage but are also neurotoxic. They are stored in the body fat of those who consume them and can remain there for decades. One square inch of sushi has been found to contain 10,000–100,000 larva of different types of worms. Toxic parasites can lay 100,000 eggs or more a day and also absorb nutrients from the body, whilst leaving their own excreted waste to further pollute the bodies of those who consume them.

Farmed fish experience more prolonged suffering than wild-caught fish and are fed with pellets which are designed for rapid weight gain. In these intensely-crowded, unnatural conditions, the fish suffer from infections, oxygen depletion, parasites, and stress. The waste that these fish produce falls as sediment to the seabed in large enough quantities to devastate and kill marine life in the vicinity as well as promoting algal growth which thereby reduces the oxygen content of the water. About 25% of wild-caught fish are used to make fishmeal that is fed to farmed fish. China produces about 70% of the world's farmed fish and is the world's biggest seafood exporter. Research shows that approximately half of the fish kept in these conditions suffer from deafness because of their unnatural, rapid weight gain. Tested farmed salmon reveals that it is one of the most toxic foods in the world. The natural red colour of wild salmon occurs because of the rich, naturally occurring, reddish-coloured astaxanthin pigment contained in the prawns and krill that salmon feed upon. Farmed salmon are naturally an unappetizing grey or beige colour because they lack access to these foods containing astaxanthin, so they are fed with red coloured pellets to induce red coloured flesh. The diet of farmed salmon can contain synthetic additives and chemical contaminants. Synthetically-derived astaxanthin and canthaxanthin can be added to their feed, which can cause eye injuries. High levels of dioxins, PCBs, and chlorinated pesticides can also be contained in their artificial diet, which can cause many health issues to those that consume them. Farmed salmon also has a substantially lower amount of Omega-3 than wild salmon because of the lack of a natural diet. Additionally, Omega-3 from fish is often rancid and nowhere near as healthy as that from plant sources. Healthy high-antioxidant and anti-inflammatory Omega-3 foods are readily available from different plant sources such as flax seeds, hemp seeds, and chia seeds so that humans can benefit from this vitally powerful antioxidant nutrient with the added benefit that sea creatures do not have to suffer.

"And God created great sea creatures, and every living creature that moveth, which the waters brought forth abundantly, after their kind, and every winged fowl after his kind: and God saw that it was good" (Genesis 1:21).

Every year many millions of crabs, prawns, lobsters, and other crustaceans are torn apart, impaled, or boiled alive, which is particularly cruel. Scientists have proven beyond doubt that crustaceans and other sea creatures do feel pain. The bodies of lobsters are covered with chemoreceptors, which makes them very environmentally sensitive. Shellfish are particularly toxic as they are filter-feeders (they filter water through their gills to collect nutrients). They were created to feed on and clean up the ocean floor to keep the oceans alive. They were not created for humans to eat. Shellfish also frequent contaminated areas of human waste disposal and as such can be a source of the hepatitis A virus, Salmonella, and E. coli. The toxins from the refuse that they eat, such as contaminated, decaying, dead creatures, are transferred to those who consume them, causing digestive and other health complications. Shellfish can also be a host to toxic parasites and other harmful infectious organisms as they do not have the appropriate filter and digestive systems to purify toxins and parasites from their bodies and are among the most well-known for causing allergic reactions. Paralytic shellfish poisoning is a serious illness caused by consuming shellfish that have been contaminated with harmful toxins produced by the dinoflagellate algae. The potency of some of these toxins can be a thousand times stronger than cyanide and the toxin levels contained in just one single shellfish can be fatal. The most common bacteria to cause food poisoning are Vibrio cholerae, which are found in shrimp. Neurotoxic shellfish poisoning is possible after consuming contaminated oysters, mussels, or clams, as they can contain potent toxins caused by viruses and bacteria. The symptoms of which will most likely be vomiting, nausea, and diarrhoea. Avoiding the consumption of these creatures will result in a healthier body.

> *By making compassionate choices, beautiful creatures do not have to suffer.*

"And whatsoever hath not fins and scales ye may not eat; it is unclean unto you" (Deuteronomy 14:10).

By making compassionate choices, beautiful creatures do not have to suffer. To reduce animal suffering, simply avoid consuming them and their products, as the consumption of animals and their products causes great suffering, not only to animals but also to humans and their loved ones. Supporting the animal product industry is supporting the enormous cruelty, exploitation, and violation of innocent, sensitive created creatures that do have feelings. But animals do have their revenge when humans get sick or die after consuming them as animals should not be ingredients.

"As the bird by wandering, as the swallow by flying, so the curse causeless shall not come" (Proverbs 26:2).

BIG PHARMA

"BIG PHARMA IS OBSESSED WITH SELLING HIGHLY PROFITABLE DANGEROUS DRUGS WHEN THE CAUSE OF DISEASE IS LIFESTYLE ISSUES."

The Rx symbol is an ancient Egyptian symbol and is associated with the claimed healing powers of sorcery that originated from the evil eye of Horus, an ancient Egyptian god of war and the father of pharmacology. The root word for sorcery is *pharmakós* (φαρμακός), which, in ancient Greek religion, had a sacrificial dimension and was a type of human scapegoat that was expelled from the community in times of disasters to appease their gods. *Pharmakós* later became *pharmakeus* (φαρμακεύς), meaning charm, spell, sorcerer, magician, poisoner, or giver of potions and drugs with magical effects to produce enchantments. *Pharmakon* (φάρμακον) is a variation of this term and is a complex expression meaning intoxicant, poison, or sacrament. It was from the word pharmakon that the terms *pharmakeia* and pharmacology emerged. This system requires millions of animals to be tortured and destroyed each year, demonstrating that the pharmaceutical drug system is still sacrifice-based. Many humans also die after using their drugs. A number of animal products from cows, horses, pigs, and fish are used in commonly prescribed drugs. Only Almighty God's natural methods bring true healing. It is interesting to note that modern pharmacology, which claims to be making war on disease, is, in reality, making war on the constitution of both humans and animals and is more interested in making huge profits. The practice of pharmacology, which is the preparation and dispensing of toxic chemical drugs, has been in existence for thousands of years and causes many deaths and severe adverse health issues. The first recorded prescriptions were discovered etched on a clay tablet in Mesopotamia that originated from around 2100 BC, and the first known drugstores were established in the ancient city of Baghdad in the eighth century AD.

"Thou shalt have no other gods before me" (Exodus 20:3).

Many toxic drugs that are made in laboratories using highly experimental chemicals are never tested on human beings before being prescribed for them,

> *Modern pharmacology, which claims to be making war on disease, is, in reality, making war on the constitution of both humans and animals and is more interested in making huge profits.*

as rapacious big pharma makes billions of dollars in profits whilst treating human beings as guinea pigs. According to the drug companies, their own studies are adequate without independent drug reviews or safety tests by the food and drug advocates who are supposed to protect the public. Drug companies are not obligated to provide any negative findings or even all of their own data but are allowed to cherry-pick their own preferred studies and bury the rest.[5] So the safety risks are transferred to consumers. Vaccines and associated pharmaceuticals are hastily put onto the market without appropriate verification or assessment. The powers that be have revealed that there is no safety data available on these drugs and vaccines and test results are obtained from consumers in lieu of clinical testing. If drugs make healthy people sick, how can they make sick people healthy?

"Let their way be dark and slippery: and let the angel of the LORD persecute them" (Psalm 35:6).

About a hundred years ago business tycoons in the U. S. devised to destroy natural holistic medicine, which has been used for thousands of years, and replace it with counterfeit unhealthy *allopathic* chemical drug concoctions that generate diseases. In the early 1900s, the oil tycoon, J. D. Rockefeller, Jr., son of the Standard Oil magnate, used his enormous political influence and immense inherited wealth to help establish the American Medical Association. Abraham Flexner, who had never even set foot in a medical school, was paid by Rockefeller to visit all U. S. medical schools and granted him the iniquitous task of creating the fraudulent *Flexner Report* in 1910, which asserted that there were too many medical schools and physicians in America and also required the standardization of medical education.

---

[5] For more information please see the following resources: Michelle Llamas, "Big Pharma's Role in Clinical Trials," https://1ref.us/1nj (accessed February 28, 2021); Ben Goldacre, *Bad Pharma: How Drug Companies Mislead Doctors and Harm Patients*, Farrar, Straus, and Giroux, 2014.

Rockefeller used his control of the media to trigger the public to protest at the report's so-called discoveries, which drove Congress to declare that the AMA was the only organization with the legal right to grant medical school licences in the U. S. Rockefeller then used the AMA to compel the government to destroy any competition and so it became the only organization that was authorized to regulate medical schools. Rockefeller extorted every medical school in the U. S. with the threat of eliminating their funding to gain control over medical licencing. The American Cancer Society was officially founded by J. D. Rockefeller Jr. in 1913, which was the same year that he made the first donation to Harvard University. Coincidently, the modern FDA and the Rockefeller Foundation were founded in the same year. The FDA works together with the AMA and the Rockefeller Foundation. Although Rockefeller only relied on traditional natural holistic medicine for himself and many of his friends at the AMA and FDA, he hypocritically decided to eliminate natural medicine for others to guarantee his monopoly of the drug market and secure the pharmaceutical industry. The FDA began an aggressive campaign to suppress natural remedies.

Following the Flexner Report, the only medical schools that the AMA endorsed were those with a drug-based curriculum with all-natural cancer cures being systematically suppressed. All nutritional education was removed from the medical schools by the AMA and only chemical drugs were allowed to be prescribed by the indoctrinated MDs who were forced to practice allopathic medicine to remain solvent. They ignored many authentic and replicated studies which verified the effectiveness of the inexpensive natural remedies and called them unapproved, untested, and dangerous. Albert Szent-Györgyi von Nagyrápolt, who discovered vitamin C, said: "The American Cancer Society tried to ruin my research foundation." Allopathic is the most profitable form of medicine, and their poison, cut-and-burn procedures are very damaging to the body. Non-allopathic schools sank into oblivion due to a lack of funding and natural holistic medicine was erroneously characterized as *quackery*. All U. S. MDs were under the auspices of the AMA and urged to promote harmful chemical drugs or lose their licence. Thereby Rockefeller secured his drug monopoly and highly profitable big pharma medicine was created, which routinely bribes doctors to prescribe their nefarious drugs.

"Let the redeemed of the LORD say so, whom He hath redeemed from the hand of the enemy"
(Psalm 107:2).

IG Farben developed Zyklon-B (hydrocyanic acid) and Carl Wurster of the German company BASF assisted in its manufacture. Zyklon-B was a powerful pesticide that was used to mass murder millions of Jews who were forced to inhale its poisonous vapours in the notorious gas chambers of Nazi Germany, which resulted in death through oxygen starvation. He also worked on highly destructive chemotherapy, a derivative of the mustard gas which was used in World War I and which is the biggest deadly destructive fraud of the century as it causes cancer rather than curing it. This gas caused terrible suffering and many deaths when released. At Hitler's command, experiments using drugs, chemotherapy, and vaccines were inexorably tested on thousands of doomed Jewish prisoners inside the Auschwitz concentration camp by members of Hitler's IG Farben drug complex (a powerful cartel comprising BASF, Hoechst, Bayer, and other German chemical companies).

After World War II, Nazi scientists, who mercilessly tortured many innocent Jewish victims in the Holocaust, were released from U. S. jails after a relatively short prison sentence for their heinous crimes, including mass murder, and were then hired and promoted by those in power and U. S. pharmaceutical and pesticide companies to fill the highest positions at BASF, Hoechst, and Bayer. Kurt Blome, of the Third Reich, who admitted to murdering Jews with gruesome experiments, was tried at Nuremberg and acquitted. He was a bacteriological warfare and biological weapons expert and was hired by the U. S. Army Chemical Corporation to work on chemical warfare in 1951. These companies (and others) produce toxic pharmaceuticals and chemicals, deadly chemotherapy, and dangerous vaccines, which have never once been proven to be safe or effective.[6] The U. S. government and huge corporations funded experiments on prisoners which included abusing them as guinea pigs by injecting them with cancer cells to try and prove that vaccines work. The sick care business creates disease with vaccines and treats the symptoms for profit, as they are more interested in repeat customers but not cures.

"Beloved, follow not that which is evil, but that which is good. He that doeth good is of God: but he that doeth evil hath not seen God" (3 John 1:11).

---

[6] Informed Consent Action Network (ICAN), news release July 13, 2018, https://1ref.us/1or (accessed June 6, 2021).

THE GERM THEORY OF DISEASE

In late 19th-century Europe, the concept of specific, unchanging bacteria types causing specific diseases became formally accepted as the foundation of allopathic microbiology and pharmaceutical controlled western medicine. Traditional western medicine practices and teaches the doctrines of French chemist Louis Pasteur (1822–1895), whose main theory is known as the *germ theory of disease*. Pasteur deliberately deceived the populace by this theory, which claims that an external source of microbe species invades the body and is the cause of infectious diseases. Pasteur's theory gave rise to the development of antibiotics, the first being penicillin in 1940, which is the poison from a fungus. An antibiotic is the poisonous waste from a *germ* which is used in an attempt to kill another. There is overwhelming evidence that the *germ theory* of disease is an unproven fallacy. This fallacy is contradicted by a significant volume of empirical evidence. No original, authoritative, scientific evidence exists that decisively and conclusively proves that any micro-organism is the definitive cause of a disease. Disease is nature's attempt to eliminate waste and diseased tissues due to improper living.

Louis Pasteur was an impostor who plagiarized the amazing work of Professor Pierre Jacques Antoine Béchamp (1816–1908), who was one of France's greatest scientists and a devout Christian who wrote several books, with the last one being *The Blood and Its Third Anatomical Element*. Unfortunately, his extraordinary accomplishments have been written out of all encyclopedias, history books, and textbooks. No doubt the *germ* theory was much more profitable for big pharma, who purports to alleviate disease with toxic pills, potions, and vaccines. Béchamp never denied that *germs* of the air or other causal factors may contribute to disease, but only that these have not been specifically created, nor are required for these purposes. *Germs* of the air will not produce disease in a healthy person. Béchamp quoted: "Nothing is lost, nothing is created ... all is transformed. Nothing is the prey of death. All is the prey of life."

Diseases are not caught but are built from an unhealthy diet and lifestyle. The presence of disease is not constituted by the presence of *germs*. Bacteria reduce dead tissue to its minimal element. The bacteria found in humans and animals do not cause disease but exist there to rebuild diseased or dead tissues. It is well known that they cannot attack healthy tissues. They are not the cause of disease and survive on unprocessed metabolic waste and malnourished, diseased, non-resistant tissue. They have absolutely no influence on live cells and by nature flourish as scavengers of dead cells at sites of disease. A similar scenario can be

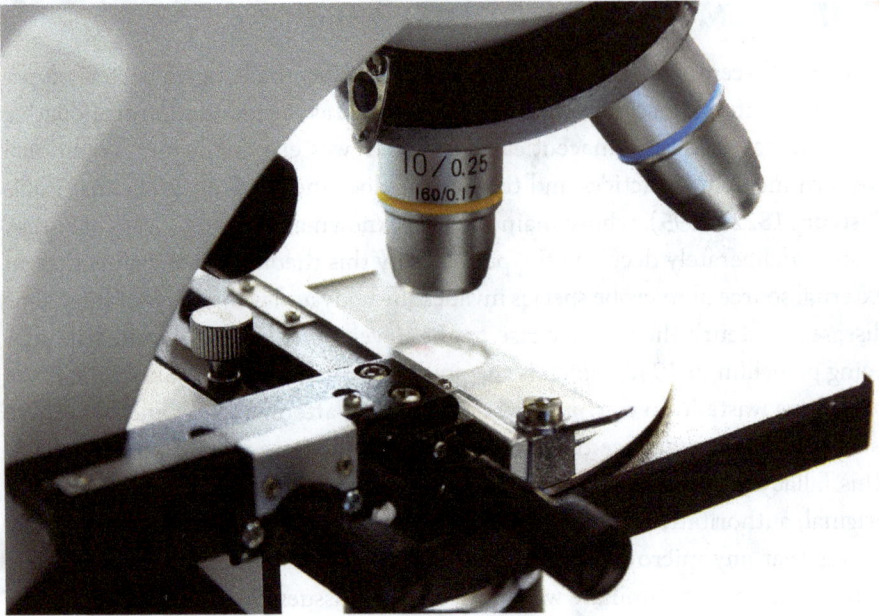

seen with flies on manure. They do not cause the manure but are attracted to the manure that is already present.

The Rife Universal Microscope, which was developed in the late 1930s and early 1940s, clearly established that micro-organisms or *germs* are the result of disease rather than its cause. If *germs* are involved, they arise as primary symptoms of that general condition. Even though *germs* do not cause disease, secondary symptoms are produced in response to their activity, which is commonly called the disease. It is not the disease-associated micro-organisms themselves that originally produce disease, but their chemical constituents enacting upon the unbalanced cell metabolism of the body that actually produces the disease symptoms.

Florence Nightingale (12th May 1820–13th August 1910) was a British social reformer. She organized care for wounded soldiers and came to prominence during the Crimean War while serving as a trainer and manager of nurses. She stated the following: "The specific disease doctrine is the grand refuge of weak, uncultured, unstable minds, such as now rule in the medical profession. There are no specific diseases; there are specific disease conditions."

"For I will cleanse their blood that I have not cleansed: for the LORD dwelleth in Zion" (Joel 3:21).

HOMEOSTASIS VERSUS ALLOSTASIS

Homeostasis is a myth and was based on a hypothesis of Claude Bernard in 1935. He proposed that everyone should have the same physiological vital signs to constantly preserve a relatively stable equilibrium of the internal bodily environment. However, studies have shown that those who consume chemical drugs to alter the natural physiology of their body to keep these signs within specific parameters, die at four times the rate of those who do not use toxic drugs. The dysfunctional allopathic model of prescribing chemicals to alter physiology is a leading cause of death.[7] Because the body is intelligently designed, constantly adapting, self-regulating, and self-healing, the more recently coined model of allostasis (stability through change) more appropriately describes the process of adjustment to the body's internal and external environment, and which keeps organisms alive and functioning in a constant state of physiologically adapting, self-regulating changes.

"Beloved, I wish above all things that thou mayest prosper and be in health even as thy soul prospereth" (3 John 1:2).

BLOOD PRESSURE

It is a myth that high blood pressure causes strokes. In 1905, physicians began monitoring blood pressure when Russian physician Nikolai Korotkov was able to measure diastolic blood pressure by using his improved version of the sphygmomanometer (blood pressure cuff). He announced this new method for determining blood pressure and different theories were hypothesized from the sounds emanating through the stethoscope as the blood pressure cuff deflated. The linear model for blood pressure has been contrived, as high blood pressure is not a disease but an adaptation of the body to circumstances that can be caused by many conditions, including toxicity, deficiencies, and pain, which causes the inner-middle, muscular layer of the arteries to decrease in size, thereby causing higher blood pressure. High blood pressure is not necessarily bad, and low (what is considered to be normal blood pressure) is not necessarily good. A huge study has shown that high systolic blood pressure actually results in lower death rates.

---

[7] B.S. McEwen, "Stress: Homeostasis, Rheostasis, Reactive Scope, Allostasis and Allostatic Load," in *Reference Module in Neuroscience and Biobehavioral Psychology, 2017,* https://1ref.us/1os (accessed June 6, 2021).

In an effort of the body to regulate itself, the blood pressure is constantly changing, depending on the circumstances. Accordingly, blood pressure readings can vary greatly depending on what a person is doing or even thinking at any given moment. It is merely a point in time of what the body is doing to regulate itself. Blood pressure increases if the arteries or tissues are damaged, as this is a self-protecting mechanism of the body. It is damaged and inflamed arteries that can be caused by many conditions, including a deficiency of nutrients, chemical toxicity, stress, toxic foods, and unhealthy blood that causes strokes and kidney damage and not high blood pressure, which is an adaptive mechanism that needs to increase to ensure a sufficient oxygen supply to the body. In the mornings it is normal to have a much higher blood pressure reading than in the evenings when the body is preparing itself for rest. Even when blood pressure is taken properly several times throughout the day it will not be an accurate measurement because many factors are involved in its regulation. These natural changes are all regulated by the nervous system and it is vitally important to stimulate its proper function. To regulate the body, the nervous system should be checked for proper functioning as any nerve interference, especially those that control the heart and lung function, will directly affect health outcomes. A good corrective chiropractor will be able to do this.

The numeric difference between the systolic and diastolic blood pressure should be around forty, and this is considered to be normal. The difference in the numbers is caused by the change in pressure, which is known as the pulse pressure. For example, the pulse pressure of 100/60 is forty, and 100/60 or 210/170 should both be considered normal as both have the same pulse pressure. The Framingham Heart Study suggests that high pulse pressure is linked to the development of atrial fibrillation, which is characterized by rapid and irregular heartbeats. Blood pressure fluctuates constantly throughout the day, and no matter what the blood pressure is, the pulse pressure should remain the same. An increase or decrease in pulse pressure is a sign that the blood is toxic. Dietary and lifestyle changes, such as regular exercising, including spinal exercises and proper deep sleep every night, will greatly improve the quality of the blood as well as the pulse pressure. The blood also supplies nutrients, regulates the pH, and core body temperature, removes waste, contains coagulation, messenger and immunological functions and more. Toxic chemical blood pressure drugs slow down these vital functions in addition to generating harmful side effects.

If the blood pressure becomes too low the arteries constrict to increase the blood pressure. There are blood vessels (vasa vasorum) that extend from the lumen (internal arterial space) of the artery that supply oxygen to the thick muscular walls of the larger blood vessels, and anything that damages these blood vessels, such as inflammation, weakens the arterial wall, which in turn can cause aneurysms and strokes. Inflammation of the vasa vasorum is called endarteritis obliterans. If damage occurs, the marvellously designed body responds by taking cholesterol and calcium from the body and laying it down where it is needed to protect the weakened muscular area.

"And He said unto them, This is my blood of the new testament, which is shed for many" (Mark 14:24).

The human body contains enough blood vessels to encircle the earth approximately three times. The heart is the first organ to function in the fetus and does so within twenty-four days after conception. It also generates the strongest electromagnetic field and the information stored in its electromagnetic field affects every organ and cell of the body. The heart and brain always communicate via this electromagnetic field and the vagus nerve system, and through this dynamic communication process, the heart can change how the brain processes information and also affects how energy flows in the body. The nervous system of the heart contains about 40,000 neurons or sensory neurites. It has been demonstrated that mentally experienced emotions will also manifest physically in the body, and feelings can affect the rhythms and beating of the heart.

The heart is a relatively small muscular organ with fairly thin walls and weighs only about 300 grams in the average-sized adult, and contrary to what is commonly believed, it is not a pressure-generating pump. The heart by itself is incapable of sustaining the circulation of the blood, and this was known to physicians of antiquity. It was first proposed to be a pressure pump by William Harvey in 1628. If it were a pressure pump, this small organ would have to perform the prodigious task of pumping approximately 8,000 litres of blood a day while the body is inactive, and much more while it is active. This blood, which is five times more viscous than water, would have to be propelled an enormous distance through millions of capillaries, some of which are narrower than red blood cells. In 1932, Bremer of Harvard filmed the movement of the blood in the very early chick embryo before the formation of the heart valves. It was circulating in a self-propelled mode in spiralling streams similar to a vortex, the pattern of which can be found abundantly in nature. The blood is propelled by a unique form of momentum boosted by the heart, and it has been noted that it very briefly comes to a halt about half-way around the system before restarting. The blood moves autonomously, and movement without applied pressure is movement with its own biological momentum, as is also profusely demonstrated in nature. Pressure is not the cause of blood flow but the result of it. This serves to explain why the brain still functions for some minutes after the heart has stopped moving as people are still alive and conscious and able to feel pain because the brain does not instantly disconnect. The medical establishment has known about this for some time and a recent study has confirmed it.[8] The inaccurate mechanistic concept of the heart being a hydraulic pump gained ascendancy and became strongly established about the middle of the nineteenth century, similar to many other *medical myths* that start with one person and are continually repeated and enlarged until they become believed as an established fact without any real scientific proof whatsoever.

"He healeth the broken in heart, and bindeth up their wounds"
(Psalm 147:3).

CELLS

A single human cell is only a few nanometers across and contains approximately two metres of DNA, which holds around 25,000 genes in about three billion base pairs. There are approximately fifty to seventy-five trillion cells in the average human body, with red blood cells comprising nearly half of that number. Every day about a billion cells die and about the same amount are created. The body is a highly-organized, awe-inspiring structure that is created with different levels, commencing with the cells. Cells are systematized into tissues which form organs, and organs are arranged into organ systems such as the nervous, digestive, and circulatory systems. The lifespan of each type of cell depends upon the workload that it endures. The body is comprised of more than 200 different cell types, with each type having its own lifespan. Within these cells, there are approximately twenty different types of organelles and structures.

> **The body is a highly-organized, awe-inspiring structure.**

---

[8] To explore this topic further, please see the following references: "The Heart Is Not a Pump" (https://1ref.us/1ot, accessed June 6, 2021); YouTube video, "The Heart Is Not a Pump!" (https://1ref.us/1ou, accessed June 6, 2021); YouTube video, "Heart May Not Be a Pump: Thomas Cowan on Cardiovascular Disease" (https://1ref.us/1ov, accessed June 6, 2021).

Some cells of the body are replaced within days, some are replaced in months, and some are replaced over years. For example, the macula of the eye replaces new cones every forty-eight hours, the stomach lining is replaced every four to five days, the colon lining is replaced about every five days (the microscopic bacteria that digest food in the intestines account for more than half of the cells in the body), the lining of the lungs is replaced every eight days, taste bud cells have a lifespan of about ten days (women tend to have more taste buds than men), the whole outer layer of skin is replaced about every thirty days (every minute approximately 30,000–40,000 dead skin cells are shed), the liver is replaced every six weeks, the red blood cells are replaced every four months, the nervous system is replaced every eight months, white blood cells live for more than a year, and the cells of the skeletal system regenerate frequently, with the complete process taking approximately seven to ten years to renew. According to a study, neurons continue to grow and change from the first developmental years well on into adulthood. Researchers have discovered that the heart continues to generate new cells throughout its lifespan.

Every year 98% of all the atoms in the body are replaced, and this occurs during REM sleep. All the cells of the body are derived from highly specialized stem cells, which are the foundation from which all parts of the body grow. They originate from an initial pool of stem cells which are formed shortly after fertilization and have the unique ability to be able to give rise to any cell type, and they self-renew by dividing or differentiating to further give rise to mature cell types. After conception, stem cells are the early cells of the foetus for the first fifty days of life and grow very rapidly prior to their differentiation into all cell types that are required by the body. These include the cells of the liver, heart, bones, skin, kidneys, pancreas, lungs and blood. Stem cells are natural repair cells that exist throughout the body for life and are replaced within the bone marrow. If damage occurs in the body, the stem cells collect in the area of damage and can differentiate into the required cells.

For optimal cell functioning, which is critical for vibrant health, cells need to be free from inflammation and cleansed of toxins. Cells have an outer lipid bi-layer. When toxins attach to this bi-layer they cause it to become inflamed. This decreases cell fluidity, which not only prevents needed substances from entering receptor sites in the cell wall but also prevents toxins from escaping, which causes the cells to lose their ability to communicate. This retention of toxins causes various adverse symptoms. Cellular detoxification occurs when cells release toxins into the bloodstream. The liver and kidneys cleanse the blood of these toxins, which are eliminated in the urine and deposited into the colon for elimination. Preventing inflammation is key to maintaining good health.

"For thou art great, and doest wondrous things: thou art God alone" (Psalm 86:10).

PROTEIN SYNTHESIS

Protein synthesis in the cell is an amazing miracle that happens in every cell about 2,000 times per second. Every bodily process takes place by way of proteins, which are constantly needed by every cell. Protein needs to be continually manufactured and this occurs in the DNA. DNA is a three-dimensional molecule that is self-replicating with each molecule able to make an identical copy efficiently and quickly. DNA is even programmed to detect and correct replication errors as special enzymes repair any DNA mistakes. The DNA is tightly constructed with about two metres of this long molecule fitting into thread-like structures called chromosomes, which are packaged into the microscopic nucleus of every cell. Each human cell normally contains twenty-three pairs of chromosomes. Twenty-two of these pairs are called autosomes which are visibly the same in both males and females. The twenty-third pair are the sex chromosomes and differ between males and females. Females have two copies of the X chromosome, while males have one X and one Y chromosome. Chromosomes have a constriction point called a centromere, which divides the chromosomes into two sections, giving them their characteristic shapes. Histones are proteins that help to condense and pack the DNA double helix into the cell nucleus in a complex known as chromatin. When cells need a protein, hormones send a message to the DNA. The enzyme proteins in the DNA take the necessary code from the DNA to manufacture the specific protein. Enzymes find the needed information to manufacture the protein by opening the relevant part of the DNA containing the code. The relevant code is extracted from a specific part of the end section of the helix where the enzymes hold it open. While this is occurring, another enzyme protein called polymerase arrives and produces a single-stranded copy of the needed section, which has been constructed inside the polymerase. This extracted copy is known as *messenger* RNA and is the bearer of the genetic assembly instructions. The copy of the code then proceeds to the ribosome, which is the site where protein synthesis occurs and the new protein is manufactured. Messenger RNA binds to the relevant part of the ribosome and prepares for the manufacture of the new protein. For production to take place in the ribosome, raw materials (amino acids) need to be brought in by *transfer RNA* and installed in line with the code. This establishes a protein chain, consisting of at least a hundred sequences each. Amino acids bind to one another with powerful special chemical bonds known as peptide bonds. Therefore proteins have a very sound structure and are not easily damaged by external factors. The arrangement of these amino acids determines the nature of the protein, and it is extremely important that each amino acid follows in the right sequence, and enzymes establish the sequence with remarkable accuracy. After a new protein chain has been manufactured it is transported to a barrel-shaped device, where it assumes its unique three-dimensional form through being folded and moulded into the precise shape that is required to perform its specific function. Without this special shape, it cannot function - even if the sequence is completely accurate. The process is then complete and a new protein has been built. Just as the newly constructed protein leaves this particular section, an enzyme arrives and transports the protein to the precise location in the cell where it is needed. This is awesome intelligent design!

"So God created man in His own image, in the image of God created He him; male and female created He them" (Genesis 1:27).

ENZYMES

It is a myth that raw food enzymes facilitate digestion. Enzymes are a special class of proteins that catalyse reactions in the body. They are essential for many crucial bodily processes at the molecular level. Enzymes increase rates of chemical reactions without changing themselves. Every cell in the body is dependent on the quality of the blood and being devoid of enzymes produces disease. A healthy lifestyle produces healthy blood that causes healthy cells which create a healthy body that can reverse disease at virtually any stage. Sufficient enzymes build healthy cells and an enzyme deficiency creates sick cells. Thousands of enzymes have been identified and thousands of chemical reactions occur in the body every second, and without enzymes, they do not take place. Water is needed for every enzymatic reaction within the body and enzymes are required for every reaction in the cells. Digestion changes the chemical structure of food and is specifically designed for the alkalizing of food in preparation for its becoming new blood and new cells. Without enzymes, food is unable to be properly digested, and if adverse symptoms arise, it is an indication that there is a problem with how the body breaks down and alkalizes nutrients for utilization. If undigested food enters into the bloodstream because of a leaky gut, toxic blood is created which causes various adverse symptoms.

There are two types of enzymes: metabolic and digestive. Metabolic enzymes are responsible for building the body and are required for structuring, remodelling, and repairing of every cell and tissue. Digestive enzymes function as biological catalysts in foods, helping to break down protein into amino acids, fats into fatty acids, and carbohydrates into sugars and starches. In the 1920s and 1930s, Edward Howell, M.D. asserted his hypothesis that the enzymes contained in raw foods break down the foods that contain them, and thereby decreases the requirement for the body to produce internal enzymes. But his analysis was largely founded on inadequate, unconvincing research. Physiology and biochemistry demonstrate that raw enzymes are not only sensitive to heat but also to the stomach pH, as hydrochloric acid denatures the enzymes consumed in raw foods. Food enzymes in raw foods are not equipped to function as digestive enzymes, as the digestive process deconstructs their enzymes into amino acids, just as other proteins are broken down into amino acids. However, raw foods do supply the body with amino acids, the building blocks of proteins.

A healthy human body, which has adequate essential nutrients and protein, contains sufficient amino acids which are necessary to construct enzymes internally. Amino acids can be used by the body as an energy source. They also perform many other bodily functions, such as the breakdown of food, tissue repair, and growth. They are classified into three groups. Essential amino acids must be sourced from foods as they cannot be made by the body. These are histidine, isoleucine, leucine, lysine, methionine, phenylalanine, threonine, tryptophan, and valine. Non-essential amino acids are produced by the body and include alanine, asparagine, aspartic acid, and glutamic acid. Conditional amino acids are generally non-essential, except during stress and illness and include arginine, cysteine, glutamine, glycine, ornithine, proline, serine, and tyrosine.

"This is He that came by water and blood, even Jesus Christ; not by water only, but by water and blood. And it is the Spirit that beareth witness, because the Spirit is truth" (1 John 5:6).

CHOLESTEROL, TRANS FAT, AND SATURATED FAT

It is a myth that saturated fats cause high cholesterol. Heart disease is one of the leading causes of death today, with cholesterol frequently being blamed as the primary culprit, but in 1900 heart attacks were almost non-existent. Recently, three large industry-funded studies discovered that cholesterol cannot possibly be the primary cause of heart disease because those with low cholesterol levels were also found to have the same amount of arteriosclerosis as those with high levels. It is only oxidized cholesterol that inflicts damage, as high levels of non-oxidized serum cholesterol are not problematic but are anti-inflammatory, protective of all cells, and essential to life. Heart disease is driven by a chronic inflammatory response, which has few apparent symptoms. The French physician and chemist François Poulletier was the first to obtain pure cholesterol from gallstones. About thirty years later a French chemist named Michel E. Chevreul named it cholesterine.

> *It is a myth that saturated fats cause high cholesterol.*

The word cholesterol (kəˈlɛstəˌrɒl) originates from two Greek words—*chole* (for *kholē*, which means *bile*) and *stereo* (for *stereós*, which means *solid*), so called because it was originally isolated from gallstones in 1784—indicating that it is part of a class of molecules that are collectively recognized as sterols (the term steroids originates from this common root word). Cholesterol is a waxy substance that is found in all cells, tissues, bile, and blood and is an important integral component of the membranes that surround all human cells and is a precursor to steroid hormones. It is so utterly vital that the body manufacturers it and without it, the body would die. That is just how critical it is. Without it, there would be no cells, muscles, bones, digestion, reproduction, movement, brain function, nerve endings, hormones, or memory. It assists beneficial molecules to pass into cells whilst keeping others out. Cholesterol is important for normal growth and repair of tissue, building brain and nerve tissue and converting UVB sun rays to vitamin D3. It also gives skin the ability to shed water.

Cholesterol is not a fat, although it travels through the bloodstream together with fats. It performs vital roles in the brain with such things as membrane function. It also keeps the brain running smoothly, helps the neurons to communicate with each other, is particularly important for cognitive function, and is necessary for normal growth and development of the brain and nervous system. The brain is the most cholesterol-rich organ of the body, with most of the cholesterol being in the myelin sheaths that surround the axons of nerve cells, thus protecting the cells and expediting the rapid transmission of electrical impulses that control movement, thought, and sensation. The brain represents only 2% of total body weight, accounts for 25% of the body's total glucose utilization, 25% of the body's oxygen, and contains approximately 25% of the body's cholesterol. The cholesterol metabolism of the brain is quite unique as it must produce its own cholesterol, on which it is highly dependent because the blood-brain barrier prevents brain cells from extracting cholesterol from the blood. Brain cells depend on HMG-CoA reductase (3-hydroxy-3-methyl-glutaryl-CoA reductase) to produce cholesterol. The brain's cholesterol has greater stability than the cholesterol in other organs, and when it naturally deconstructs it is recycled into new cholesterol inside the brain.

Cholesterol is particularly important for cognitive function, as it is needed to make neurotransmitters, which are chemicals that brain cells use to communicate with each other. Without adequate levels of cholesterol, the brain cells die. It also serves as an antioxidant and as raw materials from which vitamin D, oestrogen, testosterone, progesterone, and cortisol are made. Approximately 70% of the brain is composed of fats, 25% of which should come from healthy Omega-3 fatty acids. The three main Omega-3 fatty acids are alpha-linolenic acid (ALA), which is the precursor to docosahexaenoic acid (DHA) and eicosapentaenoic acid (EPA). Omega-6 fatty acids (linoleic acid or LA) are the precursor to gamma-linolenic acid (GLA) and arachidonic acid (AA). These two fatty acids are considered essential because the body cannot produce them so they must be sourced from the diet. When the ratio of these two omegas is adequate in the body, then ALA converts to EPA. The liver not only synthesizes cholesterol for transport to other cells but also removes cholesterol from the body by converting it to bile salts and infusing it into the bile where it can be eliminated. Cholesterol is a key player in the production of bile acid, which aids with digestion and also helps the body to regulate cholesterol, fat, and glucose metabolism.

Lipoproteins are so called because they are a mixture of fat (lipo) and protein. Cholesterol is manufactured in the liver, which synthesizes the various lipoproteins that are involved in transporting cholesterol and other lipids throughout the body and is key to the regulation of cholesterol levels. Lipoproteins are not only transporters of cholesterol, but also protein, phospholipids, and triglycerides. All lipoproteins carry all of these substances but in different proportions. As cholesterol and fat are not water-soluble, they need to be transported around the body to cells in the blood by lipoproteins to do their essential work.

The exact molecular formula of cholesterol was correctly established in 1888 by Austrian botanist Friedrich Reinitzer. There is only one chemical formula, which is $C_{27}H_{46}O$, and there are no good or bad versions of this formula. The elements in cholesterol are twenty-seven carbon atoms, forty-six hydrogen atoms, and an oxygen-hydrogen pair. This cholesterol molecule includes four rings, and its tetra-cyclic skeleton evidenced that it was extremely challenging to interpret its structure. The four hydrocarbon ring structures of this cholesterol molecule position cholesterol in the steroid hormone family and all steroid hormones are made from cholesterol. The cholesterol molecule also has hydrogen atoms that extend off rings and has a tail of carbon. Both rings and tail are non-polar, meaning that they cannot dissolve in water but dissolve in oil. The hydroxyl group is indicated by the OH, and any molecule that contains a hydroxyl group is defined as an alcohol, which is water-soluble.

HDL (high-density lipoprotein) and LDL (low-density lipoprotein) are not even cholesterol, so they cannot be either good or bad cholesterol. HDL should more accurately be termed the transporter of recycled cholesterol, and LDL should more accurately be termed the transporter of fresh cholesterol. A regular blood cholesterol test estimates LDL but does not measure it. A fasting blood cholesterol test can only measure total cholesterol and HDL. There are two other unknowns in a four-variable equation, which are IDL (intermediate-density lipoprotein) and VLDL (very low-density lipoprotein). One comparison with four variables, only two of which can be measured, is not scientific. At least one more comparison or known variable is required to evade circular referencing. Is this scientific? HDLs are frequently called good cholesterol and have various functions including transporting cholesterol from the cells back to the liver, where the liver determines whether to recycle or dispose of it as it regulates the amount of cholesterol in the body and not lipoproteins. Transporting antioxidative enzymes is another function of HDL. LDLs are frequently called bad cholesterol and they disperse cholesterol molecules to cells where they are required. VLDLs transports fats to cells in the form of triglycerides and is usually measured by a guesstimate, which is based on an assumed ratio with triglycerides. Is this scientific? They also transport cholesterol and release most of the fat; they then become IDLs. When IDLs release more fat to the cells they then become LDLs. Is this scientific? There are different types of lipoproteins which are referred to by the establishment as different types of cholesterol. This association of lipoproteins with both cholesterol and fat has led to the false assumption that cholesterol is a fat. There are several types of lipoproteins, and chylomicrons are the largest type, but they are not measured in a blood test, as the only ones that the public is being informed of are those that can be measured. Is this scientific?

In the late nineteenth century, a German pathologist named Rudolph Virchow sowed the seeds of the delusion known as the *Lipid Hypothesis* or *Cholesterol Theory*. After performing chemical analyses on arterial plaques removed from cadavers, he discovered that they contained sizeable quantities of cholesterol. He theorized that cholesterol from the blood infiltrated the artery walls and caused the plaques which he discovered there. He named this process lipid insudation. There is no interrelationship between serum cholesterol and the quantity of arteriosclerotic plaque when reviewing coronary calcium score studies or autopsy studies, proving that elevated cholesterol does not cause arteriosclerotic plaque. As a result of this misinformation, many hundreds of thousands of people have died prematurely and unnecessarily because of the deliberate suppression of this life-saving information.

A source of cholesterol is not needed to produce heart disease, but it is the trans fatty acids (synthetic fatty acids), which are present in hydrogenated or partially hydrogenated fats, that are a major cause of heart disease. Early in the 1900s, Wilhelm Normann, a German chemist, developed a process of solidifying liquid vegetable oil using hydrogenation. This process is achieved by passing hydrogen bubbles through heated oil, which chemically introduces extra hydrogen atoms to the fatty acid molecules that are present in the oil. Hydrogen is the smallest molecule in the universe. Fats that have been hydrogenated are unnatural fats that are extremely detrimental to the health of the body. They are not present in natural vegetable fats but are only present in fats that have been hydrogenated. The chemical structure of artificially, chemically hardened hydrogenated fats is different from that of either naturally hard saturated fats or naturally liquid unsaturated oils, either polyunsaturated or monounsaturated. Hydrogenated fats also have bent molecular shapes, but they are bent in the opposite direction, which is why they are known as trans-forms of naturally occurring unsaturated fats. They are triglycerides that have at least one of the three fatty acid chains as a trans fatty acid. Hydrogenated fats are difficult for the body to metabolize, and can neither be assimilated into the structures of the cells nor excreted in the normal manner. Thus, trans fats tend to remain stuck in the blood circulation and become oxidized whilst significantly contributing to an increased risk of disease. Processed foods are likely to contain trans fats. Trans fats generate enormous amounts of free radicals, which trigger inflammation and damage healthy cells, confirming the insidious link between trans fats and inflammation, as shown by hundreds of studies. Other studies prove that trans fats lead to insulin resistance, abdominal fat accumulation, and drastically raise the risk of heart disease.

Hydrogenation by the forced chemical addition of hydrogen into oils to make them firm at room temperature is also used as a process to extend the shelf life of products to keep food flavour stable. This process involves hydrogen molecules, which are used to saturate organic compounds in the presence of a catalyst. Catalysts are substances which are used to accelerate the reaction rate without being consumed in the process, and they are essential to operate this reaction. Common catalysts used during this process are metals such as platinum, palladium, and nickel. The presence of hydrogen atoms is an important requirement in the hydrogenation process and is used to remove the double or triple bond between the atoms. Hydrogen atoms turn an unsaturated hydrocarbon into a saturated one. Unsaturated hydrocarbons are compounds that contain double bonds in their structure and saturated hydrocarbons are compounds that only contain single bonds in their structure.

Trans fatty acids prevent the synthesis of prostacyclin (prostaglandin 12), which is necessary to keep the blood flowing. Conversely, thromboxane clots the blood. Those who were consuming margarine from 1910 to 1968 could not produce prostacyclin, so their blood was prone to clotting and they were liable to die from sudden death. The more solid the state that a margarine is in, the more hydrogenated it is. Both the Omega-6 and Omega-3 fatty acids build cells in the arteries that make prostacyclin and also those that create thromboxane. An ideal balance of Omega-6 to Omega-3 fats help enormously in keeping inflammation under control. Too much Omega-6 fatty acids tend to promote inflammation and Omega-3 fatty acids extinguish it. Both of these types of fats are needed in the right proportion, and most experts agree that the Omega-6 to Omega-3 ratio should range from 1:1 to 1:5 (in favour of more Omega-3), depending on health issues. The type of fat that is consumed is one of the most important dietary factors affecting the body's inflammation level because fats are precursors to anti-inflammatory and pro-inflammatory chemicals. Every cell in the body is surrounded by a lipid layer that should be just the right fluidity to allow all the necessary nutrients to pass through, while at the same time allowing critical waste material to pass out.

Good fats are the building blocks of healthy cell membranes, which are protective coverings surrounding each cell. If the diet is high in unhealthy animal fats, the cell membranes will be stiff, rigid, and unhealthy. Changing the composition of the cell membrane from healthy to unhealthy is fraught with danger, but that is exactly what unhealthy fats do. They clog cell membranes and initiate a cascade effect that finishes with a large amount of uncontrollable pro-inflammatory fatty acid eicosanoid molecules. Eicosanoids are signalling molecules that are derived from either Omega-3 or Omega-6 EFAs. Some pro-inflammatory eicosanoids, such as those that are derived from arachidonic acid, are potentially harmful if excessive amounts accrue in the body. They increase inflammation, encourage blood clotting, and constrict blood vessels. Eicosanoids compounds also include leukotrienes, prostacyclins, prostaglandins, and thromboxanes, which are responsible for many of the beneficial effects of good fats. They are a family of powerful hormone-like compounds that are produced in the body from EFAs. They reduce inflammation, inhibit blood-clotting, and dilate blood vessels. The networks of controls that rely on eicosanoids are amongst the most complex in the body. There are also Omega-7 fatty acids and Omega-9 fatty acids. Omega-7 fatty acids are unsaturated fatty acids and are contained in plant sources such as avocados and macadamia nuts. Omega-9 fatty acids are not strictly essential as they can be produced by the body and are the most abundant fats in most body cells. They are also contained in plant sources such as olives, avocados, nuts, and seeds.

Many margarine containers have 0% *trans fat* written on their labels. Manufacturers can claim that their products have zero trans fat if they contain less than one gram of trans fat per tablespoon of product. However, they deceptively make the portion size very low. This deception also applies to other foods that contain trans fats.

Sphingomyelins comprise a valuable class of phospholipids in the membranes of most eukaryotic cells. Tissues, such as the brain, ocular lenses, and peripheral nervous tissue, have greater sphingomyelin contents. Sphingomyelin is a component of five phospholipids that encircle the arterial cell to safeguard it. When oxidized fats have been consumed, the artery becomes lined with sphingomyelin. Both trans fats and oxidized fat interfere with the blood supply to the heart.

Healthy saturated fats and cholesterol have been vilified for many years as a result of Dr. Ancel Benjamin Keys' fraudulent twenty-two-country study. He was an American scientist who published an epidemiological study in 1958 comparing saturated fat consumption with the prevalence of heart disease. Data for twenty-two countries were available to him, but he picked only seven. Cherry-picking data is a means for a dishonest scientist to prove a hypothesis by choosing only the data that fits with their own criteria while ignoring the conflicting data. He was mostly funded by the sugar industry and his views were widely adopted by public health and professional organizations. He also achieved tremendous influential and professional eminence as his views formed the foundation for pursuing low-fat recommendations. Whilst demonizing saturated fats he glorified polyunsaturated fats, which has led to a very unfortunate and unhealthy path. Interestingly, refined cooking oils just so happened, by a seemingly strange coincidence, to become popular around the same time that cholesterol was demonized. Some of his following research on saturated fat and cholesterol actually undermined his own hypothesis but were never published, and as it did not support his original hypothesis, he is believed to have been responsible for its suppression.

Cherry-picking data is a means for a dishonest scientist to prove a hypothesis by choosing only the data that fits with their own criteria.

He once studied populations in Italy in the winter and Finland in the summer and hypothesized that those in Finland, who ate more of the hydrogenated and saturated fats, had more heart disease compared to those in Italy who did not eat these fats. But unfortunately, he did not differentiate between trans fats and saturated fats from animals or plants and said, in the beginning, that cholesterol was the cause of heart disease. He later retracted this and confessed before he died in 2004 that his thinking was wrong.

To unnaturally and unnecessarily lower cholesterol, the approval of the first commercial statin drug, with its many damaging effects, occurred on September 1987. Statin drugs are associated with over 300 adverse health effects and can cause the fatal nervous system disorder ALS, heart disease, memory loss, raise the risk of hemorrhagic strokes, and interfere with the production of the CoQ10 enzyme, which is vital for healthy cells. These drugs can also double the risk of diabetes as they are fundamentally diabetogenic. Common side effects include muscle problems, irritability, tingling and numbness in extremities, cognitive issues, and fatigue. Ironically, the same large, three industry-funded studies that discovered that cholesterol cannot possibly be the primary cause of heart disease also found that the claimed benefits of statin drugs are invalid, unsafe, and ineffective with misleading statistics that excluded information from unsuccessful trials. This drug has no health benefits whatsoever but has multiple adverse side effects and the risks associated with it can be deadly. A healthy diet and lifestyle is the best medicine.

"Ye shall not fear them: for the LORD your God He shall fight for you" (Deuteronomy 3:22).

Many neurons are encased in the fatty coatings of myelin sheaths. Neurons are similar to electrical wires, and myelin sheaths are similar to insulation surrounding these wires. Myelin sheaths keep electricity contained in the nerve pathways, thereby allowing signals and messages to move much quicker. Myelin is one-fifth cholesterol by weight, and a cholesterol deficiency is linked to a decline in memory and cognitive function.

The body needs a sufficient amount of full-spectrum minerals, including trace minerals. It also needs vitamins, amino acids, and omega fatty acids to function at optimal levels. A deficiency of any of these can cause adverse health issues. Cholesterol plays an integral role in the absorption of essential fat-soluble vitamins A, E, and K from food. A huge study of 150,000 people in Austria disclosed that a higher cholesterol level was associated with a longer lifespan and a low cholesterol level was associated with a shorter lifespan.

A vitamin C deficiency is one of the primary causes of cardiovascular disease, and data from hundreds of published research papers by world-class scientists specify the connection between cardiovascular disease and a vitamin C deficiency. Cholesterol adheres to artery walls in an effort to plug any damage, and a vitamin C deficiency in coronary arteries is the singular root cause of all coronary arterial blockages. Without adequate vitamin C, the body is unable to produce the collagen that is necessary to heal the arteries. While aspirin in low doses is often prescribed for people with heart conditions, aspirin causes a vitamin C deficiency, which destabilizes the elasticity and strength of arteries which can lead to brain haemorrhages.

The term *vitamin* derives from the words *vital* and *amine*, as the first vitamins to be discovered contained an amino group. High-quality healthy fats provide the important fat-soluble vitamins A, D, E, and K with high-quality cellular fuel, which every cell should be constructed of as every cell in the body uses fat as its primary fuel source. Fat-soluble vitamins are not lost when the foods that they are contained in are cooked. They must be consumed together with dietary fat to be absorbed and are first dissolved in the dietary fat. These fat-soluble activator vitamins assist with the absorption of minerals, which cannot be utilized without them. Fat-soluble vitamins are predominantly non-polar (symmetric, with no unshared electrons), and as such are soluble in non-polar solvents such as the fatty (non-polar) tissue of the body. The body stores these vitamins in the liver and adipose (fat) tissue when they are not used and are eliminated much slower than water-soluble vitamins.

The water-soluble vitamins are the B complex group and vitamin C, which are not stored in fat tissues and are quickly depleted. A deficit of healthy fats, fat-soluble vitamins, or fat-malabsorption exhibits itself in many health issues, including cancer, diabetes, memory problems and weight gain. Conversely, the consumption of healthy saturated fats from plants helps to construct good quality cell walls, which are responsive to intercellular communication, prevent cancer, benefit the nervous system, assist with weight loss, lower blood sugar and insulin levels, boost the immune system, and optimize cellular receptors. By not consuming sufficient good quality fats or consuming the wrong types of fat can cause the body to gain weight, and consuming polyunsaturated fatty acids from refined oils causes red blood cells to clump together. Without good healthy fats, the cell walls not only become rigid, but the cells function slower and become more vulnerable to inflammatory conditions. Conversely, cell walls constructed from good healthy fats means that more fat can be burned than stored. There is absolutely no correlation between heart disease and the healthy saturated fats of plants, as two major studies have recently confirmed. The body needs good healthy fats to enable it to thrive, and these fats also help to reduce heart disease.[9]

The hypothalamus is located at the base of the brain and has sensors that cause the pituitary gland, which is situated immediately below the hypothalamus, to release the thyroid-stimulating hormone (TSH). The thyroid produces T3 (three molecules of iodine) and T4 (four molecules of iodine) which binds to protein-binding globulin, the regulator of body functions. Under any type of stress, anti-inflammatory and antioxidant cortisol, which is secreted by the adrenal glands, slows down thyroid function, which decreases bodily function, and if the thyroid is depressed the cortisol increases. Cortisol, a glucocorticoid (steroid hormone), is produced from cholesterol in the two adrenal glands located on top of each kidney. The adrenal glands make everything from cholesterol, and a low thyroid function causes the adrenals to overwork. Inflammation from toxins and a low thyroid function raises cortisol, while a healthy diet and lifestyle lower it. In response to inflammation, the body secretes cortisol, which decreases

---

[9] "Monounsaturated fats from plant and animal sources in relation to risk of coronary heart disease among US men and women," *The American Journal of Clinical Nutrition,* Vol. 107:3, https://1ref.us/1ow (accessed June 6, 2021). See also "13 Studies on Coconut Oil and Its Health Effects," https://1ref.us/1ox (accessed June 6, 2021).

immune system function. To summarize, a healthy diet and lifestyle assist the thyroid while a toxic lifestyle weakens it.

One of the most toxic refined oils to consume is canola (rapeseed) oil, which often comes from genetically modified rapeseeds that have been altered to reduce toxic erucic acid levels by being processed through chemical baths before bleaching. This oil is a chemical carcinogen and health hazard that is unfit for human consumption and is used as an industrial oil that even insects avoid as it is also an insecticide. It was first used as a motor lubricant during World War II! It has been found to retard growth when included in infant formulas and also produces low infant birth rates. This oil coagulates in the blood and clogs blood vessels, increases cancer and dementia risk (including Alzheimer's disease), damages the brain and heart, increases the risk of heart attacks and strokes, decreases learning ability, reduces liver and kidney function, causes weight gain, has been proven to cause lung cancer, is an immune depressant, depletes vitamin E, causes vision loss, destroys the protective coating of the myelin sheath (which disrupts the central nervous system), causes anaemia and respiratory illnesses, triggers degenerative diseases by increasing membrane rigidity, inhibits food metabolism and enzyme function, and causes irritability of the colon.

"Be of good courage, and He shall strengthen your heart all ye that hope in the LORD" (Psalm 31:24).

It is a proven myth that saturated plant fat causes heart disease as there is no scientific evidence to support it. Not all saturated fats are created equal. In the last century, researchers thought that consuming saturated fat seemed to increase blood cholesterol levels, which was also thought to increase heart disease. Thereby, an assumption was made that if saturated fat increases cholesterol levels, which causes heart disease, then saturated fat causes heart disease. However, this was not founded on any human experimental evidence, but rather, assumptions, animal studies, and observational information. Before ever being proven to be true, this hypothesis became public policy in 1977. Many studies, involving over 643,000 participants, revealed absolutely no results connecting saturated plant fat consumption with heart disease. This has been intensely studied for decades. Studies indicate that the regular consumption of unrefined coconut oil improves the levels of lipids circulating in the blood, which potentially reduces the risk of heart disease. Studies also prove that unrefined coconut oil helps to prevent the fatty deposits that lead to heart attack and stroke. There is now sufficient

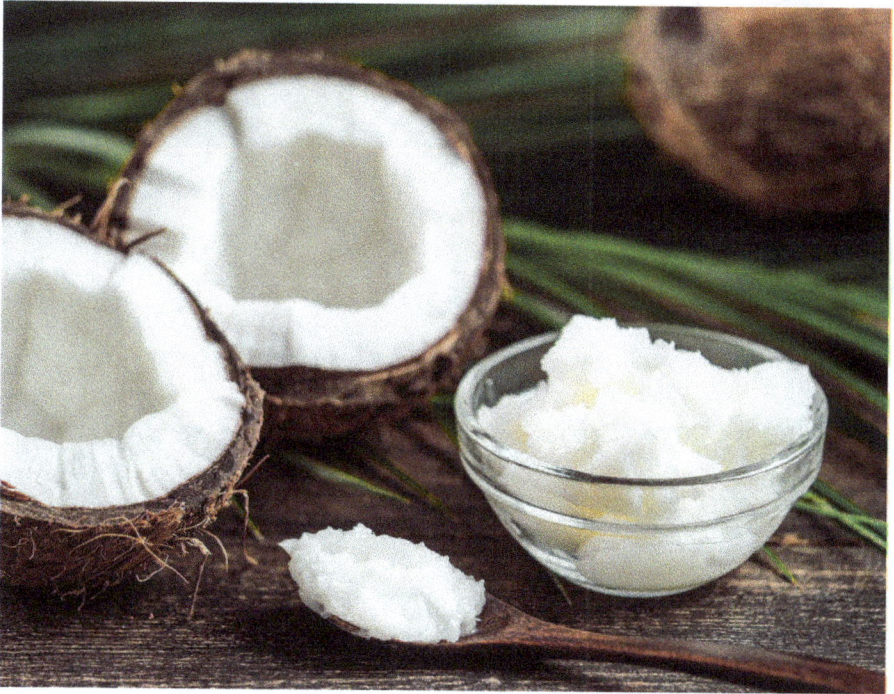

human experimental information demonstrating that the initial assumptions were erroneous, but unfortunately, the original unproven assumptions are still being propagated. Several studies that replaced saturated plant fat with polyunsaturated vegetable oils demonstrated that more participants died who were in the vegetable oil study groups. The prevalence of obesity has exploded since the low-fat guidelines were announced and this was soon followed by an epidemic of type 2 diabetes.

Fats can be identified as unsaturated or saturated. Saturated fatty acids have all of their carbon atoms fully saturated with hydrogen atoms. Saturated fats are solid at room temperature and can subsequently be divided into short, medium, long, and very-long-chain fatty acids, which have different effects in the body. Saturated fatty acids that contain less than six carbon atoms are known as short-chain fatty acids. Medium-chain fatty acids contain six to twelve carbon atoms, are absorbed directly into the bloodstream and do not appear to be stored in the body's fat tissue as easily as long-chain fatty acids are. Long-chain fatty acids contain fourteen to eighteen carbon atoms and very-long-chain fatty acids contain twenty carbon atoms.

Glycerol $C_3H_8O_3$

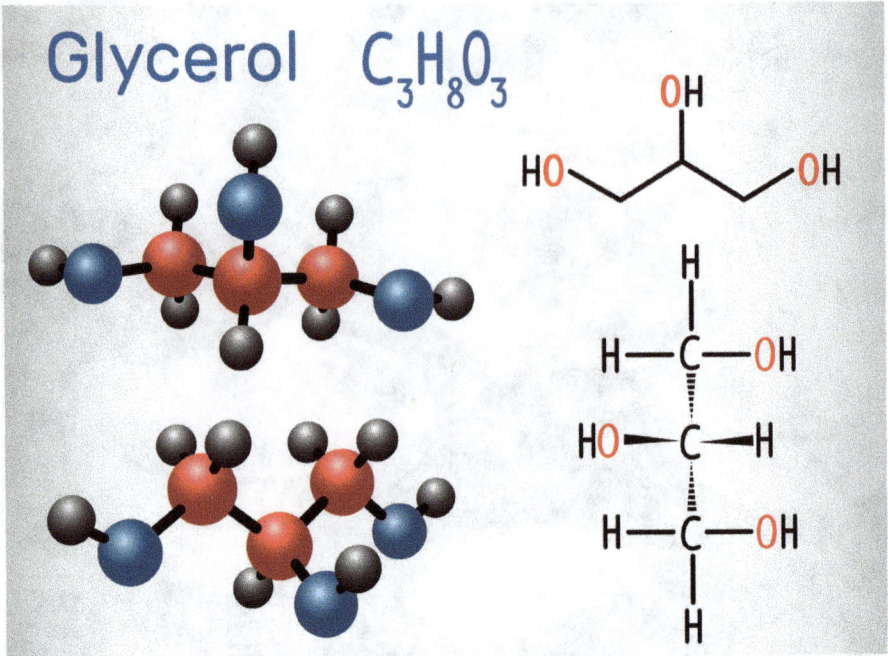

Fats contain a combination of different fatty acids, as no fat solely contains saturated fat, polyunsaturated fat, or monounsaturated fat. Fatty acids have two or more double bonds and monosaturated fatty acids have only one double bond. Unrefined coconut oil is high in healthy saturated fats that have different effects than most other dietary fats. Unrefined coconut oil has the highest concentration of rare and highly beneficial medium-chain fatty acids. The abundant medium-chain fats in unrefined coconut oil are a form of healthy saturated fat that comprises 91% of its total composition. Its 91% saturated fat content is comprised of 49% lauric acid (C12), 16% myristic acid (C14), 9% palmitic acid (C16), 8% caprylic acid (C8), 7% capric acid (C10) and 2% stearic acid (C17). Its 9% unsaturated fat content is comprised of 7% oleic acid (C18) and 2% linoleic acid.

Most other dietary fats are long-chain triglycerides. A triglyceride is an ester derived from three fatty acids and one glycerine (or glycerol) molecule, which can be either monounsaturated, polyunsaturated, or saturated. Esters are ubiquitous organic compounds where hydrogen in the compound's carboxyl group is replaced with a hydrocarbon group. Triglycerides have two primary purposes: they are either stored as body fat or transported into cells and burned for energy.

They can be formed from any combination of fatty acids. The healthy fats in unrefined coconut oil are rapidly broken down by the body, converted into energy and absorbed into the body differently than the majority of other fats. The calories in medium-chain fatty acids are unlikely to be stored as body fat as they are efficiently transformed into energy and used by the body. Unrefined coconut oil is an excellent energy source as, when consumed and digested, its medium-chain fatty acids are quickly converted into usable energy by the liver. These special fats are responsible for many of the health benefits of unrefined coconut oil and are critical structural components of cellular membranes.

Medium-chain fatty acids are metabolized differently than long-chain fatty acids and are more easily absorbed as they are transported directly to the liver for expeditious metabolisation. They can be utilized there as an instant source of energy or transformed into ketones, which can have a hunger-reducing effect and are substances that are manufactured when the liver degrades significant quantities of fat. Obesity is a well-known risk factor for cardiovascular issues. Research proves that unrefined coconut oil promotes weight loss by accelerating the metabolism and reducing the appetite. Unrefined coconut oil also stabilizes blood sugar levels and reduces insulin resistance, which leads to type 2 diabetes, as ketones and medium-chain fatty acids do not require pancreatic enzymes to be digested. Unlike other fatty acids, ketones can cross the blood-brain barrier and enter the brain, which provides the brain with an alternative energy source if the usual glucose availability is limited. Cancerous tumours rely on glucose for growth and cannot access the energy from ketones, which are produced during the digestion of unrefined coconut oil. Thereby, consuming a diet containing sufficient unrefined coconut oil is a healthy strategy for avoiding cancer.

Lauric acid is the longest of the medium-chain fatty acids. With its twelve carbon atoms it comprises about 50% of the fatty acids in unrefined coconut oil, making it one of the best natural sources of this fatty acid. Lauric acid contains the highest source of medium-chain fatty acids outside of human breast milk. When the lauric acid saturated fat is digested, it forms a monolaurin. Both monolaurin and lauric acid can kill harmful pathogens such as fungi and bacteria. These substances have also been demonstrated to help kill the dangerous Staphylococcus aureus bacteria and the yeast Candida albicans. *Scientists have discovered that lauric acid is also able to kill colon cancer cells.*

Healthy medium-chain natural saturated fats, such as anti-inflammatory unrefined coconut oil, are very protective and beneficial for the brain and

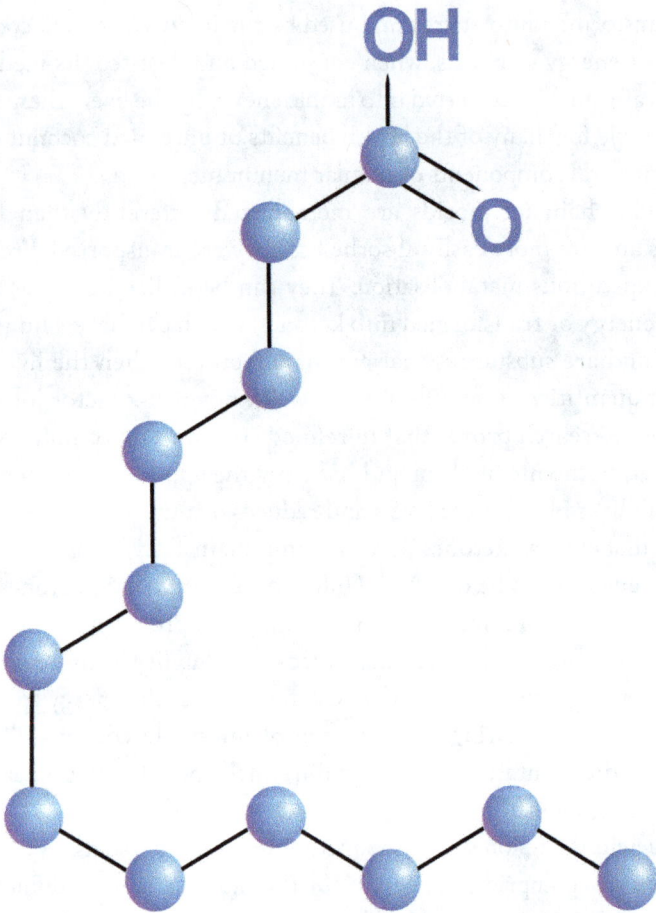

Lauric acid

immune system as well as for the rest of the body. It is also being studied for showing promising outcomes for treating Alzheimer's disease and other serious neurological issues. Healthy saturated fat is essential and nerve repair cannot occur without it. Unrefined coconut oil is not only a powerful anti-inflammatory but is also an antibacterial, antibiotic, anti-viral, anti-microbial, antioxidant, anti-cancer, and antifungal that can help to combat disease. Unrefined coconut oil is also a salve for burns and other skin issues, protects against liver damage, slows ageing, clears up kidney infections and urinary tract infections, relieves sore throats, supports healthy digestion, reduces symptoms of pancreatitis and gallbladder disease, and helps with ulcerative colitis and a leaky gut. Regular consumption of unrefined coconut oil improves thyroid gland function. Several populations around the world have thrived for multiple generations by consuming substantial amounts of coconut, replete with coconut oil, as a dietary staple.

Unhealthy saturated fat is present in all meat and fish, including chicken and turkey, even when cooked without the skin. Conversely, healthy saturated fat, such as unrefined coconut oil, as part of a plant-food diet, is extremely healthful. Unrefined coconut oil contains the most concentrated natural source of healthy medium-chain fatty acids.

"The liberal soul shall be made fat: and he that watereth shall be watered also himself" (Proverbs 11:25).

SUGAR

"EVERY TIME YOU EAT OR DRINK YOU ARE EITHER FIGHTING DISEASE OR FEEDING DISEASE."

It has recently been discovered from internal documents that, in the 1960s, the sugar industry deliberately orchestrated a campaign to downplay and falsify evidence linking sugar consumption to coronary heart disease. It was discovered that the sugar industry paid prestigious Harvard scientists a large sum of money to shift public opinion away from sugar to fat. They were asked to write a review based on studies that were hand-picked by the sugar industry and published in the prestigious J.A.M.A. The outcome was that total fats and cholesterol were vilified instead of toxic sugar (conflict of interest disclosure was not required until 1984).

Refined white sugar is known as the *white death*, and research confirms that not only does this refined sugar lead to weight gain and disease, but it has the same highly addictive effects as tobacco and other drugs, as it functions as *brain crack*. White sugar is 99.6% sucrose and 0.4% ash with no nutrient value whatsoever. It is not an innocuous substance but strips the body of nutrients, as it has had all of its nutrients and enzymes removed when processed and performs as a drug in the system. There is substantial evidence that refined sugar can promote addictive behaviours by activating the reward centre of the brain in a similar way to addictive drugs. It limits the stress hormone cortisol and quells stress signals in the brain, which can cause people to consume more in times of stress, thereby creating an addiction cycle. Consuming it removes minerals, vitamins, enzymes, and insulin from the body in order for the body to be able to process it. Depleting essential magnesium, calcium, and chromium levels in the body leads to adverse health effects and damaging reactions, including asthma, arthritis, candida, eczema, and tooth decay. In addition to promoting yeast growth, it is potentially both directly and indirectly carcinogenic as it acidifies the body. In robbing the body of essential nutrients, it limits the beneficial effects of vitamin C, as vitamin C and sugar utilize the same transporters to reach the cells, which can result in limited vitamin C absorption. This type of deficiency may result in decreased immune function and suppressed tissue regeneration.

This nutrient-depleted toxic sugar is one of the primary causes of metabolic changes in the cells of the body, which is consistent with the initiation and promotion of cancer. White sugar is acidic and cancer grows in an acidic environment. Anything that acidifies the body can cause cancer. Conversely, research indicates that depriving cells of refined sugar can reverse cancer.[10] Consuming sour foods, such as lemons, naturally curbs sugar cravings. Refined sugar is also another major dietary culprit in the development of cardiovascular disease. It is also eight times more addictive than cocaine. Eliminating refined sugar from the diet will significantly reduce the likelihood of developing cancer, as refined sugar feeds the growth of tumour cells, but healthy fats, such as unrefined coconut oil, starve them. It is refined sugar, and not fat, that drives disease, and has been found to not only to feed cancer but it also actively contributes to the transformation of normal cells into cancerous ones. Refined sugar triggers dopamine in the brain, and the regular consumption of unhealthy sugary foods and drinks causes a craving for more refined sugar. This

---

[10] "Otto Warburg Biographical," The Nobel Prize, https://1ref.us/1oy (accessed August 4, 2021).

can affect the taste buds, which also sense nutrients, and prevent them from recognizing full-bodied flavours as well as depleting their numbers.

It also affects a specific area of the brain responsible for reacting to stress. A part of the brain known as the nucleus accumbens is located near the front and bottom of the brain in an area known as the basal forebrain and is considered to be part of the basal ganglia. There is a nucleus accumbens in each hemisphere. It is mostly recognized as the reward pathway of the brain, as dopamine neurons and other types of neurons are activated during both rewarding and aversive experiences. This can increase dopamine levels in the nucleus accumbens that can lead to addiction. With addictive processes, a pleasurable experience can become overwhelming and lead to compulsive behaviour. The gut, which is teeming with microbial life, also communicates with the brain, and the link between

> *It is refined sugar, and not fat, that drives disease, and has been found to not only to feed cancer but it also actively contributes to the transformation of normal cells into cancerous ones.*

the two is known as *the gut-brain axis*. The enteric nervous system is embedded in the gut wall, which works both independently of and in conjunction with the brain. Consuming an abundance of refined sugar decimates the health of the gut, which in turn is detrimental to the brain, as changes in gut health can lead to brain disorders. A study showed that impairments in memory were directly linked to changes in gut microbiota caused by excess refined sugar consumption.

After consuming excess refined sugar, the immune system can be hindered for 1–2 hours and these effects can linger for as much as five hours. During this time too much refined sugar interferes with immune system communications and also deposits toxic substances into the body as refined sugar breaks down into toxic acids. The lymphatic and immune systems assist with the removal of these acids but it uses extra energy and resources to remove it. The body is at a great disadvantage whenever the immune system turns its attention away from a full-scale attack against pathogens. Consuming too much refined sugar also suppresses the production of immune cells such as B cells, T cells, NK cells, and specifically phagocytes, which are advantageous to the immune system and are needed to rid the body of toxins.

Scientists have discovered that mitochondrial damage and dysfunction is at the heart of practically all diseases, as damaged cells trigger nuclear genetic mutations which can cause cancer. Cancer cells are sugar addicts and have an intrinsically diversified energy metabolism and metabolic flexibility in comparison to healthy cells. Cells can produce energy either anaerobically in the cytoplasm, or aerobically in the mitochondria. Excessive levels of lactic acid are generated by anaerobic metabolism, which can be toxic, and in the presence of oxygen cancer cells overproduce lactic acid. Glucose or fat can be used as a source of energy by healthy cells, but cancer cells are metabolically constrained to consume only sugar. Tumours prefer to utilize sugar fermentation for the production of energy rather than the much more efficient oxygen-based phosphorylation. Phosphorylation is the most common mechanism for transmitting signals throughout the cells and regulating the function of protein. In addition

Mitochondrial function

1. ATP synthesis.
2. Synthesis own organic substances.
3. Education own ribosomes.

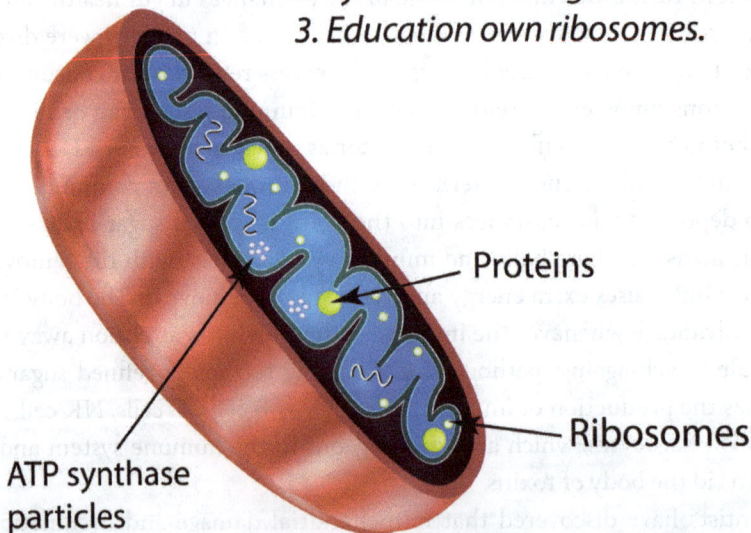

Proteins

Ribosomes

ATP synthase particles

to other building materials, all cells need adenosine triphosphate (ATP) as a source of energy. Cancer cells are antithetical to this and redirect glucose away from the manufacture of ATP to building materials that are necessary for their cell growth. These other building materials need protein and fatty acids which cancer cells take from their surroundings. This usurpation of neighbouring tissue displays how cancer spreads and metastasizes, and the driving force behind this is oxygen free-radical production, which causes random DNA damage and explains chromosomal abnormalities.

Chemical artificial sweeteners are enormously addictive and cause lesions in the brain. They are able to damage cells and vascular function, are absorbed by fat, increase the pH level in the intestines, block the absorption of nutrients, and reduce beneficial gut bacteria by 50% by damaging their DNA. A healthy gut relies on a healthy gut microbiome, which is essential for nutrient absorption, proper digestion, and immune system function. Research indicates that artificial sweeteners worsen insulin sensitivity more than refined sugar and have also been found to promote weight gain. The sweet taste of artificial sweeteners causes metabolic confusion as there are no accompanying calories. The brain releases dopamine when a sweet substance is ingested and this activates the reward centre of the brain. Leptin, the appetite-regulating hormone, is also released, notifying the brain that sufficient calories have been ingested, however, the body is disappointed. Consuming sweet-tasting substances that do not contain any calories still activates the pleasure pathway of the brain but do not deactivate it as the calories are absent. This results in cravings as the body continues to signal its need for more, and consequently there is a dramatically increased risk of obesity.

There is also a correlation between obesity and dementia as additional body fat affects the hippocampus—the memory centre of the brain. The additional body fat causes inflammation in the brain as the blood-brain barrier becomes de-stabilized and penetrated. This results in a *leaky brain*, which can cause many diseases including Parkinson's disease, Alzheimer's disease, chronic depression, stroke, autism, and multiple sclerosis.

Sucralose is not a healthy substance but is a ubiquitous, synthetic, artificial sweetener which releases toxic dioxin, dibenzofurans, organochlorine, and polychlorinated dibenzo-p-dioxins into food when heated and has been linked to a wide range of serious health conditions including cancer, endocrine disruption, and gut inflammation. It preferentially targets health benefitting gut bacteria and also accumulates in fat cells.

Xylitol is a hydrogenated and highly refined processed chemical substance that is a molecular cousin to refined white sugar. It is derived from the crushed fibres of sugar cane, corn, or birch wood, using a chemical reaction involving the use of phosphoric acid, sulfuric acid, calcium oxide, and active charcoal. The result is a sweet-tasting, bleached, powdery blend of sugar alcohols which the body cannot metabolize, and as a result, it can remain indefinitely lodged in the gut, which creates a toxic environment conducive to harmful pathogens which can adversely affect the intestinal lining. A study revealed that even small concentrations (one milligram per millilitre) of artificial sweeteners are toxic to the gut microbial system.

There is also a relationship between toxic aspartame, methanol toxicity, and the formation of toxic formaldehyde, which is formed from artificial sweeteners. It can cause vision loss, cognitive impairment, and neurotransmitter destruction in the brain while aggressively increasing chemicals that are associated with violence, anger, hatred, and fear. It can also cause the brain to be vulnerable to oxidative and chemical damage from vaccines. According to a twenty-two-year study at Harvard University, aspartame is also linked to blood cancers.

Many people who are looking for a *natural* alternative to artificial sweeteners turn to agave. Agave *nectar* is made from the starchy agave root bulb and not from the dried sap of the plant. It is not a healthy sweetener and contains about 85% D-fructose, which is much sweeter than refined sugar. This has a greater potential for provoking harmful health conditions such as insulin resistance, fatty liver disease, and dangerous abdominal fat. The concentration of fructose in agave is higher than in high-fructose corn syrup. A highly chemicalized industrial process, using GM enzymes, is required to convert the bulb into *nectar*, and is similar to the production of high fructose corn syrup. The different colours of the syrup do not vary nutritionally, with the amber-coloured syrup being refined by burning the fructose above 140° F. *Raw* agave syrup does not exist. Agave contains significant quantities of saponins, which disrupt red blood cells. This toxic steroid derivative should be avoided during pregnancy as it can provoke a miscarriage.

The sweetener high-fructose corn syrup is a very common and inexpensive sweetener used in many processed foods. The consumption of high-fructose corn syrup, even when used in moderation, has been linked to many serious diseases as it drives systemic inflammation and is a major cause of cancer, diabetes, heart disease, obesity, dementia, weight gain, liver failure, and tooth decay. A high consumption of free fructose (a monosaccharide) has been demonstrated to cause a leaky gut (where the glue protein zonulin gives way in the gut due to inflammation and consequently food can pass into the bloodstream which can then cause chaos in the body). High-fructose corn syrup and cane sugar are not processed in the same way by the body, neither are they biochemically identical. High-fructose corn syrup often contains contaminants including toxic levels of mercury, a heavy metal that the body cannot eliminate easily.

There are many other falsely-called *natural sugars* that are not much healthier than deadly refined white sugar and which also lack the important vitamins and minerals which are necessary for the digestion of sugar. When these nutrients are missing from the sugar the body must remove them from the teeth, bones, and other tissues to compensate for this lack. Sugars, such as turbinado, demerara, raw sugar, evaporated cane juice, evaporated cane sugar, organic raw sugar, and muscovado, are boiled, dehydrated into crystals, and then spun in a centrifuge to separate the crystals from the molasses. This process

The concentration of fructose in agave is higher than in high-fructose corn syrup.

is usually accomplished with chemicals and sometimes with pressure. Some of the molasses is then added back to the crystals, albeit in unnatural proportions, and this falsely-called *natural sugar* is then marketed as a health food, including Sucanat, which is made by separating the molasses from the sugars and then recombining most of the molasses back with the sugar.

In its natural state sugar cane is naturally rich in the minerals calcium, chromium, cobalt, copper, iron, magnesium, manganese, phosphorous, and zinc. It also contains vitamins A, B1, B2, B3, B5, B6, and C, which work synergistically with the minerals and polyphenols to nourish the body. Organic rapadura sugar retains all of these nutrients without the addition of chemicals or anti-caking agents. Rapadura is a Portuguese name, which refers to raw unadulterated evaporated sugar cane juice. This sugar is made by first using a press to extract the juice from the pure sugar cane. The water is then evaporated out of the juice by stirring with paddles over very low heat. This concentrated juice is dried and the resulting sugar is passed through a sieve, leaving a dark brown grainy textured sugar. Nothing is added and only the water is removed. As the rapadura is not separated from the molasses and dehydrated

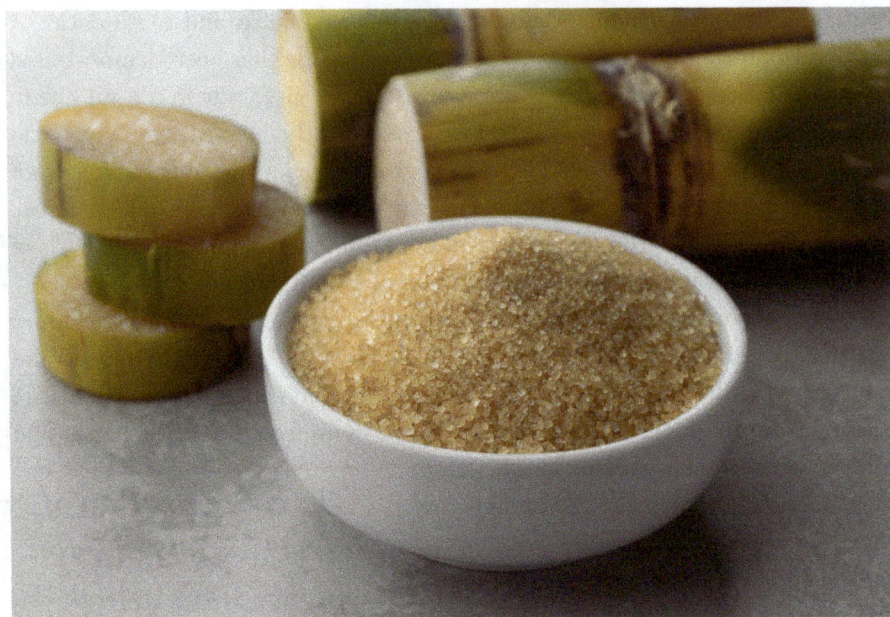

at low heat, the natural balance of vitamins and minerals present in the sugar cane is retained. This is the most important property of rapadura, which cannot be claimed by any other type of sugar.

"My meditation of Him shall be sweet: I will be glad in the LORD" (Psalm 104:34).

WEIGHT LOSS AND HAIR LOSS

For some people, gaining weight is a very unpleasant experience and losing that weight seems all but impossible, but this is not as difficult as it seems, because there are some healthy and tasty plants that encourage a high metabolic rate. Mushrooms, such as chestnut mushrooms (baby portobellas), are not only delicious but also have a meaty flavour and texture, which is especially important for those who are non-meat eaters. Although mushrooms are classified as vegetables, technically they are not plants but part of the kingdom of fungi.

Biotin (vitamin B7 and sometimes called vitamin H) boosts the metabolism which aids weight loss. It also benefits the central nervous system. Weight loss experts have found this vitamin to be highly beneficial for weight loss as it supports many functions in the body that are necessary for weight loss, such as elevating the resting rate of the metabolism. As this vitamin increases the metabolism, it can help accelerate weight loss, especially when paired with chromium, and mushrooms contain good sources of both biotin and chromium. Biotin plays a major role in helping the body convert food into usable energy. This water-soluble B complex vitamin is plentiful in a wide range of foods.

The body needs a well-balanced, anti-inflammatory diet together with regular exercise, sufficient nutrients, and good quality sleep. When the body undergoes internal inflammation from bad eating habits and stress, it is subject to accruing additional weight. Inflammation plays havoc with the hormones that control how the body processes and stores fat, which is why an anti-inflammatory diet is essential. The following healthy foods contain biotin: mushrooms, cauliflower, peanuts, hazelnuts, almonds, walnuts, pecans, pistachios, nutritional yeast, rolled oats, avocados, sunflower and sesame seeds, sweet potatoes, bananas, tomatoes, broccoli, onions, carrots, grapefruit, legumes, whole grains, leafy greens, raspberries, strawberries, and watermelon.

Medicinal mushrooms benefit the body in more ways that just encouraging a healthy metabolism. They provide the properties of immune boosting, anti-oxidation, and anti-inflammatory effects, thereby helping to protect the hair from damage and reducing hair loss.

Niacin promotes hair growth and improves blood circulation to the scalp and together with other vitamins, minerals, and antioxidants, promotes strong, healthy hair and helps to prevent hair loss and other hair problems. Flaxseed contains both niacin and biotin.

Zinc helps to prevent hair loss and the following foods contain zinc: mushrooms, nuts, seeds, legumes, whole grains, brown rice, asparagus, broccoli, wheat germ, oats, corn, and garlic.

Lentils and beans provide a source of protein, zinc, iron, and biotin. Dark green vegetables are full of vitamins A and C and help with sebum production, which are natural oils produced on the scalp. Avocados are high in Omega-3 fatty acids. They help to moisturize the hair and scalp, promoting silky, shiny hair.

Blueberries are widely known as a super antioxidant food as they are very high in vitamin C which promotes a healthy scalp. Many other fruits also contain vitamin C.

Biotin stimulates keratin production in the hair and can also increase the rate of follicle growth. Mushrooms are rich in the B vitamins: riboflavin, niacin, and pantothenic acid. This combination helps to protect the health of the heart, is also good for red blood cells and the digestive system and for maintaining healthy skin. The efficacy of mushrooms will be reduced if they are overcooked.

SALT

Science is questionably incongruent on the widely debated subject of low dietary salt, with the largest quantity of credible research targeting healthy salt as being a heart health protector, instead of something that destroys it. The notion that salt is unhealthy was initially only a hypothesis, which somehow became an *undeniable fact* around 1972 when certain government agencies decided to aggressively vilify salt and suggested its dangers. They even went to the extent of launching falsely-called *educational programmes*, condemning salt as harmful. A propaganda campaign, which lasted for decades, ultimately succeeded in sway-ing public opinion, proving the old adage that a lie can travel half-way around the world while the truth is putting its shoes on. Contrary to popular belief, science has never definitively proven that healthy salt in any respect causes abnormal pulse pressure, and much published modern scientific research has proven and supports the conclusion that healthy salt is really beneficial and safe for health, and actually suggests that salt restriction is detrimental to the health of the body. The body needs sufficient good salt to function at its maximum potential, and an insufficiency can cause much harm and even death as it is essential for the blood. *Hyponatremia* is the term for inadequate salt.

Contrary to popular belief, science has never definitively proven that healthy salt in any respect causes abnormal pulse pressure, and much published modern scientific research has proven and supports the conclusion that healthy salt is really beneficial and safe for health.

Salt is essential to life and life cannot live without it as it is fundamental to exis-tence. The misguided medical establish-ment also villainizes salt and makes no distinctions between its different types. Healthy pink Himalayan crystal salt is invaluable because of the sodium ions that it possesses, which the body uses to maintain some of its essential functions. The multitude of elements in this pink crystal salt forms a compound in which each molecule is co-dependent. This connectedness allows the components of all of the trace elements present in their natural state to be in co-operation with each other and adds to its capability of encouraging a healthy balance. This healthy salt uptakes specific nutrients from the intestines, helps to maintain fluid in the blood cells, and relays information in the muscles and nerves. The body relies on a correct balance of nutrients to maintain its vital processes, which are needed for survival. This balance is very fragile and a lack or overabundance of one mineral may affect all of the others. Sodium also affects other minerals and is as necessary to bodily functioning as potassium.

Nothing compares to pink Himalayan crystal salt with its inherent abundance of at least eighty-four minerals and trace elements in their natural mineral form. Not only does it contain an almost identical set of elements as those found in the human body, and in the same proportions as occur in the blood, but it also tastes better. Hand-mined pink Himalayan crystal salt has the most perfect geometric crystalline structure when viewed under an electron microscope. All of these trace elements and minerals are available in a colloidal form, which is more absorbable. Cells can only absorb elements that occur in an available

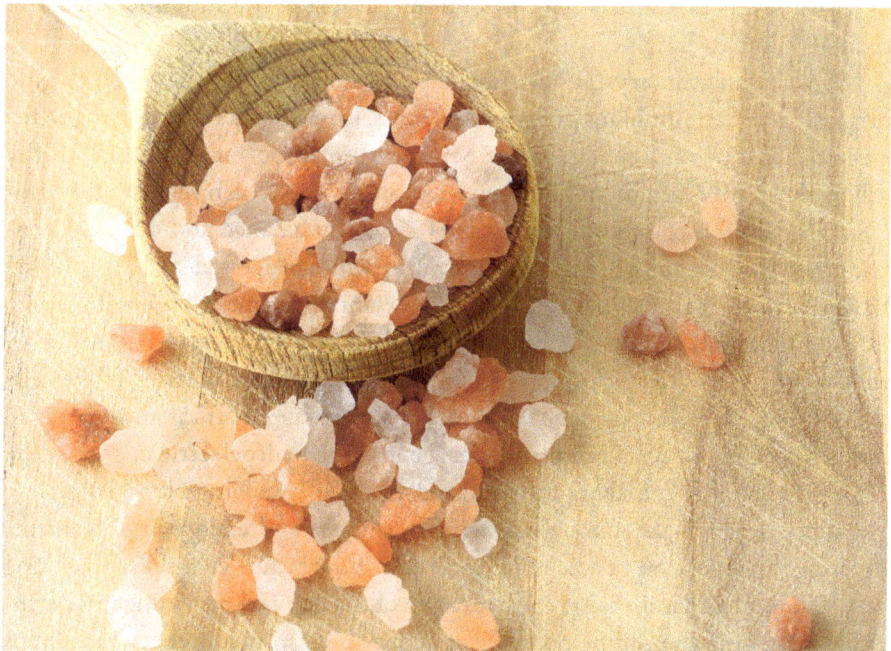

ional-colloidal form, which enables them to pass through the cell wall. These elements are available in this Himalayan crystal salt in such tiny colloidal-size particles that they can easily be absorbed and metabolized by cells.

This beautiful pink salt is mined from the Khewra Salt Mine in Northern Pakistan, which is situated at the foothills of the Himalayan Mountains about 160 km. from the capital city of Islamabad. It is the second-largest salt mine in the world. The Khewra rock salt mountain range is located in the district of Jhelum. This salt mine dates back to 326 BC, during the time of Alexander the Great. During a battle, his troops discovered that their tired and hungry horses had uncovered salt when they broke up the ground with their hooves and were licking the salty rocks. Centuries after this initial discovery the Mughal (Mogul) emperor Jalaluddin Muhammad Akbar introduced standardized salt mining in Khewra, which then became a traded commodity. This unadulterated salt is mined by hand by skilled workers using traditional methods, so there is little to no pollution or waste by-products from its manufacturing. The colours of the salt mined from Khewra include dark red, red, pink, white, and also transparent. The delicate pink colour of Himalayan crystal salt comes from iron oxides. The salt mine is nearly 0.3 kilometres above sea level and extends to approximately 3 kilometres inside the mountains. All nineteen levels of tunnels have a total length inside the mountain of more than 40 kilometres.

Pink Himalayan crystal salt does not cause hardship to the body as some other salts do, and humans are created with salt receptors on their tongue for a reason. It is very difficult for the body to absorb too much of this healthy salt as there are efficient and powerful response loops which regulate this process. This natural crystal salt encourages a healthy balance and does not contribute to adverse pulse pressure as unhealthy white processed sodium chloride table salt does. It is also needed as an important component of blood plasma, extracellular fluid, lymphatic, and amniotic fluid. Another essential function of this healthy salt is that it promotes a healthy systemic pH balance of the cells while it detoxifies. Its other health benefits also include natural antimicrobial, antifungal, and antibacterial properties; generating hydroelectric energy in the cells; transporting nutrients into and out of cells; balancing blood sugar levels; supporting weight loss by balancing hormones and energy improvement; assisting the reduction of acid reflux; increasing the brain's glial cells; regulating water content and improving the hydration of the body by providing trace minerals; increasing the red blood cell count due to its iron content, which helps to improve oxygen transportation and circulation; facilitating natural asthma treatment and reducing allergy symptoms; assisting with a balanced pulse pressure as it provides unrefined mineral-rich salt in an ionic solution, increasing performance and reducing stress; promoting sinus health and lowering the incidence of sinus problems; improving the pH balance of the stomach which leads to better nutrient absorption; stimulating digestive enzymes and salivary glands, which is important for the proper functioning of the digestive system; supporting adrenal and thyroid function; neutralizing electromagnetic radiation; naturally improving and regulating sleep by supporting hormone balance and blood sugar; increasing the elimination of CO_2 from the blood, thereby helping to prevent acidosis; replacing bodily minerals that are lost through sweating; promoting the increased absorption of food particles through the intestinal tract; acting as a powerful antihistamine; and also preventing muscle cramps by improving mineral status and supporting respiratory health. Both sodium and chloride are needed for the firing of neurons. Just one gram of this special pink crystal salt contains approximately 500 micrograms of iodine. Upon spectral analysis, pink Himalayan crystal salt demonstrates that it contains both macrominerals and trace minerals. It also contains less heavy metals than sea salt, which has been found in many parts of the world to contain minute particles of plastic from ocean waste, known as microplastics.

This crystal salt was once called *King Salt* as it was reserved for royalty. It is the purest uncontaminated salt on earth as it is sourced from a pristine area without environmental pollutants. It has an unlimited shelf life and is the highest grade of natural salt. The purity level of this rock salt can be as high as 99.3% and contains no microplastics. By analysis, its sodium-potassium ratio is 84.27% sodium and 0.77% potassium. By comparison, toxic table salt is 97.5% sodium chloride with negligible potassium, 2.5% chemicals and is dried at over 650°C (140°F). These white salt synthetic chemicals include everything from manufactured forms of sodium solo-co-aluminate, iodide, anti-caking agents, fluoride, sodium bicarbonate, toxic amounts of potassium iodide and aluminum derivatives.

Table salt is not only sodium chloride but also contains additives that have been devised to facilitate a better flow. Talcum powder, silico aluminate (which contains aluminium), and inorganic ferrocyanide are frequently included as anti-caking agents. Consuming aluminium leads to neurological disorders, especially when there is no available selenium to assist the body with chelating it.[11]

---

[11] A chelating agent is a substance whose molecules can form several bonds to a single metal ion. It's a way of removing unwanted substances from the body.

Aluminium bio-accumulates in the body, causing additional degeneration over time. Talcum powder is a recognized carcinogen and is permitted in white table salt while being prohibited in every other food because of its toxicity. According to regulations, highly-processed, de-mineralized, bleached, white table salt is allowed to contain up to 2% talcum powder.

Sodium chloride is an artificial, isolated, and unhealthy material that has no comparison to real healthy salt. Salt was once regarded as white gold but it was unfortunately transformed into white poison. Common refined white table salt has been stripped of its minerals during processing, which would otherwise help to balance the pulse pressure, and is sold instead to supplement companies. Table salt producers recognize and intentionally remove the most nutritious part of the salt, thus malnourishing their consumers whilst increasing their profits. Accordingly, instead of stabilizing the pulse pressure, this refined table salt causes fluctuations in it. This infamous danger has created a whole industry of foods with low sodium. White, refined table salt crystals are completely isolated from each other, and for the body to attempt to metabolize these white table salt crystals it must sacrifice enormous quantities of energy. When the body attempts to isolate any excess white salt that it is exposed to, water molecules encompass the sodium chloride to separate them into sodium and chloride ions to assist the body with neutralizing them. To facilitate this process, water is taken from the cells for the neutralization of the unnatural sodium chloride, which results in an unfavourable fluid balance in the cells. For every gram of sodium chloride that the body cannot eliminate, the body uses over twenty times the amount of water from the cells to neutralize it. Inorganic sodium chloride can prevent an ideal fluid balance and can overburden the systems of elimination. Sodium chloride is a hostile substance which biochemically is endlessly searching for an equalizing counterpart so that the pH of the body can always remain neutral. To produce this effect it needs its natural counterparts of potassium, magnesium, calcium, and other minerals and trace elements. These natural counterparts demonstrate, from a biophysical viewpoint, specific frequency patterns which ensure the geometric structures in the body. When these structures are missing, the body is without energy and lifeless. Well over 90% of the salt in the world is being used directly for industrial purposes that require pure sodium chloride. The remainder is utilized for preserving processes and processed denatured white table salt.

Natural chloride increases the body's ability to absorb heart-healthy potassium. Chloride helps to balance stomach acidity and sustains a healthy pH for the whole body. Chloride, in the form of hydrochloric acid (hydrogen and chloride), is also a component of gastric juice, which is invaluable for the body to digest and absorb nutrients. Potassium regulates the heartbeat, and irregular heartbeats, or arrhythmias, may occur because potassium levels are low. Adequate potassium intake controls muscle functioning, is associated with a decreased risk of strokes, and directs the transfer of nutrients through the cell membranes. Mental and physical stress can lead to low potassium levels, while heavy consumption of sugar, caffeine, and tobacco reduce potassium absorption. Processed foods are generally very high in sodium from processed, denatured white table salt, artificial flavours, and flavour enhancers. Low sodium products often contain monosodium glutamate, which is a sodium-based brain excitotoxin.

Sodium is the primary ion in the fluid outside the cells and potassium is the primary ion in the fluid inside the cells. The concentrations of sodium are more than ten times lower inside than outside the cells, and concentrations of potassium are approximately thirty times greater inside than outside the cells. The normal functioning of the body is dependent on the correct management of potassium and sodium outside and inside the cells. When consuming unhealthy, processed, denatured white table salt, intracellular water is lost. The variation in the concentration between sodium and potassium across the cell membranes generates an electrochemical gradient, which is recognized as the membrane potential and results from a separation of positive and negative charges (ions) across the cell membrane. A large quantity of energy in the body is committed to maintaining the sodium-potassium concentration gradients, accentuating the seriousness of the equilibrium between sodium and potassium in preserving life. Potassium and sodium are crucial dietary electrolytes and minerals that separate into charged particles in solution (ions), rendering them able to conduct electricity. Pink Himalayan crystal salt is life-enhancing.

"Salt is good: but if the salt hath lost its savour, how shall it be seasoned?" (Luke 14:34).

VITAMIN B12

Vitamin B12 is a term for the cobalamin class of vitamins which are not all equal in their benefits. Methylcobalamin, or methylated B12, is a most important nutrient which is created by soil-based bacteria and is the purest, active, bio-available coenzyme form of B12. All types of vitamin B12 contain the mineral cobalt. The vitamin's form depends on the type of molecules that are attached to the cobalt. In methylcobalamin, the cobalt is connected to a specific structure of molecules known as a methyl group (an alkyl derived from methane—containing one carbon atom bonded to three hydrogen atoms—CH3). This group is responsible for its impact on the body. It is one of the co-factors of B12 and is also one of the bioactive forms of B12.

Adenosylcobalamin is another co-factor and is the second bioactive form of B12. These are the only forms of B12 that are already broken down that the body is able to absorb and utilize quickly. Vitamin B12 is essential and needed by every cell of the body, and without it the body suffers and ultimately cannot survive. Research has indicated that it also has positive effects on natural sleep support due to its influence on modulating melatonin secretion, which has an impact on good quality sleep. Unfortunately, brain-altering pharmaceutical drugs are often added to the tablet form of methylcobalamin.

A B12 deficiency can affect anyone and most meat-eaters are deficient in this vital nutrient. A study of 2,999 participants—called the Framingham Offspring Study—found that B12 was low in many meat eaters as the study participants who received most or all of their B12 from meat sources had the lowest blood B12 levels. A meat eaters pH is generally more acidic than those who do not eat meat. According to Dr. Edward F. Group, "Meat is very acidic and can destroy the B12 that it contains. Even meat eating dogs and cats have been found to be deficient in B12." Animals that people eat are also fed on antibiotics and antacids. Antibiotics can also destroy B12. B12 producing bacteria are heat sensitive and killed when the animal is cooked, which makes most animal sourced B12 unusable. Meat eaters are also more than likely to have gastro-intestinal issues that inhibit the absorption of B12. A Stanford study found that taking probiotics greatly increases B12 levels and absorption, as insufficient absorption is also an issue. Most people worldwide do not get enough B12. Because the digestive system of most people is not functioning properly, vitamin B12 is a needed supplement.

Vitamin B12 is necessary for promoting nerve conduction and the repair of injured nerves, cardiovascular function, the regeneration of axonal nerves, good vision, myelin integrity, serotonin production, degenerative disorders, thyroid health and metabolism, neuroprotective activity, cell growth and replication, DNA synthesis and formation, good energy levels, diabetes and associated neuropathy, nervous system function, anaemia, dementia, brain function and mental health, adrenal function, immune system function, neuronal function and protection, proper red blood cell creation, peripheral neuropathy, nutritional support for nervous and cardiovascular systems, and an aid to converting carbohydrates to glucose. It also manifests analgesic effects, normalizes circadian rhythm, ameliorates muscle cramps, directly protects brain cells against injury from excitotoxins, and encourages the detoxification of heavy metals and toxins. The Linus Pauling Institute and Oregon State University discovered that low B12 correlates with an increased risk of breast cancer. Evidence suggests that high vitamin B12 administration can help protect against brain atrophy and destruction.

Methylcobalamin converts homocysteine to methionine, which reduces the potential for damage in the body as the reaction results in the formation of the super-antioxidant glutathione, the master antioxidant and detoxifier of the body. Methylcobalamin is the only form of B12 that acts on the nervous system and crosses the blood-brain barrier without conversion or assistance. Symptoms of a B12 deficiency include fatigue, brain fog, brain shrinkage, weight loss, depression, constipation, memory loss, Alzheimer's disease, weakness, slow reflexes, anaemia, megaloblastic anaemia, vision problems, muscle cramps, asthma, and bleeding gums. A B12 deficiency can be caused by malabsorption due to anything that results in the loss of gastric cells, any inflammatory gut issues, digestive issues, high coffee intake, stress, smoking, lack of good gut bacteria, drugs, toxins, parasites, alcohol consumption, which causes stomach inflammation and decreased stomach acid and parietal cell function.

Water-soluble vitamin B12 must be absorbed into the body with assistance. As the body cannot create it on its own, an intrinsic factor is necessary for the body to absorb B12. This gastric intrinsic factor is a very important glycoprotein. The saliva contains proteins that protect the B12 from the gastric acid in the stomach. Parietal cells (epithelial cells) in the stomach secrete the intrinsic factor which is the carrier for B12. Because of the high acid content in the stomach, B12 cannot survive the passage through it. When food is swallowed, the saliva protein, known as the R protein, protects the B12 in the stomach until it reaches the small intestine where the R protein degrades. It is then released and binds with the intrinsic factor. B12 is transported through the duodenum and the jejunum into the ileum, which has the intrinsic factor B12 receptors. GMOs adversely affect the illium and the B12 status where it is absorbed. These B12 receptors absorb the intrinsic factor which has to carry the B12 to the ileum to reach the intrinsic factor receptors. When the intrinsic factor releases the B12 it binds with the protein transcobalamin 11 for transit through the epithelial cells lining the gut and on into the bloodstream where it travels to the liver and is stored. B12 works in the cells and not the bloodstream.

Insufficient or weak stomach acid may result in a low gastric intrinsic factor. Acidic low pH conditions that are provoked by meat-eating, smoking, MSG, antibiotics, prescription drugs, alcohol, genetically-modified foods, contaminated water, coffee, and mercury have also been shown to directly decrease this intrinsic factor. Absorbing B12 requires that both the digestive system and the liver are working efficiently. Research has shown that methylcobalamin remains in the body longer and at higher levels than cyanocobalamin.

Cyanocobalamin has a cyanide group attached and robs the body of beneficial methyl groups. It should be avoided as it is commercially produced and is basically cobalamin bonded with cyanide. It is made from activated sewage sludge, or toxic ground-up cows' livers, which are overloaded with pesticides, antibiotics, and steroids. This type of B12 is produced for the purpose of cheap supposed fortification of foods and vitamins. Products sometimes contain added vitamin B12, but which type and how much B12 has been added?

"And Jesus went about all the cities and villages, teaching in their synagogues, and preaching the gospel of the kingdom, and healing every sickness and every disease among the people" (Matthew 9:35).

VITAMIN D

Vitamin D is a fat-soluble vitamin, an antioxidant, and a steroid hormone that is needed by virtually every cell of the body. Vitamin D is also known as a pleiotropic hormone, meaning that it elicits multi-faceted and diverse effects. A large number of studies have shown that low vitamin D levels can result in bone pain and deformities and is also linked to higher rates of cancer. According to research, those with low blood levels of vitamin D are at a much higher cancer risk than those with blood levels of 60 ng/mL and above. This important nutrient is a major factor in cancer prevention as it activates and boosts the immune system and has the ability to normalize and correct cancer cells. It also exerts various endocrine effects, including stimulating insulin secretion, and plays an important role in preventing a multitude of diseases as it controls 2,500 genes in the body. The vitamin D receptor complex regulates 3% of the genome, and about 10% of genes are directly or indirectly responsive to vitamin D. A vitamin D deficiency has also been strongly associated with the development of non-alcoholic fatty liver disease.

When it comes to cancer-fighting abilities there seems little doubt about the virtues of vitamin D, as it behaves more like a hormone, having receptor sites on both the cell and nuclear membranes, illustrating its all-encompassing effects. When the T-lymphocytes of the immune system discover a pathogen they immediately bind to a vitamin D molecule to activate themselves, as it enhances defences against both tumour development and invading pathogens. Vitamin D can switch genes off and on and adjust almost everything in the cancer cell, from its genetic messaging to its cytoskeleton. It can suppress cancer cell division and pacify the cancer cells so that they settle, rather than spread. Vitamin D regulates the pathway of apoptosis (programmed cell suicide) and the cell cycle, which not only suppresses cancer cell division but also induces terminal differentiation to generate specialized organ-specific cell types. Vitamin D can actually return a cancer cell to a normal healthy state, and there is more than enough research to show that it can help to prevent cancer as it also targets cancer stem cells. There are studies which show that over 90% of those with melanoma are deficient in vitamin D. Research illustrates that half of the cases of melanoma are found in locations not exposed to the sun. Other studies demonstrate that those who have regular exposure to sunshine develop fewer cancers.

Melanin (brown skin pigment) protects against skin damage from too much ultraviolet B exposure, meaning that those who were born with more melanin in their skin synthesize less vitamin D from sun exposure than those with fairer skin. Vitamin D significantly improves skin lesions in psoriasis and depigmentation in vitiligo. A recent study revealed that healthy levels of vitamin D can help considerably with conception as it can improve the possibility of an embryo being successfully implanted in the womb lining at the beginning of pregnancy. Vitamin D is extremely important during pregnancy and is known to affect the growth of a baby's bones before it is born. A study found that pregnant women with the lowest vitamin D levels were one and a half times more likely to deliver earlier than those with the highest levels. Inadequate vitamin D during pregnancy also increases the risk of childhood obesity, and obesity coupled with low vitamin D dramatically raises the risk of diabetes. Type 2 diabetes risk can be significantly lowered with sufficient vitamin D levels. Vitamin D protects against chronic inflammation, oxidative stress, and insulin resistance in those with obesity, as fat is stored in extra adipose tissue, which damages insulin signaling. It can prevent an inflammatory response of the immune system, drastically improve eyesight, and also reduce arterial stiffness.

If heavy metals, unhealthy sugars, unhealthy fats, trans fats, and other injurious substances are in the body system, they will inhibit the absorption of vitamin D. This essential vitamin enhances the absorption of phosphorus by 80% and dietary calcium by about 40%, and its physiological functions extend far beyond mineral assimilation and balance. Vitamin D cannot be metabolized if magnesium levels are low, and high magnesium levels require a lower dose of vitamin D. If magnesium levels are low, vitamin D will be stored in its inactive form, which will be of no benefit to the body. Foods rich in magnesium include nuts, seeds, figs, raspberries, bananas, legumes, avocados, and dark green, leafy vegetables. Magnesium also helps to keep calcium in the cells so that they can function more efficiently.

> *When it comes to cancer-fighting abilities there seems little doubt about the virtues of vitamin D.*

Calcium also needs to be consumed from foods in adequate levels as all these nutrients work together. An ideal ratio for magnesium and calcium is around one-to-one. A vitamin D-binding protein-derived macrophage activating factor is known as GcMAF (Globulin component Macrophage Activating Factor). Globulins are a major class of proteins in the blood that are produced by the liver and the immune system. They help to transport nutrients and play an important role in blood clotting, liver function and fighting infections. A macrophage cell is a type of phagocyte which is responsible for detecting, engulfing and destroying apoptotic cells and pathogens. GcMAF is a protein which not only improves the natural immune system response but also improves cancer outcomes. Adequate and regular vitamin D3 reduces systemic inflammation, kills cancer stem cells, and is needed by GcMAF to completely eradicate cancer stem cells and tumours.

"I will praise thee; for I am fearfully and wonderfully made: marvellous are thy works; and that my soul knoweth right well"
(Psalm 139:14).

For ensuring adequate vitamin D when sun exposure is limited, sufficient supplementation of vitamin D3 (cholecalciferol) is vital for those in regions of the world that do not have enough sunshine. Sufficient vitamin D is also beneficial for pain. This nutrient can be derived from sheep's lanolin, which is a yellowish, waxy substance that is secreted by glands in the skin of sheep.

To extract the lanolin from the wool, the wool is squeezed or rolled. This can then be used as a precursor to produce vitamin D3. To make vitamin D3 the lanolin must be purified to produce a substance called 7-dehydrocholesterol, which is the same precursor to vitamin D that is found in the skin. This substance is then converted to vitamin D3 through exposure to ultraviolet rays, which is similar to what happens when the skin is exposed to the sun. Vitamin D plays a critical role in disease prevention and maintaining optimal health.

"Truly the light is sweet, and a pleasant thing it is for the eyes to behold the sun" (Ecclesiastes 11:7).

AMALGAMS AND ROOT CANALS

It is a myth that amalgams and root canals are harmless. The use of amalgams dates back to the 1800s. Metal amalgams are formed when mercury is alloyed with other metals, the composition of which is approximately 52% elemental mercury and approximately 26% silver, with other common constituents being copper, tin, and other trace metals. Mercury exposure causes systemic harm to the body as neurotoxic mercury fillings leach mercury and mercury vapour into the body while a person is eating and drinking, as salivary enzymes stimulate the release of mercury from fillings, which mixes with the food in the stomach. When this combines with the hydrochloric acid in the stomach it produces mercuric chloride, which can damage the stomach lining and kill intestinal flora. Mercury is ubiquitous in the environment and causes a multitude of health problems involving damage to the brain, gut, heart, kidneys, and lungs together with a disruption of virtually every organ and system of the body including: the immune system, the nervous system (including the protective myelin sheath that envelopes the nerves), the circulatory system, the reproductive system, the endocrine system, and the cardiovascular pathways of the body. It also plays a considerable role in reproductive and endocrine cancers. Mercury exposure raises blood levels of homocysteine, which is a molecule associated with heart disease. It also causes an increase of pro-inflammatory cytokines, depletes essential antioxidants, triggers increased intestinal hyperpermeability, interferes with intestinal nutrient transport, and has been linked with many digestive diseases including Crohn's disease, ulcerative colitis, and an irritable bowel. Mercury can trigger a leaky gut by causing mutations to the beneficial gut flora and also dysbiosis, which is a condition in which the balance of beneficial and undesirable bacteria is disrupted. It destroys epithelial cells by damaging the stomach lining and also causes tiny holes in the intestinal lining. Research demonstrates that because mercury can induce increased gut permeability, undigested food particles, pathogens, and toxins can pass through the intestinal barrier and enter directly into the bloodstream, provoking an immune response. It can also trigger or worsen food sensitivities and allergies. Exposure to Wi-Fi radiation can amplify the toxicity of dental amalgams by increasing the release of mercury from these amalgams.

Mercury is found in the centre of tumours; it breaks the DNA and decreases liver detoxification. When mercury binds to proteins it may compromise the ability of the immune system to recognize the difference between normal cells and cancerous cells, which can result in the growth of cancerous cells as the immune system may mistake healthy tissues for cancerous ones. Mercury can also create an anaerobic environment where candida can flourish. But candidiasis and many other diseases show significant improvement when mercury fillings are safely removed and the body has undergone a mercury detoxification. High doses of vitamin C can effectively treat acute and chronic exposure to amalgams. The removal of amalgams should be undertaken by a dentist with specialized equipment that is protective of the patient to prevent mercury vapours from being inhaled while amalgams are being removed.

Pectin, the soluble fibre that is present in various fruits and vegetables, is an extremely effective chelating agent of heavy metals. Foods that are rich in pectin include citrus fruits (especially the rind and pith), grapes, pears, apples, beetroot, carrots, cabbage, and mung bean sprouts, which are particularly effective at removing lead. In a clinical trial, children with high levels of lead in their body were given pectin supplements, which increased the amount of lead expelled through their urine by over 130%.

Selenium and sulphur are associated mineral pairs which are essential to health, and garlic contains both. They both bind to a number of toxic metals including mercury, lead, arsenic, cadmium and also radioactive strontium 90, with sulphur also assisting to lower aluminium levels. Even low levels of exposure to heavy metals increases the risk of cancer and organ damage. Sulphur is not only found in garlic but also other vegetables including onions and cruciferous vegetables, with garlic having been scientifically proven to be a particularly excellent detoxifying agent. Nearly every process of the body relies on sulphur for red blood cells, hormones, nerve tissue, and enzymes. Selenium is crucial for the optimal functioning of the body and has excellent antioxidant properties which protect against the damaging effects of exposure to heavy metals and pesticides. Scientists have discovered that selenium can bind specifically to mercury and extract it from the bodily tissues for excretion.

Amino acids are effective natural chelating agents and as such are beneficial for removing high levels of heavy metals in the body. Whole plant-food sources of amino acids include carrots, spinach, turnips, plums, grapes, pomegranates, papayas, whole grains, and corn. Cilantro, also known as coriander or Chinese parsley, is excellent at removing heavy metals from the body. Toxic chemicals as well as heavy metals can also be excreted with the aid of garlic, ginger, citrus fruits, probiotic foods and crucifers, and once again nature abundantly provides natural, healthy nutrition which is needed to aid a sick and toxic body.

A tooth is dead after a root canal procedure has been performed but the remaining structure and tissue also provide an amicable environment for infection. Bacteria can then mutate into an anaerobic form, which thrives in the absence of oxygen. Dead teeth are often a source of various diseases and can relentlessly disperse deadly toxins into the body with no apparent symptoms whilst also causing a compromised immune system. The dentine, which is directly beneath the crown of the tooth, is not solid but is filled with microtubules (tiny canals). If the tubules in each tooth were placed end to end and measured they could stretch for up to about nine miles long, depending on the size of the tooth. The remaining bacteria living within the microtubules of the dead tooth can mutate into an anaerobic form and multiply into the millions, secreting potent toxins which can cause deadly diseases. When the pulp, which is beneath the dentine, is removed from the tooth, there is no longer any oxygen or blood supply, thereby rendering the tooth dead. A root canal is the only procedure that is performed on the body which leaves a dead piece of the body in place. Root canal procedures are a significant cause of cancer and heart disease, and toxicities from these root canals have been associated with most cancers. Few individuals are aware that chronic and acute illnesses may be related to mercury poisoning from amalgam fillings or to an unresolved infection involving root canal procedures.

Teeth are alive and can heal and regenerate from the inside out if the body is supplied with a healthy diet and lifestyle containing sufficient dietary nutrients, including magnesium and calcium. Tooth enamel (calcium phosphate) is transparent and can regrow. The pulp can also regenerate. The herb horsetail contains silica which can help to strengthen teeth. Silica minerals comprise approximately 26% of the earth's crust. Toxic blood is usually the reason for the origin of tooth decay and research has found that probiotics can prevent cavities. Teeth receive their colour from the underlying dentine, and the dentine (calcium phosphate and calcium carbonate) is constantly regenerating and receiving its nutrients from the underlying pulp chamber, which is located at the centre of the tooth between the crown and the root canals of the tooth. Teeth not only contain lymph capillaries but also larger conducting lymphatic vessels together with accompanying blood vessels and nerves in their course through the pulp. These larger vessels contain valves and pass through the root system.

Oil pulling originated in India and has been used as a natural health remedy for thousands of years. It has been proven to be an effective, advantageous strategy to help with oral health, including teeth regeneration and for the health of the whole body, as it effectively draws out bodily toxins. Some side effects may be experienced as toxins are drawn out. Oil pulling involves using about a level tablespoon of unrefined organic coconut oil or another healthy unrefined oil to swish around the mouth, while at the same time drawing, or pulling it between the teeth. This needs to be done for about twenty minutes first thing in the morning before anything else is put into the mouth. The oil can then be discarded, after which the mouth should be thoroughly rinsed out. It can also be performed at other times during the day when the stomach is empty. Care should be taken when carrying out this procedure so that the oil does not accidentally trickle down into the lungs, which can cause serious health issues.

Eating a healthy whole plant-food diet, including plenty of essential nutrients, keeps the teeth and gums healthy, thereby enabling the teeth to regenerate throughout life. The antioxidant vitamin E in the diet is needed to control the levels of oral bacteria as well as to regulate the oral microbiome, which is a host to various viruses, bacteria, and fungi. Odontoblasts are vital for teeth regeneration and are the cells of the teeth that produce dentin. They are a small immune system within the teeth and need vitamin D to become activated. A lack of vitamin A in the diet renders the mouth unable to make sufficient saliva, which assists in eliminating harmful bacteria and can also contribute to surface pits on the enamel. Vital vitamin C is such a powerful detoxifier that taking large doses prior to receiving dental anaesthesia renders the anaesthesia significantly weakened and may be ineffective.

Good dental care is vital for a healthy body as poor oral health can lead to serious diseases. Aluminium-free baking soda mixed with unrefined coconut oil and peppermint essential oil to taste is a safe and effective toothpaste which whitens the teeth. Baking soda can also help with a healthy oral pH and the remineralization of teeth, whereas a low pH can demineralize the teeth. Conversely, teeth whitening products that contain hydrogen peroxide damage teeth proteins, according to research.

"Blessed be the LORD, who hath not given us as a prey to their teeth" (Psalm 124:6).

EPIGENETICS

Conrad Waddington introduced the term *epigenetics* in the early 1940s. Epigenetics literally means *above* genetics and refers to external modifications to the DNA that activate or deactivate genes and determine which proteins are transcribed and how they are transcribed. It is the study of modifications to the expression of the genes to determine which genes are active and which are inactive without altering the underlying sequence of DNA. It produces a change in phenotype (genetic make-up plus environmental influences) without being a change in genotype (genetic traits such as eye colour), which affects how the cells read genes. Epigenetics exhibit how the environment and nutrients influence gene expression and DNA positively or negatively, demonstrating that nutrients are crucial for health and well-being. Genes are sections of DNA where the genetic codes are located for the production of proteins, which are comprised of nutrients and amino acids. The DNA also regulates the metabolism.

Epigenetic changes are a natural and regular occurrence which can be influenced by determinants, including diet, lifestyle, and the environment. The structures and chemical functioning of cells are formed from different proteins, which then generate every conceivable bodily action. Modification in genetic protein production affects the functioning of the body and whether or not it fights disease. Epigenetic modifications can manifest as commonly as the manner in which cells terminally differentiate to eventually become different cells, including brain cells, liver cells, and skin cells. Differentiation is the process whereby an individual cell expresses (turns on) some genes and represses (turns off) others. This causes each cell to grow and develop into a specific type with a specialized function. Studies have shown that epigenetic modifications can be passed on to multiple generations. Groundbreaking research exhibits how parental experience is epigenetically imprinted onto their offspring and also an unprecedented number of future generations. One variant of each gene is inherited from both parents and transgenerational (many past generations) inheritance of traumatic parental experiences also shapes the traits of their offspring. Negative epigenetic changes can also have damaging effects, and the expression of the genes can affect the intelligence and state of mind. Epigenetic modifications also play a crucial role in the silencing and expression of non-coding gene sequences.

At least three systems are considered to trigger and maintain epigenetic changes, and these are histone modification (histones are one of the specific proteins involved in cell division and cancer), DNA methylation (which regulates gene expression), and non-coding RNA-associated gene silencing (classified by genomic origin and mechanism of action). Epigenetic regulatory mechanisms can dynamically change in response to environmental stimuli or specific cellular conditions. Epigenetics comprises all of the components that impact the DNA and determines if specific genes are activated or deactivated. Genetic predispositions or traits must be activated before they can be expressed and this can be overridden by consuming foods which have a positive impact on gene expression, such as the foods contained in this book. This affects the methylation process and can deactivate hereditary genes. Some drugs are known to cause permanent adverse changes to the epigenome, including statins, anti-depressants, diuretics, antibiotics, anti-inflammatories, oral contraceptives, beta-blockers, anaesthetics, tamoxifen, and methotrexate. Environmental influences, such as diet and lifestyle, the physical environment, stress, and even beliefs, are primary directors of gene expression. Genes, biology, and health may be changed at any time for better or for worse.

"For the LORD is good; His mercy is everlasting; and His truth endureth to all generations" (Psalm 100:5).

GENETICALLY MODIFIED ORGANISMS

"WE NEED TO GET BACK TO THE WAY WE ATE FOOD BEFORE INDUSTRY RUINED IT."

It is a myth that GMOs are harmless. A genetically modified organism, or GMO, is an organism that has had its DNA modified or altered through genetic engineering by having foreign genes inserted into its genetic codes. In most instances,

GMOs have been altered with DNA from another organism, such as a virus, plant, bacterium, or animal and also between non-related species. MicroRNA is genetic information and has been found to pass from GM foods through the digestive process and into the blood where it attaches to the body organs and modifies the function and expression of those organs. There is no scientific evidence that GMOs provide better nutrition, greater yields, or improved drought tolerance. Some studies have shown that herbicide use has increased while yields have decreased. Short and long-term studies, completed by independent scientists, demonstrate real safety issues with GMOs. According to the latest independent research, GMOs are dangerous to health. When studies are not industry-funded the results reveal a dangerous technology with serious uncontainable and uncontrollable health hazards with no long-term safety.

Industry-funded researchers are trying to convince the world's population that GMOs are safe, when in fact they have been linked to higher death rates and many health issues and diseases, including cancer, DNA damage, liver failure, allergies, kidney damage, immune dysfunction, infertility, damage to internal organs, toxic digestive effects, and obesity. When GMOs are consumed the immune system recognizes them as foreign substances and defends itself against them by activating an immune system response in an effort to protect itself against disease. Most GM soy, corn, and canola contain a number of the same defoliant elements as agent orange, specifically, dioxin and glyphosate.

It has been shown that consuming GMOs also leads to negative genetic changes in the beneficial gut bacteria, which can also be destroyed by them. The microbiome, containing approximately 100 trillion organisms, performs important and complex tasks that regulates everything from immune function and metabolism to mental issues. Microbiome dysfunction can lead to many negative health issues, and studies have demonstrated that DNA from GM foods can indeed pass into the gut bacteria where even small changes to the intestinal flora can produce inflammation associated with bowel disease as well as many other debilitating and life-threatening diseases. GMOs are not only harmful to the human body but also to bees, as when they consume pollen from GM plants, their genes can be silenced by the double-stranded RNAs which adversely affect their survival.

"Woe unto them that call evil good, and good evil; that put darkness for light, and light for darkness; that put bitter for sweet, and sweet for bitter!" (Isaiah 5:20).

MONOSODIUM GLUTAMATE

Monosodium glutamate (MSG), also called sodium glutamate or monosodium L-glutamate, was invented in 1908 by a Japanese scientist named Kikunae Ikeda. He recognized and isolated the natural flavour enhancing substance of Laminaria Japonica seaweed and from this was able to create the synthesized, toxic, addictive MSG additive. A company for its production was formed which is now the largest producer of MSG in the world, as well as being a drug manufacturer.

MSG has absolutely no health or nutritional benefits. It is consumed worldwide and is worse for the health than alcohol, nicotine, and many drugs. As a taste enhancer, it is one of the worst food additives for causing food cravings, which can lead to obesity. MSG is used to improve the aroma and taste of many foods including baby formula, baby foods, fast foods, drinks, restaurant and processed foods, including frozen and canned foods. It causes numerous side effects and affects the receptors on the tongue, causing foods to taste much tastier than they actually are, which causes those that consume them to become addicted to these foods and drinks. MSG generally consists of 78% glutamate, 21% sodium, and almost 1% impurities.

It is known from over five hundred scientific studies that excitotoxins are substances that are added to foodstuffs to enhance their flavour and can also cause brain damage by literally stimulating brain cells to death. MSG is contained in ingredients such as aspartame, aspartic acid, plant protein extract, autolyzed yeast, textured protein, calcium caseinate, sodium caseinate, hydrolyzed protein, hydrolyzed oat flour, yeast extract, and hydrolyzed vegetable protein (such as various brown, salty, and sticky spreads). Additives frequently containing MSG include various flavourings, natural flavourings, natural beef or chicken flavourings, seasonings, maltodextrin, citric acid, malt extract, malt flavouring, stock, broth, and bouillon (bouillon cubes are sometimes hydrogenated). Other additives that may contain MSG include soy protein concentrate, soy protein isolate, enzymes (protease enzymes from different origins can release excitotoxin amino acids from food proteins), and carrageenan (sometimes extracted by hexane, a highly flammable toxic chemical made from crude oil and used as an industrial extraction solvent, which has many harmful effects on the body). MSG, in its many forms, is harmful to the body and is created when protein is either partially or fully separated into its constituent amino acids by enzymolysis, autolysis, hydrolysis, fermentation, or when glutamic acid is secreted from selected bacteria. When a protein is fragmented, the individual amino acids are freed because the amino acid chains in that protein are broken.

Hydrolyzed plant vegetable protein is a powerful excitotoxin mixture which, for maximum profits, is down-played by manufacturers as a perfectly safe *natural* substance. It is made from vegetables that are not fit for sale and are specially selected for their naturally high glutamate content. The hydrolysis extraction process involves boiling these vegetables in a vat of acid, which is then followed by neutralization with a caustic soda process. This resulting brown sludge collects on the surface and is skimmed off and allowed to dry. The final product is a brown powder that is a component of three known excitotoxins: aspartate, glutamate, and cysteic acid (which converts to cysteine). The food industry then adds this product to almost every imaginable item that they class as food.

Monosodium glutamate is a processed pharmaceutical and food additive that is not only addictive and an extremely dangerous neurotoxin (an excitotoxin) but it also kills brain cells in the hypothalamus. MSG has been linked to many unwanted health issues including cancer, inflammation, asthma, stunted bone growth, brain lesions, weight gain, depression, chest pain, nausea, rapid heartbeat, organ changes, liver and kidney damage, sterilization, tingling, seizures, migraines, numbness, arrhythmia, and other disorders. It is very dangerous for those who suffer severe reactions to it, and many people, who are very sensitive to it, experience neurological, respiratory, urological, muscular, skin, and even cardiac symptoms. How MSG may contribute to obesity is due to its effects on leptin resistance. The hormone leptin regulates the metabolism and appetite, and MSG acts primarily as an appetite stimulant. Anything that inhibits leptin increases food intake. MSG is not only confirmed to be a critical factor in the initiation of obesity but it has also been confirmed to cause liver disease. When MSG has been consumed the body releases the fat-storing hormone insulin. This insulin surge causes the blood sugar to plummet and hunger to return.

MSG becomes an altered form of the glutamic acid molecule when sodium is added. However, the poisonous part is the glutamic acid and not the sodium that negatively affects the body. Any glutamate added to processed food cannot be considered a naturally occurring substance. Processed free glutamic acid (MSG) contains D-glutamic acid and L-glutamic acid which is associated with pyroglutamic acid and other impurities. Only acid-hydrolyzed proteins contain carcinogenic dichloropropanols and monopropanols, and only reaction flavours contain carcinogenic heterocyclic amines. Food manufacturers often combine MSG with other ingredients to disguise it or use substances that are known to contain high amounts of the amino acids aspartate or glutamate. The wording *natural flavour-ings* on labels does not mean that a food additive is being used in its natural state. But instead, it means that a food additive only began with something found in nature and may contain anywhere from 20%–60% MSG.

While the glutamic acid in MSG is usually produced through the fermentation of bacteria, the glutamic acid in other ingredients containing MSG is made by chemicals (either autolysis or hydrolysis), fermentation, enzymes (enzymolysis), or a complex cooking procedure in which reaction flavours are created from an amalgamation of specific amino acids, vegetable or animal oils or fats, reducing sugars, and optional ingredients such as hydrolyzed vegetable protein.

To produce an unhealthy liquid aminos flavouring containing MSG, soybeans are treated with hydrochloric acid followed by sodium bicarbonate to neutralize any remaining acid. This creates sodium chloride which produces a salty flavour. This method takes only two days and produces a product by rapid hydrolysis and not complete fermentation. It utilizes a reactor enzyme called glutamase, and the end result is a product that contains large amounts of the unnatural glutamic acid, which is found in MSG. MSG is the sodium salt of glutamic acid.

The free glutamic acid that is found in protein and the free glutamic acid that is involved in normal body function is unprocessed, free glutamic acid which contains no contaminants. Natural glutamate in plants is known as L-glutamic acid. Another form of food flavour enhancement that is often legally labelled *natural flavours* comes from aborted human fetus cell tissues, which major food corporations use to manufacture flavour additives for a plethora of commonly consumed processed foods and drinks, including water. Many *beauty* products and vaccines also contain these aborted fetus cell tissues.[12]

"Their poison is like the poison of a serpent: they are like the deaf adder that stoppeth her ear" (Psalm 58:4).

TEA, COFFEE, COCOA, CHOCOLATE, AND CAROB

Caffeine (a methylxanthine) is a dangerous world-wide addictive psychotropic drug which affects mental activity and behaviour. It is a mood-altering drug

---

[12] For more information please see: "How Cells from an Aborted Fetus are Used to Create Novel Flavor Enhancers," https://1ref.us/1pn (accessed August 4, 2021); "Aborted fetus cells used in beauty creams," https://1ref.us/1po (accessed August 4, 2021); "Use of Aborted Fetal Tissue in Vaccines and Medical Research Obscures the Value of All Human Life," https://1ref.us/1pp (accessed August 4, 2021).

that increases the rate at which calcium is lost through the urine. Caffeine also dehydrates, is a pesticide, a poison with an underestimated lethality, and an alkaloid that the coffee plant uses to kill insects which eat its coffee beans. This toxic chemical is also used by the coffee plant to kill surrounding plants as well. Caffeine causes the termination of genetic material in live cells that come into contact with it. Coffee and tea are insidious poisons which not only contain caffeine but also thein and theophylline. These three alkaloids share some common chemical properties with theobromine, which is found in chocolate and cocoa. The tea plant not only creates caffeine but also the chemicals theophylline and theobromine as natural combatants towards insects and animals.

Caffeine is a diuretic and occurs naturally in tea leaves, coffee beans, cocoa beans and many other plants. Brain imaging studies have demonstrated that chronic coffee drinkers show the same brain degradation as patients with Parkinson's disease, cigarette smokers, and chronic alcoholics. Caffeine does not impart energy to the body but conversely removes it, as all ingested poisons activate a release of energy to effect a purge of toxic substances from the body. The habit of appetite and energy stimulation created by caffeine dependence is an addictive cycle. Any poison that is taken into the body is eliminated as soon as possible, as the body is designed to rid itself of all toxins. Drinking tea, coffee and cocoa, as well as eating chocolate, is an injurious indulgence which can cause malfunctioning of the frontal lobe of the brain, which is the seat of willpower and decision making. These substances create a morbid and stimulating action of the nervous system, and after the immediate influence of the stimulants has left the system the body drops to just below its previous position before stimulation. To compensate, people often consume more caffeine because they want to feel more energetic, thus establishing a cycle of stimulation and exhaustion which can lead to addiction and paralysis of the moral, mental, and physical powers. These substances stimulate in small doses and narcotize in larger doses, with the capability of producing paralysis in various parts of the nervous system. Hormonal systems and the lower IQ regions of the brain are activated when caffeine triggers the *fight or flight* response systems that control fear, jealousy, violence, aggression, anger, rage, paranoia, and illogical and irrational decision making, as it generates the lower powers of mental functioning and encourages very negative emotional responses. When caffeine is consumed, the limbic part of the brain is hyper-activated, meaning that the higher learning centres of the mind are inhibited. The role of the limbic part of the brain is solely to acquire food, protect territory, maintain personal safety, and engage in reproduction.

Just one cup of coffee poisons the body and activates the *fight or flight* response for three consecutive weeks on a decreasing scale, even with no other consumption of caffeine. Moreover, according to MRI images taken before and after its consumption, just one small cup of coffee decreases blood flow to the brain by over 50%.

Caffeine dependence is considered to be much stronger than marijuana and a greater addictive drug than amphetamines. Studies have demonstrated that a minimum of 100 milligrams of caffeine per day (about one cup) can produce a physical dependence that triggers significant unpleasant symptoms upon withdrawal. There is absolutely no scientific evidence that coffee provides any level of health benefits to the human body. Although tea is widely thought to be a healthier option than coffee, conventional brands of tea can be genetically modified, are mostly unwashed, and have been shown to contain high levels of toxic substances such as illegal amounts of banned carcinogenic pesticides, added flavours, and artificial ingredients which are unsafe for consumption. Kidneys filter the blood and produce urine, and as tea contains oxalates, there is an increased risk of developing kidney stones. Tea also causes brain injury and mental degeneration because of its disastrous effects on the brain. An average cup of black tea contains approximately 40 milligrams of caffeine, while an average cup of instant coffee can contain more than 110 milligrams. Caffeine can also be artificially produced, and is often added as an ingredient or as a flavouring to beverages and provides a slightly bitter taste. So-called energy drinks often contain caffeine and other questionable ingredients. Synthetic caffeine derives predominantly from large Chinese factories. It was primarily developed in 1942 by the Nazis and subsequently manufactured by Monsanto. To produce this artificial substance, urea is converted from ammonia which is then mixed with various chemicals. This potent result can be dangerous if consumed quickly in considerable amounts.

> **The habit of appetite and energy stimulation created by caffeine dependence is an addictive cycle.**

"Be not deceived; God is not mocked: for whatsoever a man soweth, that shall he also reap" (Galatians 6:7).

The consumption of caffeine considerably inhibits iron absorption, which causes anaemia. It has also been proven to cause an enlarged prostate, cancers, Crohn's disease, heart disease, colitis, IBS, PMS, strokes and TIAs (mini-strokes), heart attacks, birth defects, brain damage, depression, unnatural breathing patterns, insomnia, ulcers, learning disorders (from brain damage), behaviour disorders, carpal tunnel and other pain issues, fatigue, hyperactivity, deep anxiety, headaches, increased incidence of muscle and tendon injury, and joint pain.

Caffeine also induces weight gain, fat gain, and cellulite by constant activation of the body's *flight or fight* system (which any type of poison or threat does). Such activation aids in a metabolic shift to fat conservation and eventually changes the body's preferred primary fuel source requirement to one of fat when fighting any toxins. Caffeine also destroys muscle because, when the body is poisoned, it deliberately loses muscle to facilitate additional fat storage.

Cocoa, from which chocolate is manufactured, is naturally quite bitter and contains two main addictive alkaloid stimulants—theobromine and caffeine—which seriously and adversely affect the body. This family of chemical substances can cause cancers, birth deformities (from their mutagenic properties), sleep disturbances, obesity, acne, irritability, fatigue, chromosome damage, balance issues, a racing heart, agitation, insomnia, dizziness, bedwetting, and anxiety. Some health issues, which can be exacerbated by, and are associated with, ingesting these methylxanthines, include lowered resistance to disease, including heart disease, allergies, diabetes, stimulated heart rate, cardiac arrhythmias, stomach disturbances, and depression.

Cocoa beans are left out in the open to ferment so that they can develop their characteristic chocolate flavour, as this is part of the necessary process to produce chocolate. During this process, cancer-causing agents can form, and rodents, insects, and small animals can contaminate the fermenting cocoa beans with their excrement. These undesirable additives of up to ten milligrams of animal excrement per pound of chocolate, or up to twenty-five insect fragments per tablespoon of cocoa powder, are allowed to remain in the finished product. To mask the product's natural bitterness, large amounts of refined sugar and dairy products, such as cow's cream and milk, are added to give chocolate its flavour and texture.

"The LORD shall preserve thee from all evil: He shall preserve thy soul" (Psalm 121:7).

Naturally sweet carob (a legume), plus other tasty ingredients, can make a healthy and comparable substitute for chocolate but without the unhealthy chocolate contaminants. Unfortunately, sometimes trans fats are added to carob

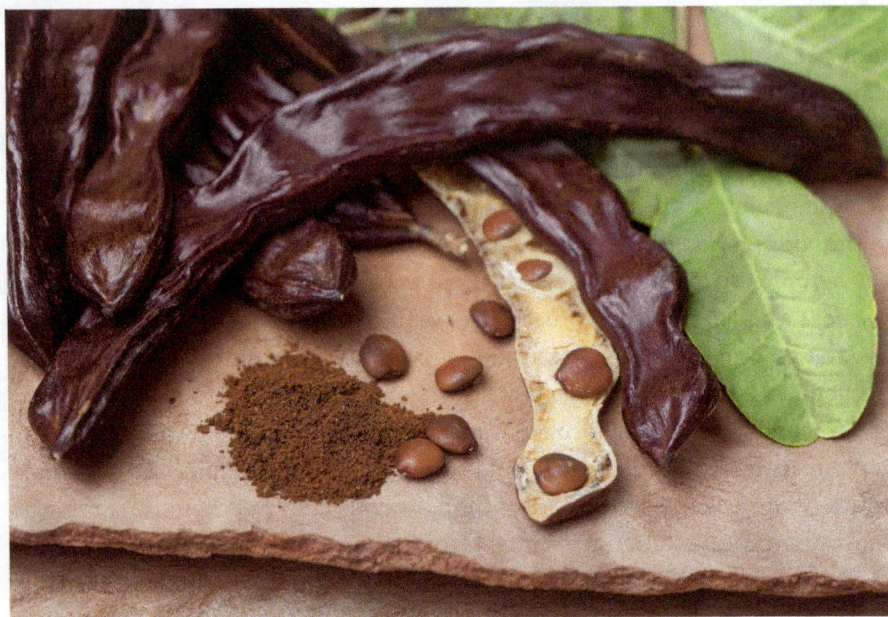

bars and carob buttons during their manufacture. Carob pods are often roasted to enhance their chocolate-like flavour and then ground into a powder, which can flavour many tasty recipes. Carob is very nutritious and contains vitamin A, vitamin B1, vitamin B2, vitamin B3, vitamin C, calcium, chromium, copper, iron, magnesium, manganese, nickel, and potassium. Carob is a God-given plant which contains many healthy nutrients.

"Pleasant words are as an honeycomb, sweet to the soul, and health to the bones" (Proverbs 16:24).

PHYTIC ACID

It is a myth that phytic acid is harmful when consumed with a balanced, nutritious diet. Nuts, seeds, legumes, beans, potatoes, and grains store phosphorus as phytic acid. Phytic acid accounts for up to 85% of the total phosphorus contained in legumes and cereals. Phytic acid is isolated in the aleurone layer of grains under the bran coat and is the single outer layer of the endosperm in most grains. It is rich in protein and comprises about 3% of the weight of the grain, about 20% of the vitamin B1, 30% of the vitamin B2, and 50% of the vitamin B3 of the grain. Phytic acid induces autophagy, which can protect against Alzheimer's disease and other neurodegenerative diseases. Autophagy is a physiological process for degrading and recycling proteins that reside in parts of the DNA that play crucial roles in controlling how organs, cells, and other tissues function. It is recognized as a principal response to cellular stress and is an important regulator of neuronal function and survival. It is also involved in the destruction and elimination of pathogens inside the cells. Phytic acid binds to heavy metals such as mercury, arsenic, and lead and safely escorts them out of the body. It is also one of the few chelating agents used for the removal of uranium.

The most striking documented effect of phytic acid is in cancer prevention as it inhibits malignant growth in many different types of cancers and only adversely affects malignant cells and not normal cells. Everyone who eats plants consumes some phytic acid. Flaxseed and wheat bran are rich sources of phytic acid. When the minerals in these foods are bound to phytic acid it is known as a phytate. It not only helps to prevent cancer but also diabetes, heart disease, osteoporosis, kidney stone formation, dental cavities, and more. As an antioxidant, it decreases inflammatory cytokines. Additionally, it increases bone mineral density, boosts immunity, suppresses tumour proliferation, induces differentiation of malignant cells, and blocks the build-up of uric acid which can help to prevent gout. By enhancing differentiation, the mature cancer cells revert back to functioning as normal cells do. The body's vitamin D status seems to influence the quantity of phytate that is retained, with a higher vitamin D level retaining more phytate and vice versa. A potential method by which phytate prevents cancer is by entering cells and helping to repair breaks in DNA strands. Most phytate is degraded in the stomach and small intestine and is rapidly absorbed from the gastrointestinal tract into the bloodstream where it is expeditiously absorbed by cancer cells and tumours throughout the body, thereby inhibiting the growth of many types of cancer cells without affecting normal cells. Phytates are anti-inflammatory (thereby preventing oxidative damage), antioxidant (which may reduce mycotoxin toxicity produced by microfungi that can cause disease and death), anti-angiogenesis, detoxifying and immune-enhancing (strengthens natural killer cell activity), which affects all of the main malignancy pathways. Phytates not only starve tumours by preventing angiogenesis, but they also disrupt angiogenesis.

It has often been advised that nuts, seeds, and legumes should be soaked, and the soaking water discarded to prevent flatulence. However, the benefits of not discarding this water far outweigh any occurrence of this. Sprouting is another healthy alternative and converts these foods to pre-digested proteins which can be utilized soon after the tiny sprouts appear. Although in the past, a high intake of phytates might have been considered to reduce the availability of dietary minerals, the latest research shows that such a concern is only valid when large quantities of phytic acid are consumed in combination with a diet poor in minerals and trace elements. This recent research has shown the opposite to be true, and that phytates are protective and not destructive, so it is more healthful to consume pulses (legumes) in their natural state with their phytates.

"Prove thy servants, I beseech thee, ten days; and let them give us pulse to eat, and water to drink" (Daniel 1:12).

CHARCOAL

Charcoal is one of the world's most powerful known antidotes. The first recorded use in history of the medicinal use of charcoal is dated to 1550 BC when, according to an Egyptian Papyrus, charcoal was used to treat intestinal disorders and decaying wounds. Recorded history also attests to Pliny and

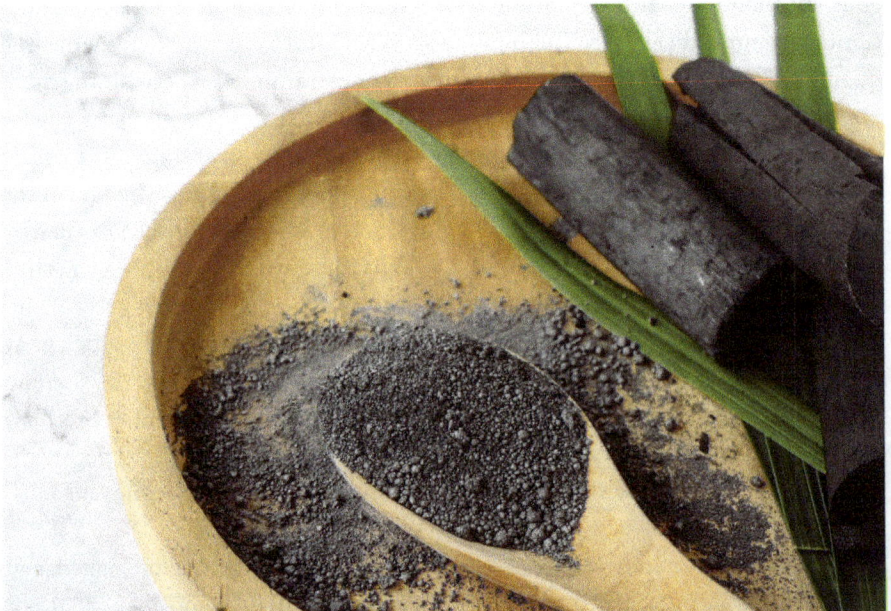

Hippocrates using charcoal in 400 BC to treat a variety of diseases, including anthrax and epilepsy.

When carbon-rich wood is burnt at a temperature of 1,000° C all of its components vapourize under high pressure except for the carbon structure. This remaining carbon skeleton is highly porous as the process erodes the internal surfaces of the carbon structure and increases its adsorption capacity by creating an internal labyrinth of invisible minute pores and tunnels (similar to a sponge) which results in a greater surface area for adsorption (adsorption is different from absorption and is a process by which a substance binds other substances onto its surfaces). Activated charcoal has a negative electrical charge that induces positive-charged toxins to adhere to it. Activated and super-activated charcoals have been treated to adsorb a much larger capacity of toxins without adsorbing nutrients from foods such as natural organic minerals and vitamins while increasing the efficiency of nutrient absorption, according to Russian researchers. Two of the best plant substances that are utilized for making charcoal are coconut shells and eucalyptus wood.

Determined to prove the antidotal power of charcoal and convinced of its efficacy, two French scientists proved how very powerful it is. In early 1813, French chemist Professor Michel Bertrand swallowed charcoal together with 150 times the lethal dosage (five grams) of arsenic trioxide, a deadly poison, and survived with no adverse symptoms. Then, in 1852, another French scientist, Professor Pierre-Fleurus Touéry, performed as daring a demonstration before a skeptical French Academy of Medicine. He swallowed charcoal together with one gram of strychnine, an equally lethal poison. This was an amount ten times higher than the lethal dose. He also survived, thereby demonstrating the amazing power of charcoal.

Natural, non-toxic, and safe charcoal powder is an extremely fine, highly adsorbent, black, chemically inert substance that has the therapeutic capacity to physically entrap other substances. It has the capability of adsorbing thousands of substances to its surfaces and can adsorb a weight of up to 200 times its own weight. Activated charcoal is a tasteless, odourless powder, and one teaspoonful of it has a surface area of more than 10,000 square feet. Charcoal performs as a powerful oxidizing agent and contains a large amount of oxygen within the microscopic holes of the carbon structure. These oxygen molecules react with most foreign substances, oxidizing and converting them into harmless matter. Once within the body, charcoal binds to toxic particles forming a charcoal-toxin complex, which restricts harmful substances from damaging tissues while the foreign particles are safely concealed within the pores of the charcoal, which then exits the body via the colon together with its toxic cargo. Its elemental nature binds to other compounds including micro-organisms, various toxins, and gases. Being an anti-microbial, charcoal can suppress and arrest disease-causing viruses, bacteria, and fungi. It is not only useful for poisoning but also pain, all gastro-intestinal issues, kidney and liver failure, systemic candidiasis (activated charcoal suppresses the growth of intestinal-based yeasts), stings and bites of all kinds, including snake and spider bites, detoxifying, and more as its applications are virtually endless. Charcoal poultices and charcoal baths can have many different applications including treating insect bites, detoxification, the removal of nicotine from smoking, chronic fatigue, skin disorders and more.

Because the porous nature of the structure of charcoal increases the surface area available for adsorption, it thereby enhances the rate and capacity of detoxification by many folds as it helps to decrease the detoxification work of the liver. Charcoal does not cause constipation, providing adequate water is drunk and the colon does not have blockages. It is very effective at neutralizing alkaloids such as morphine, strychnine, caffeine, nicotine, and theobromine, and many poisons from plants are effectively adsorbed by charcoal. However, it is not generally recommended for caustic substances such as methylated spirits, bleach, and ammonia. Some substances are not adsorbed by charcoal, and these include metals, strong alkalis and acids, alcohols, lithium, and most hydrocarbons. Charcoal powder must be stored in a tightly sealed container as it readily adsorbs impurities from the atmosphere.

To make a charcoal poultice, measure one part of activated charcoal to two parts of ground psyllium husks or ground flaxseeds. Add enough water to make a spreadable consistency. Spread it onto a paper towel and cover it with another paper towel. Flatten it out to about one-quarter of an inch thick and apply it to the area. Cover the poultice with cling wrap and secure it in place with tape or a stretch bandage. Leave it on for at least two hours, or preferably about eight hours or overnight. Do not re-use a poultice as it will contain toxins. This may need to be repeated with a new poultice. After removing the poultice, the skin can be rubbed briskly with a cold cloth. If applying a charcoal poultice to a wound area, it is advisable to wrap the charcoal poultice mixture in fabric before placing it on an open break in the skin, otherwise, the skin may heal with a tattoo effect. Multiple layers of various sizes can be made for later use by separating them with cling wrap and freezing them. Thaw before use. To apply the thawed poultice simply remove it from the cling wrap and place it on the skin.

To make an activated charcoal detox slurry add one teaspoon of activated charcoal powder to an eight-ounce glass of pure water and stir slowly. Allow it to settle and then pour the clear water at the top (slurry water) into another glass. This can be freely drunk, and especially when detoxifying from a serious disease which may require ten or more glasses per day to assist with detoxification and to ensure that the bodily organs are not overwhelmed with toxins. To make a charcoal drink add one or more tablespoons of charcoal powder to an eight-ounce glass of water or juice, stir slowly, and take as often as required. Charcoal is a great blessing which can be used for many conditions.

"For our God is a consuming fire" (Hebrews 12:29).

HYDROTHERAPY

The use of hydrotherapy is likely as old as humankind and has been widely used in many ancient cultures. Water is one of the most essential components of life and is one of the basic methods of therapy that is routinely used in natural remedies. The use of water in its various forms—as steam, water and ice, and at various temperatures—can produce different effects on different systems of the body. Hydrotherapy is the internal and external use of water for promoting health or the treatment of diseases with various temperatures, durations, pressures, and positions. Many different kinds of hydrotherapy techniques are used for various conditions and involves the use of both hot and cold water. Different delivery methods generate different immune and physiological responses. Wisely used hydrotherapy is one of the best modalities for boosting health and speeding the recovery of various health issues, especially those associated with weak immunity, poor metabolism, and blood circulation. Poor blood circulation can be observed with cold bodily extremities, which should be kept warm for good health. Hydrotherapy works much better when combined with a healthy diet and lifestyle and regular physical activity.

Water is one of the most essential components of life and is one of the basic methods of therapy that is routinely used in natural remedies.

Hot water directs the blood flow towards the surface of the body, whereas cold water stimulates the blood to flow inward toward the internal organs. Hot water

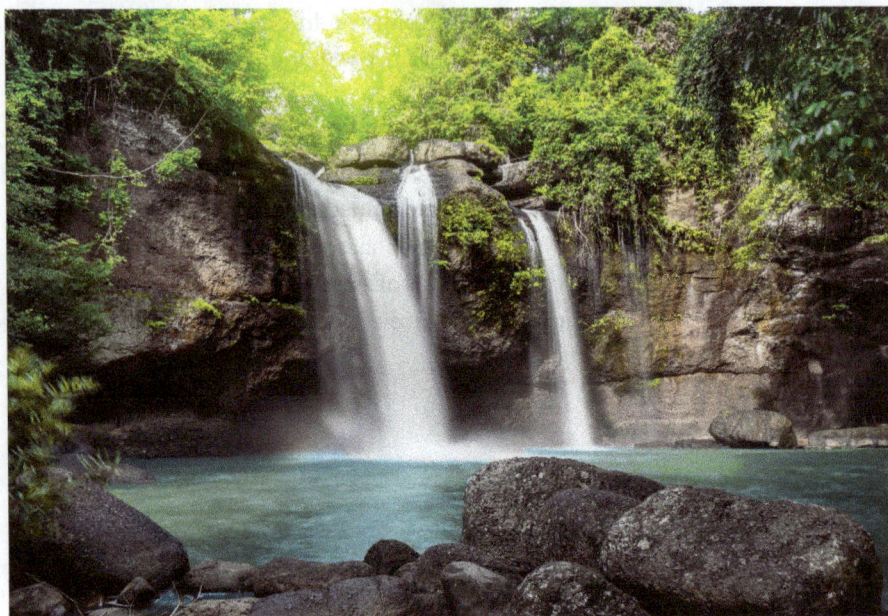

causes *vasodilation* (blood vessel dilation) whereas cold water causes *vasoconstriction* (blood vessel constriction). Therefore, alternating hot and cold treatments cause the circulation to flow out to the surface of the skin and back into the internal organs, which has a tremendously positive influence on the health of the body, as good blood circulation is one of the most important factors in preventing and treating various health issues. Because this treatment helps to open the capillaries, it increases the rate of detoxification and helps the oxygen, nutrients, and antioxidants to move more readily to various parts of the body. Physical exercise and drinking sufficient pure water are among the safest effective natural detoxifiers for the elimination of toxins.

Contrasting hot and cold showers imparts a tremendous boost to the blood circulation, improves metabolism, eliminates toxins, reduces inflammation, and stimulates the nervous and immune systems. It is beneficial to begin with a hot shower for three minutes. Then, when the body is warm, a thirty second cold shower with the temperature reduced gradually until it is very cold is considerably beneficial. For the best results, this procedure should be repeated twice more, alternating the flow of water from hot to cold, then cold to hot, and finally ending with cold. Hot and cold showers can be taken twice a day. After drying off, the feet should not touch a cold floor as this will neutralize the treatment. Keep the feet and the rest of the body warm while resting for at least fifteen minutes afterwards while being hydrated. This powerful procedure fights against any unwanted invaders as it forces the white blood cells (leukocytes) to exit some of their storage places such as the bone marrow, the spleen, and the thymus. A cold shower, which is even more beneficial than hot, will do no harm if preceded with a hot shower.

As cold water cools the body it forces it to burn more calories by activating brown body fat, which boosts fat burning. Unlike white fat cells, which store calories as fat, the brown fat cells contain many mitochondria, which gives the brown fat cells their colour and which constantly burn energy and produce heat. Brown fat is a heat-generating type of fat and can play a very important role in controlling weight as it burns energy instead of storing it. Simply put, hydrotherapy stimulates brown fat cells to burn more fat.

Saunas are very beneficial for many conditions including metabolism and skin issues, a weak immune system, poor blood circulation, and obesity. Saunas help to reverse these issues by inducing sweating and eliminating toxins. Fats become water-soluble when exposed to temperatures above 45°C (113°F). when the body is forced to eliminate water together with excess fat during the process of sweating from any source.

Drinking one to two litres of water about an hour before taking a sauna and about thirty minutes afterwards, but not during a sauna, will bring the best results for losing fat. Any hot treatments should also be frequently interspersed with cold showers. For prolonged hot treatments, very cold forehead compresses should be constantly applied as the head must be kept cool. Fainting may occur if the precaution of not rising too quickly afterwards is not observed.

Hot foot baths are excellent simple water treatments. By simply immersing the feet in a bowl of hot water, which should be as hot as can be tolerated (topping up with more hot water as needed), while applying a very cold compress to the forehead after the feet are immersed (using iced water to keep the compress very cold), results in constricting the blood vessels in the head and brings great relief. It is very helpful at relieving pain, while also reducing congestion and boosting the immunity. It has the powerful ability to move blood from the brain and other bodily areas as the hot water dilates the blood vessels in the feet and thus moves the blood away from the afflicted area towards the lower parts of the body to relieve congestion, inflammation, and other health issues. Diabetics can use a thermometer to check the temperature. Continuing to drink enough water is important for any heating treatments. Hydrotherapy is a simple God-given remedy for many applications.

"But whosoever drinketh of the water that I shall give him shall never thirst; but the water that I shall give him shall be in him a well of water springing up into everlasting life" (John 4:14).

THE EIGHT LAWS OF HEALTH

"TAKE CARE OF YOUR BODY BECAUSE IT'S THE ONLY PLACE THAT YOU HAVE TO LIVE IN."

T-R-U-S-T G-O-D is an acronym for eight natural health laws that contribute to a healthy lifestyle. These natural laws were designed by our Creator for our health and well-being. To experience radiant health, follow the Creator's handbook **THE BIBLE.**

"Trust in the LORD with all thine heart; and lean not unto thine own understanding. In all thy ways acknowledge Him, and He shall direct thy paths" (Proverbs 3:5, 6).

"T" is for TRUST GOD.

S-T-R-E-S-S is an acronym for **S**elf-**T**rust **R**estricts **E**very **S**piritual **S**uccess. Having an abiding trust and faith that God is always willing to help in times of need is very reassuring. He gives the power to break any harmful addictions and destructive lifestyle habits. He already knows our every thought but wishes us to communicate with Him who made Heaven and Earth. We are living in a stressful fallen world and in times of stress He wants us to turn to Him for help with trust and faith as He is our only hope until He returns in the clouds of glory to take those back to Heaven who have put their trust in Him. Talk to Him and put Him to the test today, as good health comes from above, and the power that made the body also heals it.

"For our heart shall rejoice in Him, because we have trusted in His holy name" (Psalm 33:21).

Constant emotional, psychological, or physical trauma causes stress. This raises the level of cortisol and creates inflammation, which causes cancer and other health issues. About 90% of all diseases are stress-related. There are three types of stress—physical, chemical, and emotional—and the body responds to all three in the same way. Prolonged or excessive stress can lead to illness and emotional and physical exhaustion. Stress can be a killer when taken to extremes. It changes the expression of the genes (via epigenetics) and the chemicals that the body produces when under stress turns genes on and off, altering such things as how efficiently the immune system functions, how quickly people age, how much fat is stored, or whether or not cancer develops. Health potential is not only determined by stress but also lifestyle, diet, environment and—more than anything else—thoughts. Every thought creates a physiological response in the body and every thought produces a physical reality. A fast heartbeat actually sends a signal to the prefrontal cortex of the brain, which handles decision making and thought processing. This signal messages the prefrontal cortex to temporarily close down to allow the midbrain to take over. Stress and the brain are intimately connected and stress can cause brain damage. Stressors can physically alter the brain which can impact learning, decision making, and memories. High-stress hormone levels damage crucial sections of the brain such as the hippocampus, which is the area responsible for memory.

The hippocampus, the amygdala, and the prefrontal cortex are three parts of the brain that are highly involved in how stressors are recognized and responded to. These areas of the brain work with the hypothalamus to regulate the production of stress hormones and related responses to stress such as an increased heart rate. The brain is not only affected by the stress itself but also controls the stress response. When feelings occur of being under abnormal emotional or mental pressure, this pressure changes into stress. When stress becomes excessive it may lead to worry, frustration, depression, anxiety, fear, anger, and an inability to cope. Stressed people behave differently and can become withdrawn, tearful, indecisive, inflexible, irritable, and aggressive. Extreme anxiety can cause heart palpitations, stomach disorders, giddiness, and headaches. It can adversely affect lives and prevent people from experiencing enjoyable pursuits. Stress is a method that the body uses to react to a challenge and it also reduces the ability of the body to detoxify and metabolize. It restricts the body and prevents it from releasing toxins, thereby adding to its burden. Research shows that stress impacts the gut function, increases the overgrowth of bad bacteria, and creates inflammation. This leads to a leaky gut, which is the result of the loosening of the tight junction barriers between the epithelial cells that line the intestines, thereby creating immune disorders and food sensitivities. Stress and the gut are closely intertwined with 95% of serotonin being produced in the gut.

Food, natural light, and exercise can affect how much serotonin is produced. Physical signs of stress can be inflammation, headaches, sleeplessness, tiredness, and an upset stomach. Stress reduces potassium levels and can also lead to disease by suspending the digestive process to preserve energy. Being stressed while eating is unhealthy and can lead to feeling nauseous. Undigested food that is suspended in the gut because of stress causes fermentation, which can lead to disease. Stress can also reduce the efficiency of the immune system and shut it down. When emotionally stressed, the body releases the hormones adrenaline and cortisol. This is how the body automatically prepares to respond to a threat, which is sometimes called the *fight or flight* response. When the body is very stressed it produces high levels of these hormones, which can give rise to symptoms of not only feeling physically unwell but can also produce serious health-damaging effects in the long term such as inflammation, which can cause many diseases including cancer, strokes, and heart attacks. Stress is also detrimental to muscles and bones. Not only is stress unpleasant, but the cascade of stress hormones produce well-coordinated and an almost instantaneous sequence of hormonal changes in physiological responses. Adrenal exhaustion, after long-term chronic stress, occurs because the brain turns off the adrenals to save itself. The adrenal medulla secretes the hormone adrenaline after receiving a message from the brain about a stressful situation. Cortisol is a glucocorticoid (steroid hormone) which is produced from cholesterol in the two adrenal glands located above each kidney and is normally released in response to acute stress. Trusting in God brings health and healing.

> **Stress is a method that the body uses to react to a challenge and it also reduces the ability of the body to detoxify and metabolize.**

"And the LORD shall help them, and deliver them: He shall deliver them from the wicked, and save them, because they trust in Him" (Psalm 37:40).

"R" is for REFRESHING WATER.

"But whosoever drinketh of the water that I shall give him shall never thirst; but the water that I shall give him shall be in him a well of water springing up into everlasting life" (John 4:14).

Water is the most abundant substance on Earth and has one of the most vitally important roles to play in maintaining a healthy body, as all life requires water for its metabolic activities.

To be sufficiently hydrated, adequate soft pure water to body weight ratio should be drunk. This can be calculated by the body weight in pounds divided by two, equaling the minimum number of ounces of water that the body needs on a daily basis for optimal health. The percentage of water in the adult body averages about 60% and adequate intake increases energy and endurance levels. For health purposes, sufficient water should be drunk before thirst is evident. If thirst is present, the body is already in a state of stress and dehydration. To improve electrical charges across the cellular membranes and vital life-saving hydration inside the cells, the body not only needs sufficient water but also electrolytes and fibre. Fruits, vegetables, grains, seeds, and herbs contain silica, which improves internal cell hydration. Some good sources of silica are bananas, mangos, avocados, green

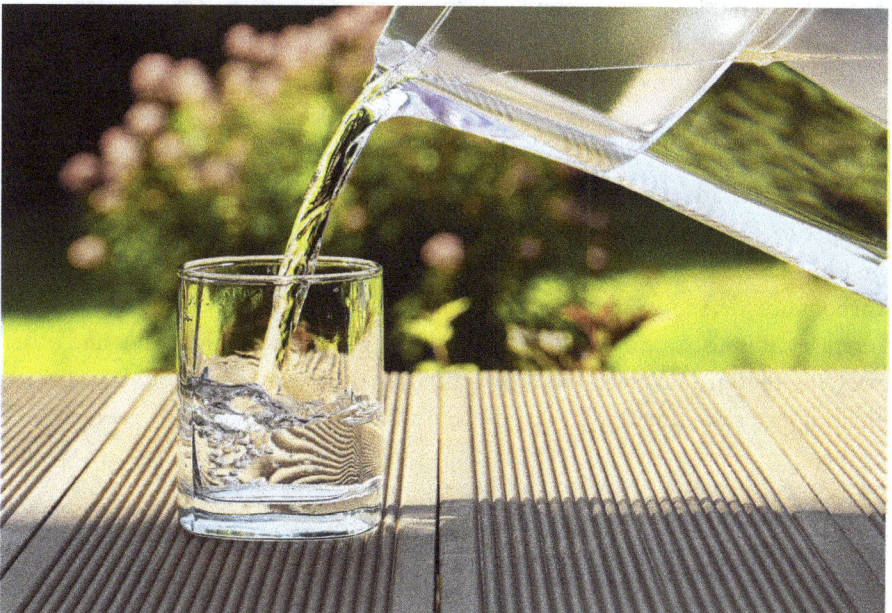

leafy vegetables, cucumbers, onions, green beans, bell peppers, parsley, Jerusalem artichokes, asparagus, whole-grain barley, rice, oats, wheat and millet, red lentils, sunflower seeds, flaxseeds, nettles, and horsetail.

The many vital health benefits of water include lubricating and cushioning the joints, protecting the spinal cord and other sensitive tissues, perspiration, bowel function and the prevention of constipation, respiration, maintenance of pH balance, regulation of body temperature, metabolism, functioning of organ systems, proper kidney function, prevention of UTIs, and urination (the urine should be almost clear if the body is adequately hydrated). Water can also generally prevent cardiovascular disorders by maintaining the correct viscosity of the plasma and blood as well as fibrinogen distribution. Fibrinogen is a protein that is essential for blood clot formation and is produced by the liver.

A healthy body should maintain a pH range of around 7.365 for proper physiological processes. This level is favourable for the oxygen uptake of the body, an optimal immune response and higher energy levels. This is attainable by consuming adequate water and maintaining a healthy diet and lifestyle. If the pH moves into an acidic state it can lead to sickness and an inability to assimilate nutrients.

The following is the percentage of water comprising various components of the body: 83% of the blood, 75% of the muscles, 74% of the brain matter, and 22% of the bones. The percentage of water in infants is much higher. It is usually around 76% but lowers to around 65% by one year of age. The composition of the body varies according to fitness levels and gender, as lean tissue contains more water than fatty tissue.

Daily bathing is not only cleansing but is also good for the circulation. Another excellent benefit of water is powerful hydrotherapy. Every system of the body requires adequate water for optimal functioning, and dehydration at the cellular level is the root cause of many diseases. Water carries nutrients, oxygen, and hormones to all parts of the body. It also provides a medium for collecting carbon dioxide, removing waste materials, dead cells, and toxins, and for dissolving gases. It is also one of the simplest and best pain relievers. Enzymes and other proteins that are involved in various fundamental processes require water for their appropriate functioning. God-given water is fundamental to the existence of life.

"And ye shall serve the LORD your God, and He shall bless thy bread, and thy water; and I will take sickness away from the midst of thee" (Exodus 23:25).

"U" is for UPLIFTING SUNSHINE.

"Then shall the righteous shine forth as the sun in the kingdom of their Father. Who hath ears to hear, let him hear"
(Matthew 13:43).

Powerful sunlight therapy dates back to the ancient Greeks who called it heliosis. It is now called heliotherapy. Sunlight is extremely beneficial for the body. The noon sunshine can deliver about 100,000 lux of light, and without sunlight, nothing can live. Light is part of a spectrum of electromagnetic energy. Ultraviolet radiation has a shorter wavelength than visible violet light, while infrared radiation has a longer wavelength than visible red light. There are seven colour frequencies in the spectrum of visible light, with each one having its own unique healing power. Ultraviolet rays are not only antiseptic but are also capable of killing viruses, moulds, yeasts, fungi, mites in water, on surfaces, and in the air. Ultraviolet is just one frequency of light, and upon entering the eyes, it stimulates the pineal gland in the brain which helps to improve thyroid function and regulates activity cycles. It also balances the hormones. Sunshine enhances the mood through the release of endorphins, thereby reducing the risk of depression.

Sunlight penetrates deep into the skin and produces natural vitamin D. It increases and enhances the volume of oxygen in the blood, which helps the body to maintain its defence against disease. It also cleanses the blood and blood vessels, thereby enhancing the capacity of the body to deliver oxygen to the tissues which increases muscular strength and endurance, with a very similar effect to that of exercise, even in those who are unable to exercise. Sunlight helps to regulate almost all the processes of the body. It has also been shown to improve sleep and increase the sense of well-being. Conversely, sun avoidance is a risk factor for death of a similar magnitude to smoking.[13] The number of both white blood cells (lymphocytes) and red blood cells (erythrocytes) increase with sun exposure and play a significant role in defending the body against infections. Sunlight is also therapeutic for depression, synchronizing important biorhythms, decreasing asthma symptoms, strengthening teeth, stomach ulcers, improving the appetite, together with assimilation and elimination, normalizing pulse pressure, dementia and brain ageing, utilizing phosphorus and calcium, raising levels of trace minerals in the blood, killing germs on the skin, increasing circulation, losing excess fat, calming the nerves, muscular development, stamina, bone health,

---

[13] "Avoidance of sun exposure as a risk factor for major causes of death," PubMed, https://1ref.us/1oz (accessed June 6, 2021).

metabolic processes, preventing and reversing tuberculosis, killing harmful bacteria, strengthening the immune system, reversing jaundice, treating many skin disorders, and helping to eliminate poisonous chemicals, heavy metals, pesticides, and other chemicals from the bloodstream faster. Conversely, it is the action of the sun on animal fats and trans-fatty acids in the skin that causes mutations that can lead to skin cancer.

Vitamin D is not only one chemical but many. It is essential for the proper utilization of calcium in the body and manages calcium in the bones, blood, and gut. Natural vitamin D is produced in the skin from the form of cholesterol known as 7-dehydrocholesterol. Ultraviolet B sunlight energy converts this precursor to vitamin D3 which is carried to the liver and kidneys to be transformed into active vitamin D. Sunbaths are also very effective in health and disease and are useful treatments for many skin diseases, being careful to avoid sunburn. Respiration, blood sugar levels, and the resting heart rate are all stabilized after a sunbath and especially if these rates are high to begin with. Sunbathing, proper nutrition, and a favourable lifestyle can reverse cancer. Vitamin D is involved in the biochemical cellular machinery of virtually all cells and tissues of the body, as virtually every cell type and tissue type throughout the body has receptors for vitamin D, which helps them to communicate properly. Many are vitamin D deficient because of an irrational fear of the sun. Sunblock stops the ultraviolet rays of the sun from creating vitamin D in the body, thereby depriving it of an element which is essential for many bodily functions. Regular sunlight exposure increases the growth and height of children, and especially babies. Many cultures throughout history have identified this phenomenon. Studies have shown that the amount of sun exposure in the first few months of life influences how tall a child will grow. Sunshine is another blessing from God.

"For the LORD God is a sun and shield: the LORD will give grace and glory: no good thing will He withhold from them that walk uprightly" (Psalm 84:11).

"S" is for SUFFICIENT SLEEP.

"For in six days the LORD made heaven and earth, the sea, and all that in them is, and rested the seventh day (Saturday): wherefore the LORD blessed the sabbath day, and hallowed it" (Exodus 20:11).

Adequate undisturbed restful sleep is essential for the proper functioning of the body. It is a good practice to avoid stressful and mentally stimulating activities before bedtime. Everyone needs regular times for rising in the mornings and for retiring at night, which should be around 9:30 p.m. if possible, as around that time melatonin, the powerful hormone that is produced in the pineal gland of the brain, is produced in response to darkness. Interestingly, the gut contains more than 400 times more melatonin than the pineal gland. Melatonin was discovered in 1958 and is an important antioxidant which is responsible for the lifecycles of cells. Low levels of melatonin are also linked to a leaky gut, and if melatonin levels are low, then the cells will live for too long and can become cancer cells, which have a different dividing mechanism. There is also a death gene that makes sure that normal cells die on time. In a study, melatonin was found to be more than 60 times more effective than vitamin C in protecting DNA from damage. Melatonin may bind to DNA, thus providing further protection beyond anti-oxidant activity. Vitamin C can become a toxic pro-oxidant when exposed to free iron, and most anti-oxidants become weak free radicals after neutralizing a free radical. But melatonin's antioxidant action involves the donation of two electrons instead of one, thereby ensuring that melatonin does not become a free radical. It boosts and strengthens the immune system and is also anti-cancer as it inhibits angiogenesis and causes cancer cell death by targeting its own oxygen and nutrient supply.

Studies have shown that melatonin also exhibits many other bioactivities besides antioxidant activity, including, cardiovascular protection, anti-inflammatory characteristics, neuroprotective, anti-obese and anti-diabetic. Melatonin easily crosses the blood-brain barrier and can protect neurons from excitotoxicity. It has also been shown to reduce cardiac arrythmias and oxidized lipids in the ischemic heart. Melatonin occurs in many nuts (especially pistachios), cereals, some kinds of mushrooms, tomatoes, peppers, legumes, and seeds. Moreover, the germination process of legumes and seeds has been proven to significantly increase melatonin levels. Sleeping in a room with light pollution, such as streetlights, bedroom lights, clocks, and watches, prevents the brain from completely switching off and may cause wakefulness on subsequent nights at around the same time. Eating a light meal no later than 5 p.m. can facilitate an empty stomach before retiring for the night, and this will help to ensure a restful sleep, during which the stomach also needs to rest. Compelling evidence demonstrates that fueling the mitochondria of the cells by eating less than four hours before bedtime, when food is not needed, increases the leakage of a large amount of electrons that liberates free radicals, thereby damaging the mitochondria and eventually the nuclear DNA. Evidence also indicates that cancer cells have damaged mitochondria. By avoiding the use of sleeping drugs, which do not induce proper sleep and are harmful to the body, a more natural sleep will result.

A lack of adequate, restful sleep is very damaging to the health and can result in many serious diseased conditions, as it is when the body is asleep that cleansing and healing occur. The harder the brain works during the day the more sleep recovery time is needed. Conversely, too much sleep is also detrimental to good health. An average of around eight hours of sleep a night is usually sufficient for adults. During sleep, the heart rate slows down and the body temperature lowers a little. Yet, while these vital signs slow down, the brain is very active. Sleep not only helps to clear toxic molecules from the brain, but sleep deprivation on a regular basis can also impair the ability of the brain to clear the nervous system. Lack of sleep not only causes tiredness but also a lapse in general neurological function, with instability and a lack of energy. If the brain does not obtain enough energy that it needs from sleep, it will often attempt to obtain it from food. Sleep deprivation can increase the production of ghrelin, which is a hunger hormone. Too much of this hormone causes the body to crave for sugary and fatty foods. Sleep deprivation can also cause leptin, the satiety hormone, to become so out of sync that the body does not recognize the signals to stop eating and can consume more of what it craves. Sleep deprivation also reduces hippocampal neurogenesis, thereby negatively altering hormone balance and cluttering the brain. Sleeping less than six hours a night can increase the risk of heart attacks by 18%. Sleeping fewer than five hours a night can raise the risk of a heart attack by threefold. High sensitivity C-reactive protein levels may increase too much if insufficient sleep is experienced and is a pre-indicative tool of a heart attack. Even if enough sleep is experienced after the level rises, it cannot easily be reduced to lower levels. Sleep deprivation for just one night is sufficient to imbalance body chemicals such as C-reactive protein and tumour necrosis factor-alpha, which can perform as toxins in the body, thereby increasing the risk of heart attacks and assisting the growth of cancer cells.

Sleep is generally categorized into several stages, these are light sleep, non-REM (rapid eye movement) sleep, and REM sleep. NREM sleep helps the body, while REM sleep assists the brain. Both should be experienced with adequate sleep. When NREM sleep occurs, pituitary hormones are discharged to repair and prepare the body. REM sleep assists with mental stability and stress and helps

112

to maintain focus. With sufficient REM sleep, the body is replaced and renewed, but without sufficient REM sleep, the body tends to break down quickly. Sleep medications do not induce REM sleep, but cause memory loss, are highly disease-causing and the duration of sleep is about the same, but not of good quality. Researchers have discovered by experiments that dreaming occurs in both REM and NREM sleep. Alzheimer's disease, Parkinson's disease, and gastrointestinal and behaviour disorders are linked to a lack of sleep, which can be caused by drugs, as every medication slows or stops metabolic processes. When the body is sick it requires more sleep to heal properly. Anabolism is anything constructive that increases the metabolism and causes the body to be healthier, and unrefined coconut oil does both. Catabolism is the metabolic breakdown and energy-burning aspect of the dismantling of structural proteins. During sleep, the cortex area of the brain, which is responsible for memory, thought and language, disengages from the senses and turns into recovery mode. The immune system produces cytokines when the body is in a state of sleep. Cytokines are proteins that are regulators of responses to inflammation, infection, immune responses, and trauma. Anti-inflammatory cytokines are protective and serve to reduce inflammation and promote healing. Conversely, pro-inflammatory cytokines promote inflammation and cause diseases to worsen. Poor sleep, which can be due to dehydration, is detrimental to the immune system and can cause significant issues with the body's ability to not only fight infections, but also many serious diseases such as cancer. Chronic sleep deprivation has not only been linked to cancer but also cardiovascular disease, depression, obesity, and an increased risk of type 2 diabetes. Also, those who have insufficient sleep tend to have hearts that have aged more. Sleep deprivation is incredibly damaging to the kidneys, affects how the brain stores memories, disrupts hormonal balance, and elevates the circulating levels of oestrogen. During tests, it has been discovered that sleep deprivation causes drivers to drive as though intoxicated.

"When thou liest down, thou shalt not be afraid: yea, thou shalt lie down, and thy sleep shall be sweet" (Proverbs 3:24).

"T" is for TEMPERANCE.

"And every man that striveth for the mastery is temperate in all things. Now they do it to obtain a corruptible crown; but we an incorruptible" (1 Corinthians 9:25).

Temperance in good health practices requires moderation and wise choices in all aspects of life. Overeating, overworking, overexercising and even oversleeping can attribute to poor health.

Overeating overburdens the liver and weakens it as a dysfunctional liver cannot efficiently filter the blood. It also stupefies the brain and aggravates other health conditions, some of which overburden the lungs, heart, and kidneys. Overeating, even of the healthiest foods, causes the liver to work much harder at detoxifying the chemical contents in foods and can lead to non-alcoholic fatty liver disease in which fatty deposits in the vessels of the liver make it difficult for it to function properly. This can cause a toxic overload to circulate throughout the bloodstream, which leads to a toxic build-up in the body. These toxins, which are usually free radicals, can damage the arterial cell membrane components of the heart. Fatty foods from animal sources thicken the arteries of the liver, which can lead to the formation of gallstones. These foods also suppress the formation of bile, hinder the process of fat digestion, and encourage weight gain. It is estimated that 10%–20% of those with a fatty liver will develop cirrhosis. Choline plays a vital role in non-alcoholic fatty liver disease and is also an essential nutrient for a healthy brain, nervous system and cardiovascular function. It is necessary for DNA synthesis, for making the important neurotransmitter acetylcholine and is used in the synthesis of phospholipids such as phosphatidylcholine, which is needed for the composition of cell membranes. Choline is also required for cell structure, cell messaging, metabolism, and fat transport as it is needed to carry cholesterol from the liver. A deficiency of choline may cause fatty liver diseases. It is contained in spinach, green peas, cauliflower, shiitake mushrooms, broccoli, asparagus, cabbage, Swiss chard, Brussels sprouts, and collard greens. Obesity is one of the leading causes of liver damage in most affluent countries. Those with fatty liver disease can die from complications which are related to cardiovascular health difficulties and not necessarily as a result of cirrhosis of the liver.

> *Temperance in good health practices requires moderation and wise choices in all aspects of life.*

Being a workaholic is definitely a hindrance to optimum physical and mental health. Studies show that overwork in any area doubles the risk of heart attack and stroke and significantly increases the risk of depression. According to studies, overworking generally is antithetical to a healthy mind and body, and the

Vitamin B$_4$

Choline

VECTOR OBJECTS
EPS 10

Molecular Formula of Choline:

$$C_5H_{14}NO^+$$

Structural Formula of Choline:

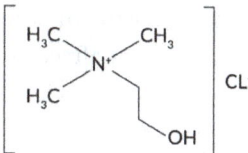

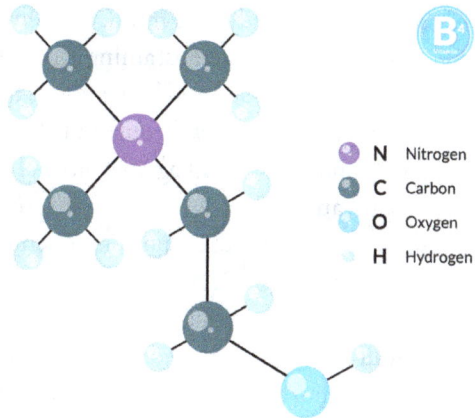

N Nitrogen
C Carbon
O Oxygen
H Hydrogen

greater the number of hours worked per year, the greater the likelihood of a poor quality of life and premature death. Stress and overwork not only cause new illnesses but also exacerbate pre-existing conditions and can cause life-threatening health issues.

Exercising incorrectly or excessively can injure health in a number of ways. The tissues can break down, microscopic tears in muscle fibres can occur, and the stress hormone cortisol can be released, which can contribute to a weakened immune system and chronic disease. Scientific studies have warned that extremely strenuous workouts can damage the heart. Intense endurance exercises may be cardiotoxic and can cause permanent structural changes to the heart, which can exacerbate the risk of heart arrhythmias or even sudden cardiac death.

With a sleeping duration of more than nine hours per night, studies have shown an increased risk of Alzheimer's disease and dementia, obesity, diabetes, heart disease, angina, strokes, memory impairments, degenerative diseases, headaches, decreased cognitive function, persistent depression, inflammation, and pain. Sleeping for more than eight hours per night correlates with a 50% higher stroke risk, whereas those who sleep for over eight hours and who also have drowsiness during the daytime have a 90% higher stroke risk. Oversleeping is not usually due to the body requiring extra sleep but is often linked to exhaustion from mental, physical, emotional, or spiritual deficiencies.

Abstaining from all harmful and addictive indulgences including caffeinated soft drinks, tobacco, tea, (except herbal teas) chocolate, coffee and alcohol contributes to a healthier body and mind. Abstemiousness is the moderate use of that which is healthful while abstaining from substances that are harmful. To obtain a balanced mind, body and lifestyle, it is beneficial to utilize both the mental and physical powers equally throughout the day.

The temperance movement against alcohol began around the 1820s. Alcohol is a deadly drug and a class A1 carcinogen, regardless of its type; it is also an endocrine disrupter and a toxic poison which can have lethal consequences. It also has a very acidifying effect on the pH and robs the bloodstream of oxygen. The long and short-term effects of this dangerous toxicant can affect not only the body but also the lifestyle and mental health. If a large amount of alcohol is consumed in a short space of time, the concentration of alcohol in the blood can prevent the body from functioning properly. Alcohol consumption depletes nutrients, slows down the functions of the brain and especially adversely affects the higher functions of the frontal lobe. The resulting dehydration can also cause permanent brain damage. It affects the nerves that control breathing and heartbeat and can stop both. Beneficial gut bacteria are also affected and are killed as soon as alcohol enters the gut. The consumption of alcohol also increases the risk of developing cancers and other diseases. Heavy consumption of alcohol is very costly to the liver and can lead to a variety of problems including inflammation, fibrosis, cirrhosis, alcoholic hepatitis, and a fatty liver. Chronic alcohol drinking prohibits the ability of the pancreas to absorb vitamin C, which renders the pancreas vulnerable to diseases. Alcohol causes the pancreas to manufacture noxious substances that can cause pancreatitis.

Consuming too much alcohol can weaken the immune system, which makes the body more vulnerable to disease, while also depleting the body of vitamin C. Drinking a substantial amount of alcohol over a long period of time or too much on a single occasion can damage the heart, causing arrhythmias, cardiomyopathy, and stroke.

"Who hath woe? who hath sorrow? who hath contentions? who hath babbling? who hath wounds without cause? who hath redness of eyes. They that tarry long at the wine; they that go to seek mixed wine" (Proverbs 23:29, 30).

Jesus Christ did not drink alcoholic wine, even when He was suffering excruciating pain on the cross. The Bible mentions two types of grape juice. One being fermented (alcoholic) and the other is new wine, which, from the Hebrew language, means fresh grape juice. Temperance is vital for good health.

"Wine is a mocker, strong drink is raging: and whosoever is deceived thereby is not wise" (Proverbs 20:1).

"G" is for GOOD NUTRITION.

"And Jesus said unto them, I am the bread of life: he that cometh to me shall never hunger; and he that believeth on me shall never thirst" (John 6:35).

A varied healthy whole plant-food diet will include fresh fruits and vegetables, grains, nuts, seeds, beans, and legumes. Frozen and dried foods, as well as sprouts, can also be healthful and organic produce is the healthiest, especially if it has been grown in mineral-rich soil. The original God-given diet was comprised of whole plant-foods. Many people do not consume adequate healthy nutrient-rich foods, and as a consequence, their health suffers, as sound nutrition is of the utmost importance to good health. Using a healthy salt, such as Himalayan pink crystal salt, will furnish the body with more minerals, which are essential for a variety of bodily functions. Consuming adequate protein is not problematic with this diet, but the consumption of animal products has been linked to many diseases, including cancer. Diets high in protein cause more calcium to be lost through the urine, while the mineral boron may slow the loss of calcium from the bones. Many whole plant-foods contain an abundance of boron including potatoes, chickpeas, apricots, almonds, green leafy vegetables, red grapes, carrots, bananas, prunes, walnuts, oranges, onions, avocados, raisins, peanuts, red apples, broccoli, legumes, prunes, pears, beans, Brazil nuts, and honey. Carbohydrates originate from the photosynthesis of plants and take the form of sugars, starches, and cellulose. Carbohydrates provide energy to living cells and are comprised of carbon, oxygen, and hydrogen. Avoiding refined and adulterated oils, but consuming adequate amounts of healthy saturated fat, such as medium-chain unrefined coconut oil, and other coconut products which boost the metabolism, plus olives, nuts, seeds, avocados, and Omega-3 fatty acids, are extremely beneficial for health, and especially brain health, as the brain needs healthy fats. Heating any oil to its smoke point will render it carcinogenic, and different oils have different smoke points. Unrefined coconut oil has a smoke point of 176°C (348.8°F).

Many different bioactive phytochemical nutrients are contained in different fruits and vegetables and they bind to specific cell receptors and proteins. There are four types of cell receptors and there are specific cell receptors for specific fruits and vegetables. It is beneficial to have a wide variety of these foods, as many phytonutrients are not distributed evenly amongst different plant families. Different fruits and vegetables can lower the disease risks of different bodily parts or organs. For example, crucifers are associated with a lower colon cancer risk in the middle and right side of the body, whereas apples, pumpkins, and carrots can help to alleviate the risk of colon cancer on the lower left side of the body. Intestinal intraepithelial lymphocytes are critical cells which are a defence against pathogens. They are covered with receptors that act as locks and the key to opening these cell sensor receptor locks are plants, such as crucifers. Crucifers contain high levels of nutrients that are transformed by stomach acid into a critical key that fits the receptor lock on these lymphocytes, leading to their activation to boost immune function. Cells are uniquely created and designed to assimilate plant nutrients. Habitual consumption of fruits and vegetables have positive effects on many functional aspects of the body, including DNA repair. Green vegetables are most essential for health and are specifically required by the body to maintain a large population of these lymphocytes. Avoiding the consumption of fruits and vegetables at the same meal helps to facilitate proper digestion, as when they are combined together in the stomach they can cause fermentation, which produces alcohol.

It is healthier to refrain from eating than to do so hurriedly or under stress, as the digestive process can become impaired. Taking sufficient time to eat helps to avoid overeating. Avoiding the following items is beneficial for good health: MSG, processed white table salt, all refined sugars, aluminium and non-stick cookware, all artificial sweeteners, alcohol (inhibits calcium absorption), irradiated and microwaved foods (microwaving renders foods denatured and harmful), and denatured grains, which have the most nutritious parts of the grain removed (the bran and germ) and are often bleached. Vinegars are also unhealthy. Pure vinegar has a pH of 2–3. Apple cider vinegar is made by combining apples with yeast and is slightly more alkaline than pure vinegar as it contains more alkaline nutrients. However, it is still acidic. The yeast converts the sugar in the apples into alcohol. Bacteria are then added to the mixture, which ferments the alcohol into acetic acid.

"But my God shall supply all your need according to His riches in glory by Christ Jesus" (Philippians 4:19).

"O" is for OUTDOOR AIR.

"And the LORD God formed man of the dust of the ground, and breathed into his nostrils the breath of life; and man became a living soul" (Genesis 2:7).

Pure fresh air, with its life-giving oxygen, is of vital importance to good health and well-being. It is a precious boon from Heaven and fresh country air is especially invigorating. Cancer cannot exist in the presence of oxygen, which is continuously replenished by plant photosynthesis, which uses the energy of sunlight to produce oxygen from carbon dioxide and water.

The depletion of 35% of oxygen to the body's healthy cells can change them into cancer cells within just a couple of days so that some cells can survive in the acidic environment in the absence of oxygen.

The heart beats approximately 100,000 times a day and consumes a large amount of oxygen, but an acidic body prevents oxygen from being transported to the cells. A supply shortage means that the heart cannot use blood as effectively, and diminished heart function leads to poor circulation of oxygen in the blood.

The lungs contain 300–500 million alveoli and approximately 1,500 miles of airways. Bad breathing habits reduce the ability of the body to deliver oxygen to the cells and can cause many negative effects on health and well-being as well as limiting the energy that is produced because every process of the body is dependent upon oxygen. The average amount of breaths that people take every day is about 25,000. A shortage of oxygen causes the brain to perform slower and also affects the regulation of many other bodily functions. Fresh, oxygenated air is vital for good health and provides a steady supply of oxygen, which is needed by the brain and every cell of the body and which cannot survive for more than a few minutes without it. Daily exercise in the fresh air promotes circulation and floods the body with oxygen. Windows should be opened regularly and bedrooms should always be well ventilated while sleeping, even in the winter months. Polluted indoor air is a huge health hazard, as it not only causes many health issues, including mental health, but it also affects the intelligence.

The average resting bodily intake of air is approximately 11,000 litres per day. During normal breathing, this inhaled air travels at about eighty kilometres per hour, but during a cough or a sneeze, it can reach speeds of 1,200 kilometres per hour. The inhaled air is about 20% oxygen, and the exhaled air is about 15% oxygen. Which means that about 5% of the air volume is consumed in each breath and converted to carbon dioxide.

A large deep breath of air through the mouth at a temperature of minus 45°C (-49°F) is capable of killing a human being, as the lungs can freeze almost immediately. However, if air at the same temperature is breathed in through the nose, the air temperature changes from minus 45°C. to body temperature by the time the air travels just two inches up the nostrils. Conversely, very hot air has the same reaction and can kill those who breathe it in through the mouth. But if breathed in through the nose the hot air becomes body temperature by the time it travels just two inches up the nostrils.

It is best to breath in and out through the nose, which prepares the incoming air to be used by the body as effectively as possible. This is very beneficial for asthmatics. Breathing in through the mouth inhales unfiltered air, which can be full of bacteria and viruses. It is advisable to avoid smoke, including paraffin wax candle smoke, incense burners, aerosol sprays, chemical air fresheners, and other chemicals. Indoor plants help to improve the quality of indoor air by producing oxygen and absorbing carbon dioxide from their surroundings. Some plants can even remove toxic pollutants from the air.

The diaphragm is the primary breathing muscle and contracts during inspiration. It moves down into the abdominal cavity, thereby creating a negative pressure in the thoracic cavity which forces air into the lungs while simultaneously increasing the intra-abdominal pressure, which distends the abdominal wall. This facilitates the gas exchange of oxygen and carbon dioxide and also massages the stomach, liver, and intestines. Standing tall and sitting up straight allows for the expansion of the lungs which enables them to take in sufficient oxygen.

Fresh air stimulates the appetite and helps food to digest more efficiently. It assists with clearer thinking; changes brain levels of serotonin, which helps to improve the mood and promotes a sense of happiness and well-being; improves concentration; supports and strengthens the immune system by supplying it with the oxygen that it needs to fight off disease more effectively; helps with better sound sleep at night; aids with improving the heart rate, pulse pressure, and metabolic rate; soothes the nerves and imparts a feeling of being more relaxed and refreshed; improves the cleansing action of the lungs; helps to clear the mind; aids the body to rid itself of accumulated impurities; and helps the airways of the lungs to dilate more fully. Fresh air is a blessing from God.

Improper breathing can negatively impact the mood and bodily functions, including digestion, sleep, the heart, the nervous system, the brain, and the muscles. A shortage of oxygen also has a negative effect on stamina, as without enough the muscles tire and tense up. Conversely, correct breathing can impact bodily functions in a positive way, including the stimulation of brain neurons, improved health, more energy, better harmony, less anxiety and fear, better relationships, and feeling happier. Breathing in a way that is physiologically optimal for the body is the way that the body was designed to breathe. A breath of fresh air is an invigorating thing to take and a much more rewarding thing to be.

Through experiments, using a lung of a living mouse, scientists have recently revealed that the lungs make blood and produce more than ten million platelets (tiny blood cells) per hour. The lungs have a previously unrecognized role in blood production and produce more platelets, or required blood clotting components, than bone marrow. They also identified a previously unknown pool of blood stem cells, which are capable of restoring blood production when the bone marrow stem cells are depleted. It was previously assumed for decades that bone marrow produces all of the blood components.

"Then we which are alive and remain shall be caught up together with them in the clouds (of angels), to meet the Lord in the air: and so shall we ever be with the Lord. Wherefore comfort one another with these words" (1 Thessalonians 4:17, 18).

"D" is for DAILY EXERCISE.

"Know ye not that they which run in a race run all, but one receiveth the prize? So run, that ye may obtain" (1 Corinthians 9:24).

Daily morning walking in the fresh air is the best exercise and is very beneficial for the body, as the important aspect of the impact of the feet touching the ground not only affects the muscles and heart but also increases the blood supply to the brain by sending pressure waves through the arteries, demonstrating that walking is more beneficial than cycling or swimming. These benefits can be life-saving and have been demonstrated to halt cancer as well as benefitting mental and physical health, including greatly improved blood circulation, increased oxygen to the brain, and better sleep. It is the best remedy for diseased bodies as it imparts strength to the muscles. A short leisurely walk after a meal is beneficial for the digestion, as all the organs of the body will be brought into use. Walking helps the body to stay fit and lowers the risk of stroke and death from cardiovascular disease by more than half. Regular walking promotes good

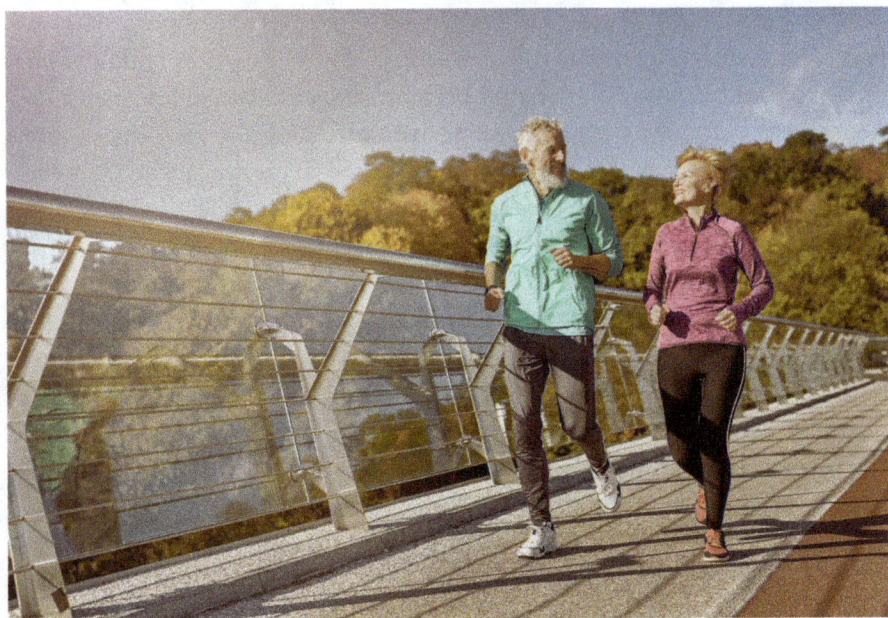

health, strengthens the immune system, and not only attributes to an increased blood flow but also healthier cells. It also releases endorphins into the system and improves the disposition. During inclement weather, the use of exercise equipment is very useful, and if exercise is conducted in the fresh air it is even more beneficial. Exercise slows bone loss and is one of the most important factors in maintaining the health of the bones. Cells need four essential things to live and function efficiently: oxygen, nutrition, water, and cleansing.

Various studies have shown that cardiovascular exercise can create new brain cells (neurogenesis) and improve overall brain performance. An exercising session can subsequently improve creativity for up to two hours afterwards. Regular physical activity boosts memory and the ability to learn new things and can also help with addiction recovery.

One of the most common psychological benefits of exercise is stress relief, and working up a sweat can help to manage psychological stress. Exercise increases concentrations of norepinephrine (also called noradrenaline), which is a chemical that can moderate the response to stress in the brain. Studies have shown that exercise can also help to alleviate the symptoms of depression, type 2 diabetes, and arthritis. It not only builds stronger muscles and bones but also encourages better digestion. Exercising can increase free radical damage if the body is lacking proper nutrients. The brain releases dopamine, which is a reward chemical, in response to any form of pleasure, and this chemical is released during and after exercise. Exercise releases endorphins, which can generate feelings of euphoria and happiness. Dopamine and endorphins are both types of neurotransmitters, which are chemicals that travel between neurons and relay information. Dopamine is a monoaminergic (diminutive) neurotransmitter, which is part of the primary reward pathways in the brain. It is also a neuromodulator, which modulates other neurotransmitter behaviours. Some neurotransmitters make neurons less likely to fire and some make them more likely to fire. Dopamine tends to be involved in reinforcing behaviour, while endorphins are involved, among other things, in sleep and wake cycles and numbing pain signals. Endorphins (peptides) are larger molecules which are related in structure to proteins and comprise of a whole category of neurotransmitters with a variety of molecules that have comparable functions and shapes. There is no inherent property in these chemicals themselves but rather in the brain circuits that they are involved in. These circuits comprise of millions of neurons that have receptors for these neurotransmitters. Exercise creates a healthier body if not taken to extremes.

Having an attitude of gratitude is a great blessing.

"But they that wait upon the LORD shall renew their strength; they shall mount up with wings as eagles; they shall run, and not be weary; and they shall walk, and not faint" (Isaiah 40:31).

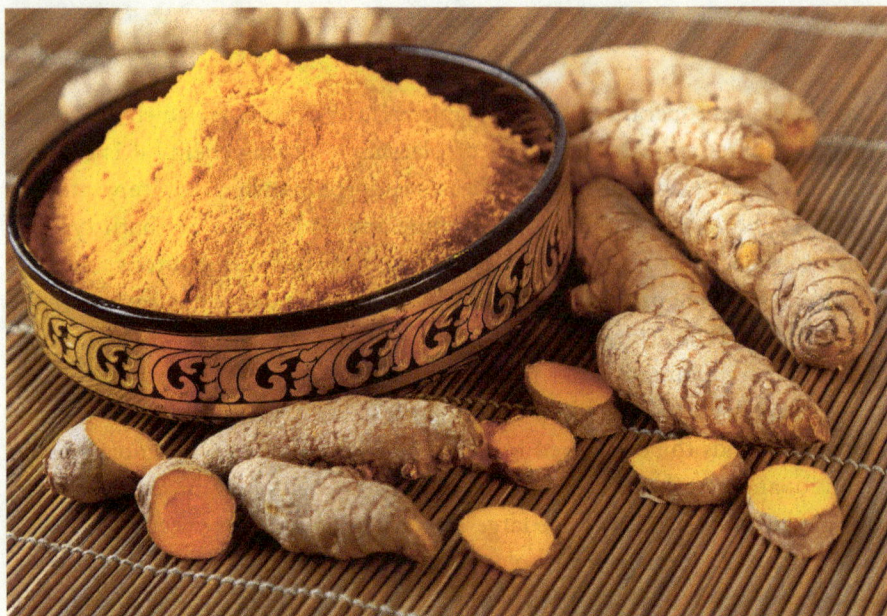

Chapter 3

Turmeric

"EVERY DRUG THAT THE FDA HAS RECALLED WAS FIRST PROVEN BY THEM TO BE SAFE AND EFFECTIVE."

Turmeric is one of the most thoroughly researched plants in existence today. It is also one of the most powerful, versatile, and beneficial medicinal plants in the history of the entire world. Its name derives from the Latin words *terra merita* (*meritorious earth*), a term that refers to the colour of the ground plant, which resembles a mineral pigment.

This powerful, prized orange root is a member of the Curcuma longa botanical group, which is part of the ginger family of plants called Zingiberaceae. Turmeric grows mainly in tropical and sub-tropical climates and has been revered for its therapeutic properties since time immemorial. The plant grows to a height of about one metre, has lengthy oblong leaves, and to thrive it needs a considerable amount of annual rainfall and a growth season with temperatures between 20° and 30°C (68° and 86°F). As many as 133 species of Curcuma have been identified worldwide and are used traditionally as a spice or medicine.

Turmeric is native to Indonesia and southern India, with India, where it is known as *Indian saffron*, continuing to be the world's largest producer, consumer, and exporter of turmeric. The quality of Indian turmeric is considered to be the best in the world market.

In its whole state as a rhizomatous herbaceous perennial, turmeric appears in one of the earliest known surviving records of the use of medicinal plants. It was reportedly listed in the Ebers Papyrus from Egypt, circa 1500 BC, for the healing of wounds and as a dye. The Assyrians were also familiar with turmeric, and it is believed to have been cultivated in the hanging gardens of Babylon. This phenomenal and cherished rhizome was described in a herbal remedies book from 600 BC and has been used as a medicine, flavouring agent, and dye at least since that time. In 420 BC, Hippocrates, a Greek physician and philosopher who was renowned as *the father of medicine,* said: "Leave thy drugs in the chemists' pots if thou cans't heal the patient with food." There is no cure in any chemical drug, only additional poisoning and suppression of symptoms, as poison does not equate to wellness. The following amusing hieroglyph was found in an ancient Egyptian tomb that reads: "One-quarter of what you eat keeps you alive. The other three-quarters keeps your doctor alive." An ancient proverb says: "When diet is wrong, medicine is of no use. When diet is correct, medicine is of no need." The Greek physician Pedanius Dioscorides utilised turmeric in the first century AD while serving as a physician for the Roman Empire. Turmeric was recorded in the Tang Materia Medica, which was compiled in China in AD 659 and which is considered to be one of the world's first pharmacopoeias. There is also evidence that it was used in Chinese medicine about 1,000 years ago. Around AD 1280, Marco Polo was introduced to turmeric during his voyage to India and China and described it as a plant with all the qualities of saffron while being a root vegetable. Arab traders introduced it into Europe in the thirteenth century, and during the fifteenth

> *Turmeric is one of the most thoroughly researched plants in existence today. It is also one of the most powerful, versatile, and beneficial medicinal plants in the history of the entire world.*

century, the Portuguese explorer Vasco de Gama visited the Indian subcontinent, bringing turmeric and other spices of the Orient with him. During the period of British rule over India, turmeric was combined with other spices and named *curry powder*. By the eighteenth century, it had made its way to Jamaica and other places with tropical climates.

Turmeric is an incredibly potent, accessible, affordable, time-tested, and generally safe plant that has been closely interwoven with human culture for thousands of years. It is so intensively supported by scientific investigation as to be unparalleled in its proven value to health and well-being. Turmeric owes its many medicinal benefits to its active primary polyphenol ingredient—curcumin (also found in ginger), which is also responsible for its distinctive colour and spicy, bitter flavour. Curcumin has amazing therapeutic qualities and is a very potent property of turmeric. The turmeric rhizome is comprised of 70% carbohydrates, 6–9% oil, 7% protein, 4% minerals, at least 4% essential oils, 1% resin, and also vitamins and other alkaloids. Its health-benefiting essential oils are cineole, curlone, curumene, p-cymene, and termerone. Turmeric has hundreds of molecular constituents with each possessing a variety of biological actions. It is lipophilic (fat-soluble) and has at least twenty-three molecules that are antibiotic, fourteen known anti-carcinogenics, seventeen anti-tumour, thirty-seven anti-inflammatory, and at least twenty-seven anti-oxidants.

"For one believeth that he may eat all things: another, who is weak, eateth herbs" (Romans 14:2).

A statistical analysis of over 3,000,000 published scientific studies has revealed that curcumin is the most widely researched phytochemical in science today, as it is the most frequently mentioned phytonutrient. Its medicinal properties can simultaneously modulate over 150 biological pathways in the body and have been the subject of nearly 6,000 peer-reviewed and published biomedical studies, exhibiting its therapeutic value in over 800 distinct, preventative, and therapeutic health applications, in addition to 175 distinct beneficial physiological effects, establishing it as one of the world's most significant non-toxic plants. Curcumin is only one of the hundreds of biomolecules found in turmeric and is capable of modulating over 2,000 genes simultaneously within a cancer cell line with positive results. A cancer cell line is the study of cancer cells that constantly divide and grow over a period of time under specific laboratory conditions and which are used in research to study the biology of cancer. Curcumin has been the subject of extensive research that has demonstrated its ability to kill both cancer cells and cancer stem cells, with over 1,500 studies relevant to over 100 distinct cancer types, including twenty-four studies demonstrating its anti-pancreatic cancer properties which have revealed that curcumin kills highly lethal pancreatic tumours. It has been proven, in various human studies, that curcumin is extremely safe where it is not contraindicated and does not produce any known side effects.

"I will instruct thee and teach thee in the way which thou shalt go: I will guide thee with mine eye" (Psalm 32:8).

Whole turmeric has been the subject of over 15,000 studies and carries a wider range of therapeutic compounds than curcumin alone. These compounds include alpha-curcumene, alpha-pinene, alpha-terpineol, api-procurcumenol, ar-turmerone, azulene, beta-pinene, beta-sitosterol, beta-turmerone, bisdeme-thoxycurcumin, bis-(4-hydroxy cinnamoyl)-methane, borneol, caffeic acid, caryophyllene, 1,8-cineole, cinnamic acid, curcuminoids, dehydrodurdione, demethoxycurcumins, diferuloylmethane, eugenol, feruloyl-4-hydroxycinnam-oyl-methane, furanodiene, germacrone, limonene, linalool, procurcumenol, protocatechuic acid, quercetin, salicylates, sodium curcumate, stigmasterol, tet-rahydrocurcumin, and vanillic acid. God did not create isolates, and when these compounds are composed together they gain beneficial synergistic effects, as the whole plant is more powerful than an isolated part of it. Although curcuminoids show promising results, isolates can have side effects as they were created to work synergistically in the whole plant. If a nutrient is extracted out of its natural whole food state, it performs less like a nutrient and more like a drug.

"Such knowledge is too wonderful for me; it is high, I cannot attain unto it" (Psalm 139:6).

This amazing golden plant is truly unique in its exceptional efficacy and safety, as has been demonstrated by many thousands of studies. The roots and rhi-zome stems, which are highly antiseptic and aromatic, can be either eaten fresh, crushed and powdered into ground turmeric, or the fresh-cut root can be freeze-dried and ground into powder. These are used worldwide and are the source of its natural curcumin component, which is responsible for it biological activity.

"The hay appeareth, and the tender grass sheweth itself, and herbs of the mountains are gathered" (Proverbs 27:25).

Phenomenal turmeric contains vitamin B2, vitamin B3, vitamin B6, vitamin C, vitamin E, vitamin K, choline, fibre, and folate. It also contains very good amounts of calcium, copper, iron, magnesium, manganese, Omega-3, potassium, and zinc. *Calcium* has many benefits, including building and maintaining strong bones and teeth, proper heart function, muscles, cells, the brain, and nerves. Calcium-rich whole plant-foods are protective and can be found in cabbage, broccoli, kale, collard greens, bok choy, watercress, nuts, figs, oranges, and white beans. The health benefits of *copper* include the efficient utilization of iron, increased red blood cell formation, proper body growth, regulated heart rhythm, increased energy production, balanced thyroid glands, maintenance of blood vessels, prevention of premature ageing (including greying of the hair), bone integrity, proper enzymatic reactions, and improved health of the connective tissues, eyes, and hair. Sufficient amounts of copper in the blood are also required to maintain proper oxygenation. Healthy copper-rich foods include sunflower seeds, cruciferous vegetables and dark leafy greens, almonds, asparagus, lentils, organic blackstrap molasses, and dried apricots. *Iron* is an essential protein co-factor component for cytochrome oxidase enzymes at the cellular level metabolism in the mitochondrial membrane. It is essential for the proper growth and development of the body. Its main health benefits include the reduction of iron deficiency anaemia, assisting to metabolize proteins, and performing an important role in the production of red blood cells and haemoglobin, thereby providing life-giving oxygen to organ systems. Haemoglobin is the iron-containing oxygen-transport metalloprotein in the erythrocytes (red blood cells). Approximately two-thirds of the iron in the body is found in the haemoglobin. Good sources of iron-containing foods include healthy dark green leafy vegetables, sunflower seeds, whole grains, lentils, organic blackstrap molasses, nuts, and beans. Non-haem, or plant iron, causes less damage to the body than iron from meat. Adding toxic metallic iron filings to foods such as cereals and calling them *iron-enriched* has been a pervasive strategy throughout the food industry for many years. This can easily be demonstrated with a magnet. *Magnesium* is an essential mineral and is required for over 300 biochemical reactions in the body. The multiple health benefits of magnesium include body temperature regulation, detoxification, energy production, the transmission of nerve impulses, and the formation of healthy teeth and bones. High magnesium-containing foods include dark leafy greens, nuts, seeds, beans, whole grains, avocados, bananas, pumpkin seeds and dried fruit.

Magnesium, calcium, and zinc are three of the most important minerals that are essential for good health. Magnesium aids in the absorption of calcium and zinc, actively supports the immune system and is protective against strokes. The essential trace mineral *manganese* is used by the body as a co-factor for the antioxidant enzyme superoxide dismutase, making manganese a powerful antioxidant that helps to protect cells against free-radical attacks. Good sources can be found in green leafy vegetables, whole grains, fruits, legumes, and nuts. Manganese also contains a small amount of brain-nourishing and highly anti-inflammatory Omega-3 fatty acids, which can improve blood flow in the brain. *Potassium* is an important component of the cells and body fluids that helps to normalize the pulse pressure and heart rate. Foods high in potassium include dark leafy greens, avocados, bananas, mushrooms, potatoes, squash, beans, coconut water, and sweet potatoes. *Zinc* is an essential trace element. It is found in cells throughout the body and is needed for cell division, cell growth, wound healing, proper functioning of the immune system, the breakdown of carbohydrates, and for the senses of smell and taste. It is found in napa cabbage, dried apricots, peaches, prunes, whole grains, chia seeds, peanuts, toasted pumpkin seeds, sesame seeds, beans, flax seeds, mushrooms, corn, sunflower seeds, and watermelon seeds. Zinc is also found in nuts such as cashews, pine nuts, pecans, Brazil nuts, almonds, walnuts, hazelnuts, pistachios, macadamias, and coconuts.

Riboflavin (vitamin B2) is involved in energy metabolism and has recently been found to affect iron metabolism in important ways. It is contained in healthy plant-foods such as leafy greens (including spinach), grapes, cabbage, carrots, beetroot leaves, peppers, mushrooms, root vegetables and leaves, cauliflower, asparagus, squash, celery, green peas, broccoli, sweet potatoes, almonds, Brussels sprouts, green beans, and maple syrup. *Niacin* (vitamin B3) is an important nutrient and is needed by every part of the body to function efficiently. It also acts as an antioxidant, assists with dermatitis, performs a role in cell signalling, and the making and repairing of DNA. As with all of the B vitamins, niacin helps to convert food into energy by assisting enzymes to work. It boosts brain function as well as being of extreme significance in dealing with mental disorders. Healthy sources are found in peanuts, mushrooms, green peas, potatoes, sweet potatoes, squash, corn, peas, and parsnips. *Pyridoxine* (vitamin B6) is used in the treatment of homocystinuria, radiation sickness, and sideroblastic anaemia. Its healthy whole plant-food sources include pistachios, sunflower seeds, bananas, prunes, avocados, and cooked spinach.

One of the important factors of *vitamin C* is its role in collagen synthesis. Collagen provides important functions in the blood vessels as it both comprises and imparts integrity and strength to the walls of the capillaries, veins, and arteries, which is very important for preventing aneurysms and strokes. *Vitamin E* is an antioxidant, and thereby reduces inflammation. It helps to prevent and treat diseases of the blood vessels and heart. It is contained in whole grains, parsley, nuts, papaya, seeds, avocados, broccoli, green leafy vegetables, and olives. *Vitamin K* is a fat-soluble vitamin that activates the protein that clots the blood and fights inflammation. A deficiency can lead to cancer, heart disease, tooth decay and weakened bones, as it is needed for the synthesis of bone proteins. There are two types of vitamin K: type 1 and type 2. Vitamin K1 is found in vegetables, whereas vitamin K2 is produced by gut bacteria. Whole plant sources are green leafy vegetables, broccoli, cabbage, Brussels sprouts, prunes, cucumbers, and cultured vegetables (using a starter culture of vitamin K2-producing bacteria). *Choline* is a water-soluble micronutrient that is important for nerve and liver function, the maintenance of healthy metabolism and energy levels, muscle movement, and normal brain development. It is involved in important processes many times every day and is contained in Brussels sprouts, dark leafy greens, asparagus, bok choy, cauliflower, mushrooms, split peas, navy beans, lima beans, lentils, chickpeas, sunflower seeds,

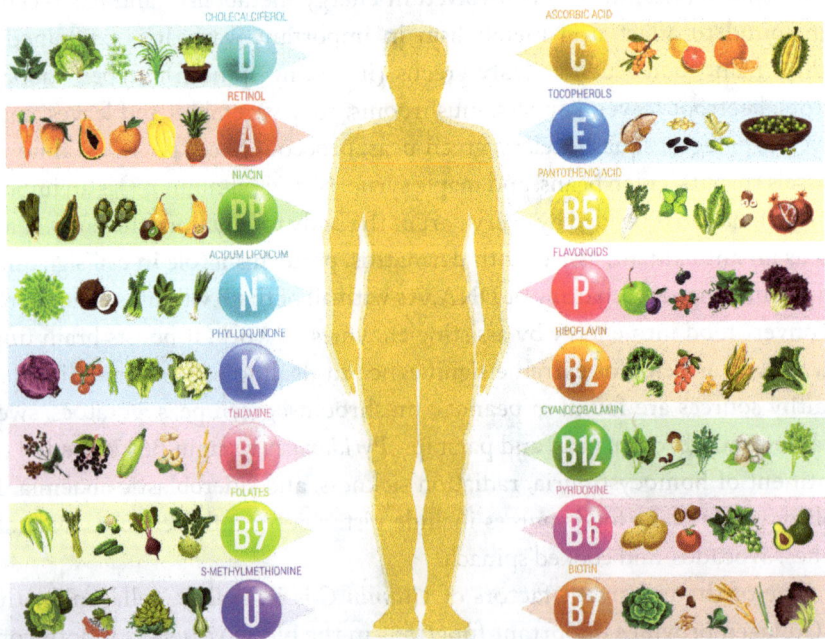

pumpkin seeds, sesame seeds, flaxseeds, almonds, pistachios, hazelnuts, macadamias, pecans, Brazils, walnuts, cashews, pine nuts, and coconut. It is also related to the vitamin B complex and folate.

"For God so loved the world, that He gave His only begotten Son, that whosoever believeth in Him should not perish, but have everlasting life" (John 3:16).

The therapeutic advantages of turmeric and curcumin are almost too numerous to list, as they have been shown to exhibit powerful biological effects including: adaptogenic (uniquely adapts to the needs of the individual), alterative, analgesic, anti-ageing, anti-allergenic, anti-amyloidogenic, anti-angiogenesis, anti-arthritic, anti-asthmatic, anti-atherogenic, antibacterial, antibiotic, anti-carcinogenic, anti-cytotoxic, anti-depressant, antidiabetic, anti-fibrotic, anti-flatulent, anti-fungal, anti-hepatotoxic, anti-infective, anti-inflammatory (painkiller), anti-ischaemic, anti-malarial, antimicrobial, antimutagenic, antioxidant, anti-parasitic, antiphlogistic (prevents or relieves inflammation), anti-psoriasis, anti-rheumatic, antiseptic, antispasmodic, anti-tumour, anti-ulcer, antivenom, antiviral, anxiolytic, apoptotic, astringent, cardioprotective, carminative, cholagogue (promotes the discharge of bile), cytotoxic (to microbes and cancer stem cells), detoxifying, digestive, diuretic, epigenetic, hepatic-protective, immune-protective, immunomodulatory, insect-repellent, metal-chelating, neuroprotective, neurorestorative, remyelinating (proven nerve-regenerative), spasmolytic, stimulant, vermifuge (causes expulsion of worms), and vulnerary (aids in wound healing).

"Oh that men would praise the LORD for His goodness, and for His wonderful works to the children of men!" (Psalm 107:8).

Potent turmeric has been proven effective in treating many ailments afflicting the world today. These include many forms of cancer, multiple sclerosis, diabetes, arthritis, rheumatoid arthritis, leprosy, edema, bronchitis, Crohn's disease, colds, coughs, flu, asthma and respiratory support, tendonitis, ringworm, hepatitis, toothache, gout, conjunctivitis, fibromyalgia, bursitis, anaemia, inflammation, diarrhoea, heartburn, angina, stomach pain and bloating, anthrax, flatulence, immune diseases, jaundice and liver issues, Alzheimer's disease, headache, bronchitis, lung infections, cystic fibrosis, pneumonia, chest congestion, pain, infections, meningitis, anorexia, urinary tract infections, kidney disease and infections, rabies, tetanus, gallstones and gallbladder disorders, osteoarthritis, hemorrhoids, liver disease, ulcerative colitis, acne and skin blemishes, haemorrhage, athletes foot, colic, allergies, bursitis, cardiovascular disease, gonorrhea, neurological and mental issues, epilepsy, bloody urine, burns, endothelial and epithelial dysfunction, candidiasis, sexually transmitted diseases, prostatitis, ringworm, mumps, inflammatory bowel disease, indigestion, parasites, smallpox, chickenpox, eczema, shingles, ulcers, including aphthous (mouth ulcers), malaria, tuberculosis, fibromyalgia, measles and rubella, depression, macular degeneration, cataracts, brain and spinal chord injury, loss of appetite, scarlet fever, nail fungus, water retention, trauma, amenorrhea and other menstrual issues, fevers, sore throat, lower back and abdominal pain, poor circulation, injuries, food and heavy metals poisoning, bruising, snake and leech bites, abscesses, including dental abscesses, eyesight and eye infections, surgery, infected wounds, and soreness inside of the mouth. Turmeric is also myocardial infarction protective, thrombosis suppressing, an electromagnetic radiation protector, a blood thinner, destructive of cancer cell mitochondria, a kidney and liver protective, a wound healer, a beneficial gut bacteria promoter, stroke and aneurysm protective, disruptive of the cancer cell cycle and its signalling pathways, a mosquito repellent, protective against DNA damage, a potent antifungal agent against many types of fungi, helpful for pregnancy, childbirth, and balancing of the female reproductive and lactation system. The voluminous research of the potential of turmeric to prevent and treat multi drug-resistant cancers including metastasis, serious infections, neurological problems, and chronic degenerative conditions as well as hundreds of other diseases, is well known. Turmeric is a super-herb that has a high antioxidant value which boosts the immune system, which is the first line of defence for the body. Turmeric is one of the paramount plants on a list of herbs and spices with the highest antioxidants.

> *"And said, If thou wilt diligently hearken to the voice of the LORD thy God, and wilt do that which is right in His sight, and wilt give ear to His commandments, and keep all His statutes, I will put none of these diseases upon thee, which I have brought upon the Egyptians: for I am the LORD that healeth thee"* (Exodus 15:26).

Natural, healthful foods, herbs, and healing have not simply been forgotten by the modern-day medical system, but vilified as dangerous and intentionally erased, as it requires the belief in the incurability of the body to perpetuate enormous profitability for big pharma. Pharmageddon is the death of natural, healthful healing through drugs, as all drugs either poison an enzyme or block receptor sites on cells—causing a negative reaction in the system. The word medicine originates from the Latin word medico, which means, *cure or heal,* and from the Greek verb μέδομαι (médomai), which means, *think, take care of, execute with great art.* Drugs never cure, but are prescribed to alter symptoms, which are often made worse by their use. The body has amazing self-regenerative capabilities if encouraged by a healthful whole plant-food diet and lifestyle, which, if publicly acknowledged, would cause the entire superstructure of the drug-based paradigm to implode. To become empowered, safe, inexpensive, and very effective natural plants can be utilized, which are much more powerful than unsafe, expensive, and ineffective pernicious chemicals that are the antithesis of good health.

"The wicked shall be turned into hell, and all the nations that forget God" (Psalm 9:17).

Ionizing radiation treatments use high-powered X-rays, which are inherently damaging to the DNA. According to scientific evidence, approximately 78% of cancers are caused by this type of accumulative radiation intervention. Radiotherapy wavelengths actually transform non-cancerous cells into cancer stem cells, which can enrich the production of tumours, as it damages the genes in the cells that control how cells grow and divide. Radiation has been found to induce cancer stem cell-like properties in breast cancer cells—essentially increasing their malignancy and tumorigenicity by thirty-fold. Conventional protocols do not kill cancer stem cells but are promoting agents of post-treatment malignancy. DNA damage is one of the detrimental effects of ionizing radiation as it not only induces cancers but also secondary cancers and a wide range of serious adverse effects such as causing damage to glands, organs, nerves, and the brain. A woman whose breasts have been irradiated is more prone to develop lung cancer, and ironically, its effects may be much worse on the primary cancer that it was supposed to treat. Radiation not only promotes malignancy in cancer cells instead of destroying them, but it also promotes cancer regrowth with an even greater lethality.

"For evildoers shall be cut off: but those that wait upon the LORD, they shall inherit the earth" (Psalm 37:9).

Laboratory tests have revealed that turmeric is antimutagenic, meaning that it has the potential to help prevent new cancers by inhibiting chemotherapy and radiation-induced chromosomal damage caused by these conventional treatments. Lethal chemicals, dangerous surgery, and devastating radiation are not justified as the first standard of care for cancer treatment, and a significant body of evidence implicates these interventions as worsening the prognosis and driving cancer stem cell enrichment in tumours. These very expensive, dangerous drugs and protocols induce extremely damaging consequences within the whole body system, some of which are irreparable. Conversely, curcumin inhibits radiation-induced chromosomal damage. Cost-effective, harmless foods and herbs exercise only health-restoring properties, as God's *farmercy*, which comes from the ground, is a much healthier natural choice between *farmerceuticals* or toxic chemically comprised *harmaceuticals*.

"For thy merchants were the great men of the earth; for by thy sorceries were all nations deceived" (Revelation 18:23).

Radiation exposure from Wi-Fi, cell phones, and smart meters causes leakage to the blood-brain barrier, which is the brain's first line of defence against toxic chemicals and infections. Red blood cells coagulate after only about fifteen minutes of exposure to an engaged mobile phone. This red blood cell formation is known as rouleaux and restricts the oxygen-carrying blood flow to all body tissues. Radiation from cell phones increases the risk of miscarriages by 50%. Even the weakest levels of exposure to wireless radiation results in the greatest effect, causing the blood-brain barrier to leak, which results in degenerated and shrunken neurons. Consuming a teaspoon of bentonite clay every day helps with radiation poisoning.

"It is better to trust in the LORD than to put confidence in man" (Psalm 118:8).

A healthy lifestyle and good health choices should be a decision that is made available to everyone. Those who do not have their patients' well-being as their primary concern, but rather, their own profits and that of the big pharma industry, should not use pressure and despotic tactics to force nefarious, dangerous, and toxic conventional methodologies upon sufferers. There are no big profits to be made in natural plants, which cannot be patented, but there is clearly a monetary inducement to promote their ravaging treatments that often bring pain and death much sooner than if their courses were not followed, as every drug slows or stops a metabolic process. Insidious chemotherapy and radiation (including mammography) are proven carcinogens which destroy the body and spread cancer while creating many other new adverse health issues. Cancer often returns aggressively with a vengeance for an overwhelming number of cancer patients after being informed by their oncologist that their cancer is in remission, when in reality, the cancer that returns is often the same cancer, as cancer stem cells are untouched by their toxic methodologies and once again the cancer proliferates, but with heightened lethal outcomes. Cancer tumour cells grow back more aggressively while the body becomes resistant to chemotherapy, which damages the healthy cells and also causes them to secrete a protein, dubbed WNT16B, that accelerates the growth of cancer tumours. Research has shown that this protein is utilized by cancer cells, which then causes them to grow, invade, and resist subsequent protocols, and also explains why cancer tumours grow more aggressively following chemotherapy poisons, which are very effective at damaging the gastrointestinal and immune systems as well as causing enormous harm to the rest of the body. Thalidomide, a toxic drug that was developed in the 1960s and was often prescribed for morning sickness in pregnant women, is often used today together with chemotherapy and has many toxic side effects. Chemotherapy does not target cancer stem cells but kills far more normal cells than cancer cells whilst toxifying many of the surviving normal cells. Researchers discovered that chemotherapy increases intravasation, which is the entry of cancer cells into the vasculature, thereby increasing the risk of death. It has been well known for many years that these toxic cocktails kill the body by depleting it of nutrition and oxygen, thereby causing it to become severely inflamed and highly acidic. When enough poisons are consumed or injected, the systems of the body fail and death inevitably results. This is iatrogenic death (iatrogenic is Greek for physician-created) and describes death that is caused by the result of a conventional physician's diagnosis, drug reactions, and interventions of conventional methodologies and is the leading cause of death, including cancer and heart disease. When the immune system has been severely compromised by these orthodox destructive protocols, it is very difficult for the body to return to a resemblance of normality, as the body cannot be poisoned into health with drugs, radiation, or chemotherapy, which are themselves cancer-causing, as their own product information, included with these agents, discloses.

Surgery can also severely compromise the immune system while causing metastasis of cancer cells and damage to heart cells. Statistics show that nine out of ten oncologists refuse the same treatments for themselves and their loved ones because they know of the ensuing failure rate and misery. Patients are often bullied into receiving these perditious treatments, whilst also being misinformed that natural methods do not work and are not even an option. When a diagnosis of cancer is given to a patient without their receiving knowledge of effective healthful, natural alternatives, it is well known, and has even been studied, that this devastating news and harbinger of death has such severe effects on them, and they become so highly stressed from this death fright, that they go into a state of shock reaction in a very short space of time from which they succumb to and never recover from, and they die from a cancer that they would not normally die from because their body functions become paralysed.

Chemotherapy is not only known to cause heart failure but exponentially exacerbates pain and suffering. It is so toxic that, when medical staff administer it to patients, they have to protect their skin from exposure, and it is a sad reality that medical staff have often succumbed to being a victim of its horrendous effects after administering these life-threatening substances. Devastating chemotherapy drugs can cost 4,000 times more than their weight in gold. Researchers discovered that many patients undergo physically and emotionally harmful chemotherapy, surgery, and radiation in the last month of their lives. These types of methodologies at the end of their life are not only physically and emotionally harmful to patients, but they are also emotionally harmful to the patients' loved ones. A large study revealed that aggressive and inimical conventional treatments were used on approximately three-quarters of cancer patients in their final month of life when greater endeavours could have been made to enhance their quality of life instead of keeping them on aggressive and dangerously destructive interventions that clearly do not work. And to add insult to injury, patients are charged exorbitant fees as big pharma handsomely rewards doctors and psychiatrists with incentives for pushing their profiteering agenda onto an unsuspecting public. Patients are often compelled into succumbing to these devastating and unnecessary protocols, which make their final months agonizing and miserable with tremendous suffering, while oncologists promote the same one-size-fits-all vicious treatments, which ravage whatever is left of their languishing bodies.

"And GOD saw that the wickedness of man was great in the earth, and that every imagination of the thoughts of his heart was only evil continually" (Genesis 6:5).

Curcumin exhibits a profound level of complexity and targets and kills cancer stem cells by modulating numerous molecular pathways simultaneously. Conversely, the key element of conventional cytotoxic chemotherapy is nitrogen mustard, which is, by design, a lethal poison derived from deadly mustard gas used in chemical warfare. Nitrogen mustard is incapable of such delicate and intelligent behaviour, as it preferentially targets fast-replicating cells by damaging their DNA during the vulnerable mitosis stage of cell division, regardless of whether they are healthy, benign, or cancerous cells. Mitosis is part of the cycle of cell division that is instigated when more cells are needed for the growth and replacement of worn-out cells. For mitosis to occur, firstly the cells must duplicate their DNA before segregating the helix and ultimately dividing its nucleus in two. The purpose of mitosis is to produce two cells that are identical to each other. Unlike the non-selective cytotoxicity of chemotherapy, the selective cytotoxicity of curcumin targets the dangerous cancer stem cells whilst leaving the normal cells unharmed.

"Whoso sheddeth man's blood, by man shall his blood be shed: for in the image of God made He man" (Genesis 9:6).

Cancer stem cells are the most lethal and tumourigenic of all cancer cells and are resistant to chemotherapy and radiation. They may also be provoked towards increased invasiveness through surgical intervention and are widely believed to be responsible for tumour recurrence and the failure of conventional treatments. This can drive a primarily benign tumour into greater invasiveness through increasing the number of intrinsically resilient cancer stem cells while defeating the harmless offspring cells. When the tumour regrows, it often becomes more invasive and conventional treatment-resistant, resulting in rapid demise and death, which is often written off inaccurately or disingenuously as non-treatment

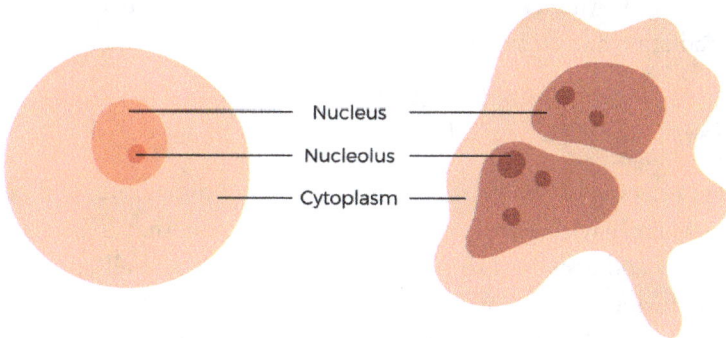

Normal cell	Cancer cell
- Round or elliptic cell shape	- Irregular cell shape and size
- Spheroid shape, single nucleus	- Multiple irregular shape darker nucleus
- Single nucleous	- Multiply nucleous
- Large cytoplasmic volume	- Small cytoplasmic volume
- Controlled grows	- Uncontrolled grows
- Remain in their intended location	- Can spread to different locations (metastasis)

Nucleus
Nucleolus
Cytoplasm

related. Recent research has demonstrated that turmeric is much more effective at eliminating cancer stem cells from the body than dangerous chemotherapy and radiation but without the toxic side effects.[14]

"Fret not thyself because of evildoers, neither be thou envious against the workers of iniquity. For they shall soon be cut down like the grass, and wither as the green herb" (Psalm 37:1, 2).

Whilst the conventional concept of cancer assumes that the majority of the cancer cells within a tumour possess self-renewal capacity to varying degrees, the concept of cancer stem cells as the source of cancer proposes that the initiation, preservation, and perpetuation of a tumour is driven by a minor population of cancer stem cells. It is these stem cells which undergo continuous self-renewal and differentiate to heterogeneous cancer cells, forming new tumours and recapitulating the parental tumours, while the majority of cancer cells lack self-renewal capabilities. Only cancer stem cells are capable of producing all the other cells within a tumour. Specifically, the cancer stem cells are at the pinnacle of a hierarchy of cells within a tumour and are the progenitors of the various offspring cells that comprise it, most of which are intrinsically benign. With conventional treatments, cancer stem cell populations are often overlooked or even enriched as a result. Normal stem cells are essential for health because they are responsible for differentiating into the various types of cells that are required to replace damaged or unhealthy ones. Curcumin provides a compelling alternative to toxic radiation and chemotherapy, as it renders no harm to normal cells.

"That thy way may be known upon earth, thy saving health among all nations" (Psalm 67:2).

Malignant cells import much more curcumin than normal cells, and curcumin alters the micro-environment of the cells in such a way that is adverse to cancer stem cells and beneficial to normal stem cells. Amongst all other nutrients, curcumin, turmeric's primary bioactive compound, indicates the most evidence-based information endorsing its use as a cancer support agent. Curcumin not only directly attacks cancer stem cells, but it can also encourage them to differentiate into non-lethal benign cells. The approximate amount of curcumin contained in one teaspoon of fresh or ground turmeric is 200 milligrams, depending on its origin. For anti-inflammatory effects, 500–1,000 milligrams

---

[14] Kirk Stokel, "Curcumin Starves Cancer Cells to Death," https://1ref.us/1p0 (accessed June 6, 2021).

of curcumin is needed per day for adults. Safe, time-tested, natural substances are superior to dangerous, synthetic ones. It is advantageous to use non-irradiated, 100% certified, organic turmeric on a regular basis, as it is usually expelled from the body soon after ingestion. Curcumin metabolizes quickly in the gut and degrades rapidly in the body as it is not suspended in the blood for very long because the liver quickly breaks it down.

Black pepper is the cultivated, partially-ripened, dried fruit of the flowering vine Piper nigrum. Its impressive array of health benefits include anti-tumour, anti-inflammatory, antioxidant, anti-infective, and immunomodulatory. Piperine (or piperin) is the major active constituent of black pepper and is a white insoluble crystalline alkaloid with the chemical formula of $C_{17}H_{19}NO_3$. Black pepper is advocated together with turmeric because the bioactive, adjuvant piperine contained in black pepper appears to inhibit an enzyme that breaks down curcumin in the body, thereby helping to prevent the liver from prematurely degrading the curcumin so that it remains in the blood for longer. As curcumin is not readily bioavailable, consuming turmeric with a tiny amount of freshly ground black pepper will significantly enhance its bioavailability, and just one-twentieth of a teaspoon of black pepper can significantly boost the bloodstream levels. Much research has shown that with the addition of piperine the amount of curcumin in

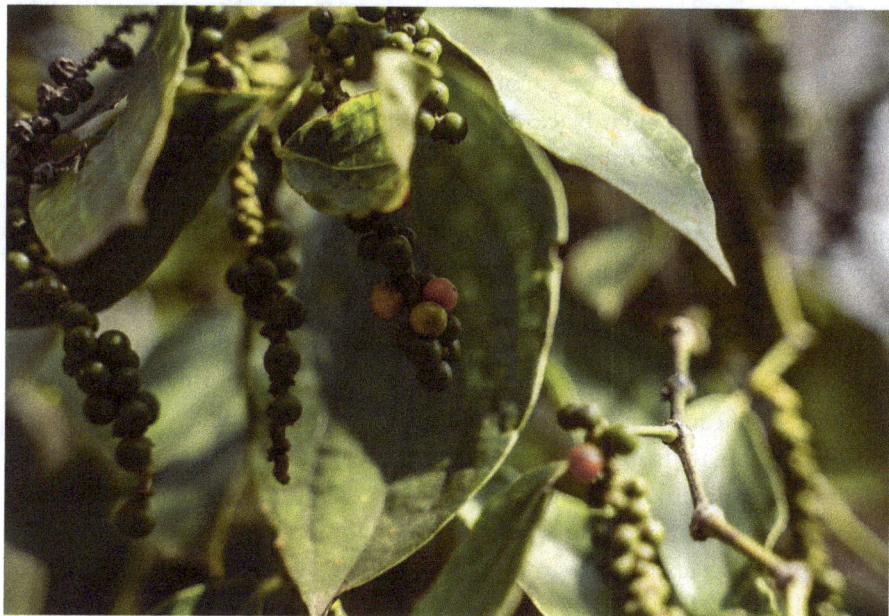

the bloodstream is significantly bioavailably increased by about 2,000%. Piperine not only protects the liver but also enhances the bioavailability of a broad range of nutrients including numerous vitamins, minerals, and amino acids. It accomplishes this by inhibiting specific metabolic enzymes.

Curcumin undergoes glucuronidation when ingested. Glucuronidation is the metabolic process whereby substances are combined with glucuronic acid to form further water-soluble compounds that are more easily excreted by the kidneys or bile. Piperine is a known inhibitor of intestinal and hepatic glucuronidation and is known to exponentially increase the bioavailability of curcumin. Piperine also has a significant effect on hydrochloric acid as it stimulates the stomach to increases its secretion by up to 22%, which helps with better digestion and absorption of nutrients. The whole contents of the stomach are more thoroughly broken down when consumed with black pepper, which traditional medicine has long considered to be an aid to digestion. These broken down components are more easily absorbed when they reach the small intestine and there is less substance for the large intestinal bacteria to consume, thereby producing less bloating, as black pepper is considered to be an effective carminative (discourages flatulence) and can also help to increase beneficial gut bacteria. The most abundant nutrients in black pepper are vitamin K, which is critical for blood clotting, and manganese, which activates enzymes, some of which are necessary for processing vitamins B1 and C. Piperine can also increase the absorption of the vitamin B complex, beta-carotene, selenium, and other nutrients and supplements including a rich amount of glutathione peroxidase and glucose-6-phosphate dehydrogenase. Although black pepper could be a stomach irritant for those with a very sensitive stomach, turmeric has a strong protective effect against foods that are stomach and intestine irritants. Black pepper increases serotonin and dopamine in the brain and also helps to relieve pain, nausea, headaches, poor digestion, seizures, and many other health issues. Research has demonstrated that black pepper inhibits several types of pathogens including E. coli, Staphylococcus, and parasites. Black pepper contains about the same amount of piperine as turmeric contains curcumin. A study found that consuming piperine and curcumin together significantly enhanced neurotransmitter activity and decreased depression effects due to its neurochemical and biochemical activity. Curcumin alone did not have this effect. Upon comparison, curry powders tend to contain very little curcumin compared to whole turmeric powder, which works synergistically with ginger and freshly ground black pepper to provide even more potent antioxidant benefits. It is the piperine in black pepper that gives it its pungent flavour and piperine also has the ability to target cancer stem cells. Piperine has been determined to be one of the significant compounds which attack the cancer stem cells of breast tumours. Black pepper and turmeric together also aid weight loss. Curcumin prevents fat accumulation and assists with fat burning. Piperine has thermogenic properties which increases the metabolism. A study has found evidence that curcumin can change fat cells by inducing the browning of white fat cells, meaning that the cells produce heat and burn it instead of storing fat. Turmeric needs to be consumed with healthy fats to achieve more potency. Heating turmeric also makes it more bioavailable. When consumed with healthy fat, curcumin can be directly absorbed into the bloodstream through the lymphatic system, thereby, in part, bypassing the liver. Although consuming unrefined coconut oil with turmeric will increase its bioavailability, it is even more effective with the addition of black pepper.

> *The whole contents of the stomach are more thoroughly broken down when consumed with black pepper, which traditional medicine has long considered to be an aid to digestion.*

> *"And the LORD shall guide thee continually, and satisfy thy soul in drought, and make fat thy bones: and thou shalt be like a watered garden, and like a spring of water, whose waters fail not" (Isaiah 58:11).*

Free radicals are atoms or groups of atoms that have an unpaired number of electrons (normal atoms are paired) and can be highly reactive with other cellular structures. They can be generated from normal metabolic processes, and once formed these highly reactive radicals can start a chain reaction. The biggest danger occurs from the damage that they can inflict when they react with important cellular components such as DNA or cell membranes. If this reaction occurs, the damaged cells may function poorly, or they may cause diseases such as cancer, or they may die. There are two different types of DNA inside the cells. One is cellular DNA and the other is mitochondrial DNA. Mitochondria create 95% of the body's energy in the form of ATP, and they are also responsible for apoptosis. Some cells can contain around 2,500 mitochondria, which are able to replicate inside each cell, but mitochondrial DNA, which only women bequeath, is much more susceptible to severe oxidative damage than cellular DNA. Maintaining a healthy diet and lifestyle assists mitochondrial function and also helps to prevent premature ageing. All diseases are caused by increased oxidative stress in the body as a result of pro-oxidant toxins, which can be either fat-soluble or water-soluble. This causes electrons to be removed from biomolecules, thereby oxidizing them. Conversely, antioxidants donate electrons to help repair oxidative processes and to prevent free-radical damage as the body has a defence system of antioxidants. Phytochemicals found naturally in foods enable the body to create antioxidants that fight against free radicals. Nrf-2 (nuclear factor-erythroid 2 related factor 2) is a protein messenger within the cells that binds itself to DNA and is a master regulator of the body's activated antioxidant response element gene signalling pathway in the cellular defence against oxidative stress. After a nutrient is broken down and metabolized, it only provides nutrition if it has antioxidant powers. Conversely, when a pro-oxidant reaches the cellular level it has a toxic effect. Curcumin is rich in important disease-fighting antioxidants, which are molecules that can safely interact with free radicals and terminate a chain reaction of damage to vital molecules.

Most fruits are high in antioxidants and are quite acidic (pH 1–5). If something is acidic, it means that it has a greater isolated hydrogen iron concentration and does not have an electron. The following fruits are alkalizing and anti-oxidant: apples, apricots, avocados, bananas, cantaloupe melons, cherries, coconuts, dates, figs, grapes, grapefruits, honeydew melons, lemons, limes, mangos, oranges, papaya, peaches, pears, pineapples, rhubarb, tangerines, and tomatoes.

"Who forgiveth all thine iniquities; who healeth all thy diseases"
(Psalm 103:3).

The pleasurable taste phase of nutrition, or the actual experience of tasting and consuming food, profoundly affects the physiology of digestion and assimilation. The assimilation of nutrients from the process of digestion plays a pivotal role in health and wellbeing. The enjoyment of eating appetizing food prompts the parasympathetic nervous system to trigger a relaxation response. This system also relaxes the muscles in the gastrointestinal tract and increases digestive juices. Because eating delicious food is pleasurable, this satisfaction turns off the drive to eat more than is needed. It also aids in triggering good digestion and can impart a feeling of satisfaction even if less food is eaten. Conversely, consuming unappetizing food can hinder digestion and cause gut issues and fat storage. If the food that is eaten is not pleasurable, the brain relates this experience as hunger and the body will crave for more. Meals should be eaten slowly and chewed thoroughly. If a whole meal is quickly gulped down without adequate chewing, overeating can occur. Eating healthy, delicious foods that are full of nutrients imparts strength to the body. The human ability for sensing natural flavours inhabits more DNA than any other system of the body. For thousands of years, natural flavour compounds have provided humans with crucial information concerning the nutritional composition of foods. Hundreds of years ago, when sailors at sea were plagued with scurvy, they were obsessed with insatiable cravings for fruits

Curcumin is rich in important disease-fighting antioxidants, which are molecules that can safely interact with free radicals and terminate a chain reaction of damage to vital molecules.

and vegetables, which are now well known to cure scurvy because of their abundance of vitamin C. Animals and insects utilize natural flavour chemicals to ascertain the differences between foods and poisons.

"For the body is not one member, but many"
(1 Corinthians 12:14).

Diseases are generally caused by an acidic condition of the body, which is reversible. The parietal cells of the stomach not only produce the intrinsic factor for the assimilation of vitamin B12 but also secrete hydrochloric acid to an approximate range of 1.5–3.5 pH. This highly acidic environment has important functions and is very corrosive outside of the human body. Different organs have slightly different pH requirements. The pH of the small intestine is approximately 8, the pH of saliva should be at least 7 or above, and the pH of healthy urine should be between 6.5 and 7.25. A pH reading of 5.9 is ten times more acidic than 6.9, and at 4.9 it is 100 times more acidic than a pH of 6.9. One of the functions of the kidneys is to eliminate strong acids from the body. If the pH of the urine is in the alkaline range, the body is effectively processing acids and contains enough reserves of alkalizing minerals. Conversely, if the urine pH is in the acid range because the diet and lifestyle are acidic and insufficient water is drunk, the kidneys will suffer from having to process strong acids, which can be seriously corrosive and deplete mineral reserves. Nutrient deficiencies can lead to kidney failure.

Normal blood pH should be within a narrow range of 7.35–7.45 to enable the body's metabolic processes to function efficiently and deliver the correct amount of oxygen to the tissues. Usually the body maintains the blood pH close to 7.40. The kidneys and lungs are the major organs that are involved in regulating the blood pH. Many disease conditions can cause the blood pH to fall outside of these healthy limits. Alkalosis occurs when the blood pH rises above 7.45, indicating a reduction in hydrogen ion concentration. Acidosis occurs when the blood pH falls below 7.35, indicating an increase in hydrogen ion concentration. Both of these conditions trigger alarms and produce actions intended to restore the balance and to return the blood pH to its normal range.

When blood starts to acidify, the body deposits these acidic toxic substances into cells to allow the blood to remain slightly alkaline. These deposits cause the cells to become even more toxic and acidic, resulting in DNA damage, hypoxia (decreased oxygen levels), and the destruction of respiratory enzymes. Acidic environments also encourage pathogens to thrive. Hydrochloric acid plays an essential role in the digestion of proteins by activating digestive enzymes which further aid digestion. It also protects the body by killing any pathogens that may be present. Contrary to popular belief, strong stomach acid is vitally important for good digestive health, and food cannot be digested properly without this unique substance. It is capable of breaking down difficult to digest substances and proteins into a digestible form of amino acids by the activation of the pepsin enzyme. Turmeric inhibits enzymes that negatively impact stomach health. If the production of stomach acid is low, the whole digestive system can malfunction, which can lead to inadequate nutrition and numerous disease processes. To help facilitate more stomach acid, it is very beneficial to drink warm fresh lemon water with ginger and cayenne pepper to taste about half an hour before a meal.

"And Jesus said unto them, I am the bread of life: he that cometh to me shall never hunger; and he that believeth on me shall never thirst" (John 6:35).

Gastric juices include a combination of hydrochloric acid, mucus, pepsinogen, and various enzymes. The inner lining of the stomach is protected from its own acid by a thick mucus layer, which is secreted by the goblet cells. Situated in the stomach lining are the chief cells, which secrete pepsinogen to aid digestion, and this is converted to pepsin in the presence of hydrochloric acid. To protect the cells from the damaging acidity of hydrochloric acid, the parietal cells, which are

Parietal cell

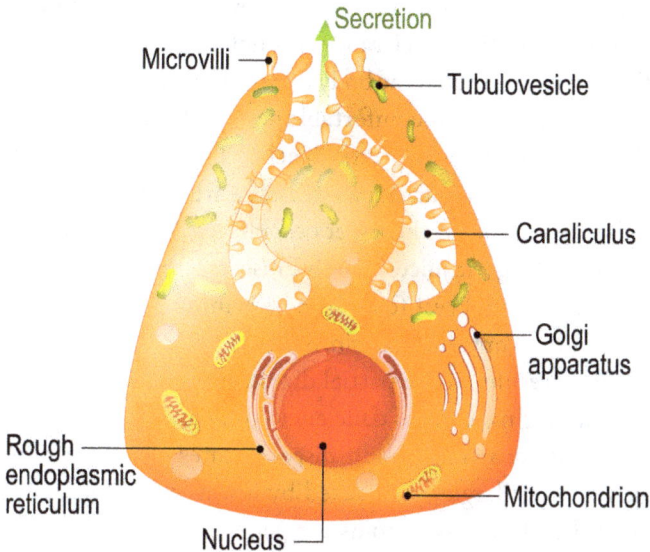

Microvilli — Secretion — Tubulovesicle

Canaliculus

Golgi apparatus

Rough endoplasmic reticulum

Mitochondrion

Nucleus

situated in the gastric pits of the multiple folds of the stomach lining, produce the components of hydrochloric acid separately.

Carbon dioxide from the blood vessels enters the parietal cells and combines with water. Together they produce carbonic acid with the assistance of the catalyst carbonic anhydrase. The carbonic acid divides into two, with one part being hydrogen and the other part being bicarbonate. The hydrogen is pumped into the stomach in exchange for potassium. This pump is called the hydrogen-potassium adenosine triphosphatase (ATPase) pump, with only one ATP molecule working the pump. The bicarbonate returns into the blood vessels. It is another remarkable feat of creation and chemistry that chloride exits the blood vessels and combines with hydrogen molecules in the gastric gland duct to form hydrochloric acid, which is then secreted into the lumen of the stomach for the digestion of food.

"He hath made His wonderful works to be remembered: the LORD is gracious and full of compassion" (Psalm 111:4).

It is a myth that heartburn is caused by too much stomach acid. The stomach has two sphincter valves: the pyloric sphincter, which is situated at the bottom of the stomach and opens only one way, while the lower oesophageal sphincter, which is situated at the top of the stomach, is a two-way valve designed to open both ways and is identified with dopamine receptors. When there is too much pressure in the stomach, but the optimal pH range has not been reached to facilitate the opening of the pyloric sphincter, the body is forced to release the pressure into the oesophagus, which results in uncomfortable heartburn symptoms as the oesophagus is not designed to cope with stomach acids. This pressure may be caused by overeating. It is low stomach acid that causes heartburn symptoms and not an abundance of stomach acid, as the lower oesophageal sphincter does not open to allow the backflow of gastric juices, which cause heartburn symptoms, if there is sufficient stomach acid to digest food. If there is insufficient stomach acid, there is insufficient acidity to optimize pepsin, a digestive enzyme which requires a pH of around 2.0. This results in the partial digestion of food, which leads to many health issues including nutritional deficiencies, diarrhoea, constipation, bloating, flatulence, rheumatoid arthritis, skin diseases, intestinal disorders, and many other diseases. Many allergies are caused by low acid production in the stomach. Those with heartburn symptoms are generally prescribed antacids which contain aluminium. These drugs not only greatly increase the risk of kidney disease and failure but are also alkaline and raise the gastric pH which neutralizes stomach acid, and food cannot digest properly without stomach acid. By eating and drinking wisely, and at the right time of the day, heartburn symptoms can be avoided and food can be properly digested.

"O give thanks unto the LORD, for He is good: for His mercy endureth for ever" (Psalm 107:1).

The stomach should be empty when retiring for the night because this overworked organ also needs to rest, as quality sleep is difficult while the stomach is still working. For proper digestion of food and the assimilation of nutrients, meals should be taken at regular times. If meals are not taken at regular intervals, the stomach does not know when it needs to regulate stomach acid secretion to properly digest and assimilate food. If meals are eaten before or after stomach acids are available in the stomach, the food will not be adequately digested or assimilated and indigestion and nutritional deficiencies may occur. When digestion fails, the rest of the body systems do likewise, but turmeric can contribute to healthy digestion. Meals should be well spaced out during the day without snacking on anything in between and leaving sufficient time for the previous meal to be fully digested. Eating the most substantial meal of the day in the morning will help to facilitate better digestion as the body has more energy at that time of the day. Two meals a day is preferable to three, and if enough of the right nutrients are consumed, meals will be satiating.

By eating and drinking wisely, and at the right time of the day, heartburn symptoms can be avoided and food can be properly digested.

One meal can be a selection of various healthy foods such as fresh fruit, healthy desserts, home-made popcorn, healthy cakes, nuts, and more, while the other can be a vegetable meal. If any amount of food is taken into the stomach while the previous meal is still digesting, the previously undigested meal will be mixed with the latest meal, and the whole amount of food in the stomach can ferment and produce alcohol, which can cause disease. Overeating, even of healthy food, restricts the stomach from digesting properly, because a stomach that is too full does not have adequate room to mechanically churn and needs enough room to do so for proper digestion. Furthermore, if emotional stress occurs, the stomach will not have adequate digestive enzymes to digest the food, which can also interfere with the digestive process. However, if indigestion or any other gastrointestinal upsets do occur, then one heaped tablespoon of activated charcoal in a glass of water will remedy the situation, as it is a valuable quick remedy for any digestive upsets. Vinegar suspends digestion, and because of its destructive effect on ptyalin, an enzyme in saliva that helps with the predigestion of starches, even a small amount diminishes the digestion of starch. Water extinguishes stomach acid 175 times faster than some drugs, which is why it should not be drunk with meals. The stomach is an organ that needs to be greatly respected, as its abuse can result in many negative health outcomes. To abuse the stomach is to abuse health and life.

"A man's belly shall be satisfied with the fruit of his mouth; and with the increase of his lips shall he be filled" (Proverbs 18:20).

The body prefers to retain food in the stomach until it reaches an adequate pH level. Insufficient stomach acid causes food to remain in the stomach for longer without adequately breaking down the nutrients, and ultimately the stomach has to move its contents into the small intestine through the pyloric sphincter valve. Insufficient stomach acid is also a cause of digestive problems in the small intestine as the pH level is not able to be at an optimal range. As a result, the small intestine is unable to break down large undigested food particles which can impact the system in a negative way, especially if the small intestine has a susceptible permeable lining which allows undigested food particles to pass through and enter the bloodstream. This negatively impacts the body, as the immune system recognizes these food particles as foreign bodies and activates a systemic immune response, which causes a considerable amount of inflammation and subsequent malabsorption of minerals and vitamins, and especially the B vitamins, in the first part of the small intestine. This resulting deficiency of B vitamins then causes a vulnerability to elevate homocysteine levels. Elevated homocysteine levels can cause vasospasms (blood vessel spasms similar to muscle cramps). The large intestine may also encounter malabsorbed food particles, leading to a disruption in normal gut flora and causing a variety of health issues, including inflammation and an irritable bowel. Undigested food particles may be seen in the faecal matter if food is not properly digested. Compounds in turmeric aid with the digestive process.

"Who giveth food to all flesh (mankind): for His mercy endureth for ever" (Psalm 136:25).

The Greek physician Hippocrates (460 BC–370 BC) said: "All disease begins in the gut." An unhealthy gut environment produces an unhealthy bodily state, including detrimental effects on the thyroid. The unique action of turmeric assists the entire gastro-intestinal system by increasing beneficial intestinal flora and generating healthy digestion. It prevents the release of histamine in the stomach, thereby quelling a nervous stomach and counteracting food allergies. Turmeric is also useful for weak stomachs, poor digestion, dyspepsia, parasites, abdominal cramps, normalizing the metabolism, assisting with the digestion of protein, the breakdown of fats to increase absorption, and the ability of the stomach to withstand digestive acids. Plants that treat digestion are often the most important of all because good digestion is the basis of mental and physical health. A diet that has few fruits and vegetables reduces the gut microbiome, thereby increasing the likelihood of inflammation. Plant fibre, which is the best prebiotic of all, is a non-digestible carbohydrate and is extremely important for good health. A high-fibre diet can help to lower the risk of premature death from any cause. Plant foods contain both insoluble and soluble fibres in differing amounts and are found in abundance in whole grains, nuts, seeds, beans, legumes, fruits, and vegetables. Insoluble fibre does not absorb water but adds bulk to the waste, which helps food to pass quicker through the stomach and intestines. This fibre is not broken down by the gut or absorbed into the bloodstream and is found in fruits and vegetables, nuts, seeds, and whole grains and specifically in the skins, seeds, and stalks of these foods. Soluble fibre is hydrophilic (attracts water). It is a soft fibre that forms a gel-like substance with the water that it attracts during digestion, which slows down the digestive process. It is found in psyllium husks, whole grains, nuts, seeds, avocados, beans, lentils, fruits, and vegetables. It helps with satiety, regulates blood sugar levels, and boosts the population of the beneficial gut microbiome, which is associated with improved health. Studies have shown that processed foods decimate gut bacteria diversity and worsen health outcomes such as inflammation, repressed mental acuity, allergies, and suppression of the immune system. Other studies have revealed that a whole plant-food diet feeds a positive gut environment, while animal products feed a negative gut environment. When fibre is removed from foods, many of the minerals that alkalinize the body, together with any beneficial fats, are also removed.

Fibre intake has been shown to not only lower inflammation throughout the body, but it also makes a significant difference in the brain. The digested fibre produces short-chain fatty acids together with the by-product butyrate, which preserves brain function by reducing inflammation in the brain's microglia. Microglia account for about 15% of all the cells in the brain. There is approximately 100 times more genetic material in all of the micro-organisms in the gut than there are in the cells of the body, and the

> *"All disease begins in the gut."*

weight of these micro-organisms can be around 1½–2½ kilos (3–5 pounds). This translates into the fact that the microbiome has a larger role to play in the health of the body than inherited genetic material. A newborn baby inherits a transgenerational microbiome, which affects health outcomes. The average body contains hundreds of different strains of yeast and bacteria, and when these bacterium are properly balanced, they can essentially promote efficient digestion and nutrient absorption. Approximately 80% of the immune system is located in the gut and a gut imbalance has been linked to increased risks of cancer, type 2 diabetes, obesity, neurodegenerative disease, liver disease and cardiovascular disease. There are beneficial and harmful bacteria in the gut and the key is achieving a balance, as death begins in the colon. The gut also contains around 100 million neurons and hosts over thirty types of neurotransmitters.

Multiple studies have exhibited that the bacteria in the digestive system not only have a direct impact on weight management but also on the metabolism. Metabolism is not only a term used specifically to refer to the breakdown of food and its subsequent conversion into energy but also the elimination of waste, the transport of substances into cells and all of the chemical reactions that occur in the body. The digestive system is a highly complex and fragile ecosystem that contains over 100 trillion bacteria, which control every facet of the digestive process. Turmeric is one of the best carminatives, which is a substance that helps to decrease flatulence and distention. It is very balanced and does not aggravate if taken in reasonable amounts. As a vulnerary (herbs or natural remedies used to promote wound healing), it also helps to nurture and heal mucous membranes, as it has a strong protective effect against foods and materials that are corrosive to the stomach and intestines.

"Give us day by day our daily bread" (Luke 11:3).

Turmeric exhibits the utmost efficacy in managing a whole host of inflammatory intestinal conditions including Crohn's disease and ulcerative colitis, which are types of inflammatory bowel disease. Being astringent, it can help to seal the digestive tract lining and the bowel, thereby reducing the risk of a leaky gut. It also contains an anti-spasmodic property, which helps to relax the smooth digestive muscles that help to keep digestive spasms at bay. This helps food to pass gently through the bowel and discourages bloating and flatulence. Curcumin facilitates the healing and regeneration of colonic crypts, which are glands that are found on the inside surface of the colon. The average person can retain up to nine kilograms of trapped rotting undigested waste in their digestive system, which makes an enormous negative impact on the health of the entire body. Colonics can be undertaken by those who have not been consuming a healthy diet as trapped undigested waste is the most significant source of poisoning to the body. Waste needs to be expelled from the bowel at least once daily for every meal that has been consumed.

A healthy bowel transit time should be twelve to eighteen hours for a hydrated body. The sewage system of the colon can become a cesspool by abuse and neglect. Most disease-causing toxins enter the body via the intestines. These toxins make their way into the bloodstream, thereby causing toxaemia, which overworks the liver. Following this, every type of tissue is infiltrated with these toxic elements. This alimentary autointoxication poisons every organ of the body including the brain, the nervous system, the lungs, the heart, the digestive organs, and also the blood, thereby causing a myriad of ailments. The colon walls are covered with nerve endings which connect with different areas of the body, and if the contents of the colon are toxic and have poisoned the nerve receptors, then deterioration and pain will occur in seemingly unconnected bodily areas. All of the vital absorption of essential minerals, vitamins, and other nutrients occur during the digestive process in the gut, which is also responsible for fighting infections and diseases. If the gut is burdened with poisonous waste, then its ability to absorb nutrients becomes impeded and nutrient deficiencies and many other negative health issues may result. Even slouching can seriously impede digestion and contribute to constipation. Chewing on gum, which contains questionable substances, also has adverse health effects upon the body as it unnecessarily stimulates the secretion of digestive enzymes, which can also deplete these enzymes. Fibre was created as a medium to lock in oils and other nutrients, and it is by thorough chewing that these nutrients are released. Thorough mastication combined with saliva is the key that opens the door to good digestion, which is so vitally important.

When nutrients are released from the fibre, the fibre is then able to absorb toxins from the system and transport them out of the body. The word *digest* (di-gest) originates from two words—di (for *dis*, which means *apart*) and gest (for *gerō*, which means *to carry*), and means, in this instance, separating the nutrients from the fibre. Fibre causes a slow release of nutrients into the bloodstream, making it easier for the body to utilize and break them down. It also cleans and sweeps out the colon, thereby helping to prevent a vast array of adverse health issues. Juicing fruits and vegetables removes an abundance of nutrients as they are locked in together with the fibre. For optimum nutrition, consuming them whole, as they were created, is much more advantageous for good health. Juicing is not a healthful practice as it can cause the body to crave for the missing nutrients, and drinking too much liquid of any kind can overburden the kidneys. Peristalsis refers to the involuntary, progressive, wave-like constriction and relaxation contractions of the circular and longitudinal muscles that occur from the oesophagus to the intestines, and which facilitates the movement of food through the entire gastro-intestinal tract. If food is not sufficiently chewed this peristalsis movement does not occur properly. Taking sufficient time to chew food thoroughly until it becomes almost liquid also enables each morsel of taste and texture to be thoroughly savoured and thereby exposes a greater surface area of the food to digestive enzymes, which facilitates better nutrient absorption, as poor digestion is worse than poor nutrition.

The digestion of carbohydrates begins in the mouth with ptyalin, which is a form of the enzyme amylase that is present in saliva. Ptyalin catalyses the hydrolysis of starch into sugars. Drinks should also be mixed with saliva before being swallowed. Drinking iced water with meals changes the temperature of the contents of the stomach and causes the body to use more energy to warm it. It also inhibits the production of stomach acid and slows down digestion. Insufficient stomach acid (achlorhydria) causes inadequate digestion and microbial overgrowth. Sufficient stomach acid sterilizes food, is essential for the proper absorption of vitamins and minerals, kills pathogenic organisms such as parasites, bacteria, and yeasts, maintains bacterial balance in the intestines, and activates pepsin and the intrinsic factor for vitamin B12 absorption. It also helps to stimulate the release of digestive enzymes from the pancreas and bile from the liver and gallbladder. To naturally improve stomach acid production and upper digestive function, drinking herbal teas such as fresh root ginger, hops, or dandelion root are effective. Adding fresh lemon juice and cayenne pepper will also be beneficial when drunk about half an hour before meals. However, some herbal teas are not suitable when gastritis and ulcers are present. Duodenal ulcers can result from having a higher pH in the first section of the small intestine. A mass of partially digested food and digestive secretions are formed in the stomach and intestine during digestion. Digestive juices in the stomach are formed by the gastric glands. Food in the small intestine stimulates the pancreas to release fluid containing a high concentration of bicarbonate. This fluid neutralizes the highly acidic gastric juice, which would otherwise damage the membrane lining of the intestine, resulting in a duodenal ulcer.

"Death and life are in the power of the tongue: and they that love it shall eat the fruit thereof" (Proverbs 18:21).

Intestinal health can exert a profound influence on mental health and vice versa as the gastro-intestinal system is also known as the second brain, having a large semi-autonomous nervous system (enteric nervous system), which is the largest outside of the brain. It is in constant communication with the minuscule epithelial cells which perform a remarkable amount of critical functions including communication with macrophages, immune T cells, B cells, trillions of microbes, and also determines multiple attributes of food digestion and vitamin production. The enteric nervous system lies below the epithelial layer of cells. Leaky gut occurs when the intestinal lining barrier becomes damaged and the barrier of epithelial cells that line the gut wall, which normally adhere together with the protein zonulin, becomes separated. Zonulin is the physiological modulator of tight intercellular junctions which are highly regulated by cytokines. Recent research implicates zonulin as a master regulator of intestinal permeability, a condition that is linked to the development of chronic inflammatory disorders. Chronic inflammation is caused by an accumulation of oxidative compounds within the cells and the bloodstream. The amazing intestinal epithelium, which is only one cell thick (unilayered and columnar) despite the need for an impregnable defence, is the only barrier that keeps food particles and micro-organisms in the intestine from entering into the bloodstream, and these epithelial cells exist to protect the bloodstream.

Inflammation loosens the tight junctions that bind the epithelial cells together and allows undigested food particles, yeasts, viruses, and bacteria to pass through gaps in the intestinal membrane and into the bloodstream. Vasodilation, which accompanies inflammation, leads to increased blood flow and additional immune cells can enter the inflamed tissues. However, once the inflammatory pathogen is no longer present, the loose zonulin junctions close up to become tight junctions again.

There is a spectrum of diseased states that have the common effect of breaking down endothelial and epithelial barrier functions. Unrefined coconut oil has been proven to improve these functions as it is anti-inflammatory and inhibits platelet coagulation. Conversely, transfats increase disease-causing inflammation. The epithelium is an avascular tissue, meaning that it has no blood supply as it has no blood vessels to transport blood. The epithelial cells obtain their nourishment through the diffusion of water and nutrients from capillaries, which are found in the nearest underlying connective tissues. Essential functions of the epithelium are selective absorption, protection, selective transcellular transportation, detection of sensation, and secretion. The epithelial cells that form the epithelium not only cover the outside of the body, such as the epidermis (the outermost layer of the skin), but they also provide a coating to all the internal organs of the body, such as the inner surface of the liver, the lungs, the stomach, the large and small intestines, the bladder, the urethra, and other bodily organs. The process that allows particles to pass through the epithelial cells of the intestinal wall, is also the same process that occurs with the endothelial cells of the blood-brain barrier and the blood vessel walls when inflammation is present. Turmeric is anti-inflammatory. A healthy diet and lifestyle with adequate vitamin C, Omega-3, turmeric, and other anti-inflammatories effectively halt these

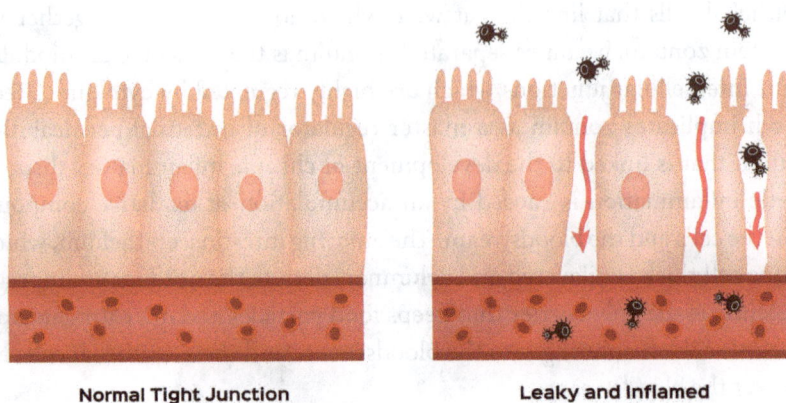

Normal Tight Junction   **Leaky and Inflamed**

inflammatory processes. The inner intestinal lining has one of the fastest growth and replacement of all bodily cells, with the epithelium regenerating about every five days due to the intestinal epithelial stem cells rapidly renewing the intestinal epithelium. This is needed due to its constantly being worn away by the breaking down of food, nutrient absorption, and waste elimination. Therefore a healthy whole plant-food diet can soon facilitate a healing process in this area.

"And Jesus went forth, and saw a great multitude, and was moved with compassion toward them, and He healed their sick"
(Matthew 14:14).

The action of turmeric assists all body systems and immune cells, which, together with the rest of the body, are continually trying to be free of toxins, chemicals and waste products, which mainly circulate in the lymphatic system. If organs are overburdened because they are no longer eliminating toxins as quickly as they are generated, they are then forced to accumulate them elsewhere in the fluid surrounding the cells. Bacteria that decompose undigested food produce substances that are poisonous and putrid, which, when present, force the body to protect itself from these substances. The intestines, being protective of themselves, divert the worst poisons to the lymphatic system in an attempt to neutralize these metabolic waste products and harmful substances. The immune system can become overburdened with trying to deal with these accumulating poisons, which makes it more difficult for them to be removed. If the immune system is incapable of breaking them down, they will be surrounded or absorbed by fat cells, which increases fat growth, or they will be surrounded or absorbed by fluids, which increases fluid retention. The body retains these substances to protect itself, and weight gain begins in the gastro-intestinal tract before spreading to the rest of the body.

"Oh that men would praise the LORD for His goodness,
and for His wonderful works to the children of men!"
(Psalm 107:15).

There are several hormones that control hunger and the main two are leptin and ghrelin. The main role of leptin is to suppress the appetite, whereas ghrelin is the hunger hormone. These two hormones exert a considerable influence on the balance of energy, with leptin being a long-term energy balance regulator and ghrelin being a fast-acting hormone. The word leptin is derived from the Greek word *leptos*, which means thin. It is produced and secreted from fat cells and helps to regulate body weight by suppressing food intake and thereby induces weight loss. It has been established that those who are obese are leptin-resistant. The word ghrelin (also known as lenomorelin) is derived from the words g(rowth) h(ormone) rel(easing) + in, and is a hormone that has numerous functions with levels typically rising before mealtimes when the stomach is empty, and decreasing when the stomach is full. An important function of ghrelin is that it enters and travels through the bloodstream, signalling the hypothalamus of the brain that the body needs food. The hypothalamus governs the appetite and the hormones. Ghrelin is a peptide hormone that is produced and secreted predominantly by the stomach (when empty) with small amounts also being released by the brain, pancreas, and small intestine. It is termed the hunger hormone because its primary function is to stimulate the appetite, and the higher the level of ghrelin, the higher the experienced level of hunger. Conversely, the lower the levels of ghrelin, the less food will be desired, as it plays a key role in regulating caloric intake and body fat levels. It also affects the sleep and wake cycle, carbohydrate metabolism, reward-seeking behaviour, and taste sensation.

"I am that bread of life" (John 6:48).

The amygdala and the hypothalamus are situated near the brainstem, or the lower brain. The amygdala is responsible for regulating emotions and the hypothalamus is responsible for regulating the appetite, sleep, temperature, behaviour, attitude, mood, and many other functions. The functions of the lower brain are often referred to as the lower human nature or the carnal nature. The frontal lobe (which comprises about one-third of the brain) is responsible for the conscience, intellect, and reasoning. If the appetite is the governing factor, the portion of the brain that has more control is the carnal nature. If the appetite is overindulged because the lower brain is allowed to take control and make decisions rather than the frontal lobe, incoming information bypasses the frontal lobe and bad decisions are made based on the carnal nature and therefore the appetite is in control. Tanycytes, which are located in the centre of the region of the brain that controls body weight, respond to the amino acids in foods which utilize the same receptors on the tongue that detect flavour, and when they react with lysine and arginine, which are two of these amino acids, they send satiety signals to the brain. Amino acids in the brain following a meal is of important significance as a sensation of fullness is imparted. Lysine and arginine are particularly prevalent in certain foods, including walnuts, pistachios, almonds, tahini, sesame seeds, dates, figs, apricots, plums, lentils, aubergines, and sweet potatoes.

"They shall not hunger nor thirst; neither shall the heat nor sun smite them: for He that hath mercy on them shall lead them, even by the springs of water shall He guide them" (Isaiah 49:10).

Gluten is a naturally occurring protein that is found in wheat and is often blamed for being the cornerstone of a leaky gut and brain-causing inflammation, as science has discovered that the blood-brain barrier can become just as permeable as the gut lining. When whole grains are introduced into the body, symptoms of gluten sensitivity can arise and cause inflammation, which degrades the body's essential barriers, permitting viruses, yeasts, bacteria, and proteins to penetrate and enter the bloodstream of the brain as well as the gut. There are two types of gluten proteins present in the endosperm of the wheat berry:

> *If the appetite is the governing factor, the portion of the brain that has more control is the carnal nature.*

glutenin and gliadin. During breadmaking, these gluten proteins form the structure of rising bread. Conversely, a gluten-free diet may adversely affect the gut health in those without gluten sensitivity or celiac disease. It may also harm the immune function and the gut flora and cause an overgrowth of harmful bacteria.

Whole organic grains can protect the body against diseases caused by oxidation, which is involved in all major chronic diseases. Grains must be thoroughly cooked as raw grains are unhealthy and their uncooked starch can cause health issues. When refined grains are consumed, the body extracts the missing nutrients from its own deposits to compensate for the missing nutrients in the food, thereby causing nutrient deficiencies in the body. When the gut microbiome becomes disrupted through contact with herbicides, pesticides, chemicals, drugs and unhealthy foods and drinks, the gut flora is altered, which makes it more sensitive to its reactions to gluten. What is often termed as a gluten intolerance, or an allergy to gluten, is often the result of consuming toxic substances that have been sprayed on grain products and legumes. Non-organic grains, legumes, and sugar cane are generally sprayed with glyphosate, polyethoxylated tallow amine (a surfactant which enhances glyphosate's activity), or other herbicides, germicides, and pesticides, which are also used as desiccants and harvest aids. Polyethoxylated tallow amine assists glyphosate to penetrate human skin and is then stored inside the bone marrow and can cause lymphoma. Symptoms of gluten sensitivity are a fairly new phenomenon that did not exist thousands of years ago and which are now prevalent and likely due to the coincidental practice of applying herbicides just prior to harvesting to prevent spoilage and yield loss. Wheat quality deteriorates if it is harvested and stored at a high moisture content, and this influences its pricing and grading factor. Wheat with more than 15% moisture content must be dried before it can be stored, and desiccants are used to lower its moisture content. Toxins on grains can activate strong zonulin inflammatory signalling, leading to increased permeability to macromolecules. It is much safer to consume organic wheat and avoid bread and other wheat products that contain toxic additives.

"But He answered and said, It is written, Man shall not live by bread alone, but by every word that proceedeth out of the mouth of God" (Matthew 4:4).

Toxic glyphosate, an organophosphorus compound used as a weed killer, is used world-wide as a broad-spectrum herbicide and is carcinogenic and genotoxic. Over 80% of GM (genetically modified) crops grown worldwide have been engineered to tolerate the spraying of glyphosate, which was reputed to kill all plant life apart from the crop, but weeds quickly became resistant to glyphosate and farmers are now turning to older and even more potent herbicides. Grains are generally sprayed with more glyphosate than most fruits and vegetables. Glyphosate is a mineral-chelating agent in the body, and a mineral deficient body cannot utilize vitamins. Commensurate to the mercury in vaccines, it also destroys the master anti-oxidant glutathione. Fortunately, consuming high antioxidant foods can raise not only glutathione levels but also another significant antioxidant: superoxide dismutase. Glyphosate is a very selective and powerful antibiotic that kills beneficial but not pathogenic micro-organisms in the soil and intestines. Beneficial gut bacteria boost immunity by assisting in nutrient absorption. They also neutralize toxins and produce fatty acids and vitamins.

It is significant to note that the prefix *anti* means *opposing* or *killing*, and *bios* is the Greek word for *life*. Consequently, the word *antibiotic* literally means *life-destroying*. In 1949, scientists confirmed that turmeric is a natural probiotic. Food manufacturing processing techniques cause gut dysbiosis, which is the disruption of healthy gut flora. Very high levels of herbicide poison residue are permitted in foods, and this is an important factor in the development of multiple chronic diseases. Glyphosate is linked to a serious form of non-alcoholic fatty liver disease. The beneficial human oral microbiome is also subject to this harmful pesticide exposure. Organic food is much healthier to consume than pesticide-sprayed crops, which take up systemic toxins through their roots. These toxins can prevent nutrients in the soil from being absorbed by the plant, providing that the nutrients are in the soil, as some soils are nutrient deficient and need enriching. Plants only contain nutrients if they are in the soil that they are grown in.

> *What is often termed as a gluten intolerance, or an allergy to gluten, is often the result of consuming toxic substances that have been sprayed on grain products and legumes.*

"How oft is the candle of the wicked put out! and how oft cometh their destruction upon them! God distributeth sorrows in His anger" (Job 21:17).

Glycine is an amino acid which the body produces on its own and is also contained in high protein foods such as legumes. Glycine eliminates glyphosate from the body via the urine. If required, glycine powder can be taken in doses of four grams twice a day for a few weeks and then one gram twice a day, which forces the glyphosate out of the system, according to Dr. Dietrich Klinghardt, an expert in metal and environmental toxicity.

"See, I have set before thee this day life and good, and death and evil" (Deuteronomy 30:15).

ANATOMY OF GRAIN

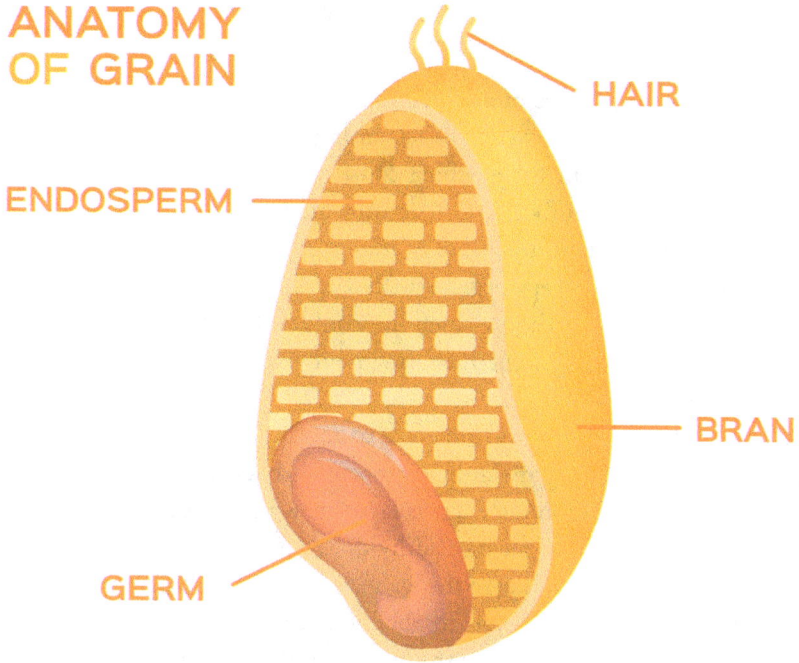

HAIR

ENDOSPERM

BRAN

GERM

Each grain of wheat contains about 83% endosperm (potential white flour), about 2½% wheat germ, about 14½% bran, and approximately one microgram of wheat germ agglutinin, which is a glycoprotein that is classified as a lectin. Lectins were discovered in 1888. The very low levels of naturally occurring toxins in lectins are a defence mechanism which protects raw plants from being eaten by animals and insects, as is shown profusely in nature. Lectins are carbohydrate-binding proteins that are pervasive in many foods and play a protective role against external pathogens such as fungi and other organisms. They are extensively and diversely distributed in nature in plants, animals, crustacea, insects, bacteria, fungi, and viruses. Plant foods such as legumes, fruits, vegetables, kidney beans, black beans, spices, nuts, seeds, and grains can contain relatively high concentrations of a variety of lectins. Animal products such as meat, dairy, and seafood also contain high concentrations of lectins. The current data on the health effects of cooked lectins do not show adverse health effects as they lose their binding activity when they are denatured by heat. The consumption of foods containing wheat germ agglutinin has been shown to significantly reduce the risks of cardiovascular disease, cancers, and type 2 diabetes.

"For the bread of God is He which cometh down from heaven, and giveth life unto the world" (John 6:33).

Turmeric is a good source of vitamin B6, which can be used to lower homocysteine levels and prevent it from becoming too elevated. High homocysteine levels can be a silent killer which causes blood vessel damage. It is also a sulphur-containing amino acid and an intermediate product of an important cellular process called methylation. Methylation is an amazing vital metabolic process that occurs in every organ and cell of the body more than one billion times per second and without which life could not exist. This basic biochemical process occurs when a chemical fragment called a methyl group (an alkyl derived from methane containing one carbon atom bonded to three hydrogen atoms—CH3) passes from one molecule to another. This results in creating significant matter including melatonin, phosphatidylcholine, carnitine, CoQ10, and creatine. Methylation instructs cells to grow into a specific body part, and it is adversely affected by an unhealthy diet, the consequences of which can lead to methyl groups binding to the wrong place and making mistakes because of bad instructions, which leads to abnormal cells becoming a disease. Blood levels of homocysteine tend to be the highest in those who eat largely of animal protein and consume few fruits and green leafy vegetables, which provide the folate (vitamin B9) and other B vitamins that help the body rid itself of excess homocysteine, as a folate deficiency has been linked to elevated homocysteine levels. Beans, legumes, beetroot, oranges, bell peppers, asparagus. papaya, potatoes, green leafy vegetables, cauliflower, parsley, turnips, broccoli, avocados, brewer's yeast, nuts, and seeds are good sources of folate, which is a critical glutamic acid B complex vitamin that has long been recognized as an important nutrient for health. Low folate intake can have devastating adverse effects on health, including blood diseases, birth defects, and cancers. Sufficient amounts of folate also help to support the function of the nervous system and are necessary for the production of red blood cells. Adequate vitamin B12 levels of methylcobalamin are also able to reduce homocysteine levels.

"Now therefore, our God, we thank thee, and praise thy glorious name" (1 Chronicles 29:13).

The word *smallpox* derives its name from the Latin root word for *spotted* (*maculosus*) and refers to the pustular raised spots that occur on the face and body of those that are affected. The first recorded smallpox epidemic occurred during the Egyptian-Hittite War of 1350 BC. The earliest evidence of smallpox was not only found on the faces of mummies from the eighteenth and twentieth Egyptian dynasties, but also on the famous, well-preserved mummy of the fourth pharaoh of the twentieth dynasty of Egypt, Ramses V, who died of smallpox in 1141 BC. Variolations (inoculations) were deliberate contacts of pustular matter from the smallpox virus with uninfected persons. Variolations originated in the magical potions of sorcery with the early Egyptian priest-physicians. Before 200 BC this practice was carried along trade routes to India and much later to China, where the variolation process was developed in the tenth century. Exploration records from the 1500s show that Indians were variolating dried pus from smallpox pustules as a regular practice, which they no doubt obtained from ancient Egypt. In the mid-1500s, Francis Xavier (1506–1552), who co-founded the iniquitous Jesuit order with Ignatius Loyola (1491–1556), spent ten years in India from which, it is claimed, he adopted this practice to silence the opposition of the protestant reformation. He later introduced it to Southern Europe. Lady Mary Wortley Montagu (1689–1762) is credited with introducing variolation to Britain in 1717, as the Jesuits introduced this religious rite from India by using her as a smokescreen. Smallpox is a disease which primarily occurs as a result of progressive gastrointestinal putrefaction. Too much putrid food in the intestinal tract, especially animal products, causes enervation and systemic toxaemia of the body. This causes the body to quickly eliminate the toxic poisons through the skin. The use of drugs both prolongs and worsens the outcome.

There was an old English superstition that said that if one contracts the cowpox then smallpox would not develop. This led to some dangerous and life-threatening experiments. In 1776 Benjamin Jesty used a stocking needle to transfer cowpox lesion pus from the udder of a cow to just below the elbow of his pregnant wife's arm, inserting it under her scratched skin. Understandably, his wife became extremely ill with a high fever and her arm became very inflamed. Fearing for the safety of his wife and unborn child, a doctor was summoned to treat the fever.

Twenty years later, Edward Jenner, who was both a Freemason and a Jesuit, took this idea even further. History books disclose that Edward Jenner (1749–1823) was a con-man who bought a fake medical degree in 1790 from the University of St. Andrew's for the sum of £15. He used his spurious credentials to introduce the first vaccine for smallpox to the world, which was worse than the smallpox itself. This did not work and killed his very own ten-month-old firstborn son when the baby was used as a test subject. The smallpox vaccine often caused much harm and many people succumbed to vaccine-induced deaths.

Through deception and political fabrication, he conducted additional experiments with the commendation of the English government.

Edward Jenner's first experiment with inoculation was on May 14th, 1796, when he tested his hypothesis for smallpox. A young dairymaid named Sarah Nelms had fresh cowpox lesions, and Jenner inoculated eight-year-old James Phipps, the son of his gardener, using pus from the pox of Sarah Nelms. Cowpox is a similar virus to smallpox, which is caused by the variola virus, and exacerbated by poor nutrition, poor lifestyle and poor hygiene habits. Jenner coined the word *vaccine* from the Latin *vacca* for cow, and a whole new very profitable deadly business was born.

When Jenner invented his variolae vaccinae (smallpox of the cow) he sowed the insidious seed that both animals and humans shared the same diseases and therefore must have a common ancestor. This paved the way for injecting animal diseases into humans. Vaccinations are immoral and unethical because vaccines are produced through great suffering of poisoned animals. Charles Darwin (1809–1882) stole his monkeys to men evolution (devilution) fable from the Egyptians, where variolations were practiced. Coincidentally, variolations appeared around the same time as Darwin's *Origin of Species*.

> *When hygiene, sanitation, and nutrition were adopted, the disease rate significantly declined. The anti-vaccine movement, with its alternative solutions, was vindicated.*

In England, victims of variolation were abundant, including the son of King George III, who was lost to this procedure. In 1840, it was condemned as a criminal offence by an act of parliament. Then, in 1853, the UK compulsory vaccination act was imposed, which was inspired by the Epidemiological Society of London. Following this strict enforcement, statistical analysis disclosed a dramatic increase of epidemics. There were three distinct epidemics resulting in nearly 79,000 deaths. Vast numbers of those who were vaccinated contracted the disease long before the unvaccinated were affected. Smallpox has statistically been five times more likely to be fatal in the vaccinated than in the unvaccinated.[15] According to reliable records from nineteenth-century England, epidemics

---

[15] Alfred Russel Wallace, "A Summary of the Proofs That Vaccination Does Not Prevent Small-pox but Really Increases It," https://1ref.us/1p1 (accessed June 6, 2021).

occurred due to populations receiving the compulsory vaccines, and many thousands of people died from vaccinations that would not have died from the resultant illness, from which vaccinations were supposed to protect them. This strict enforcement led to a vaccination rate of 97.5%, which was the highest rate of vaccinations ever achieved in England, and this high rate also coincided with England's worst smallpox epidemic. Smallpox was already declining before the introduction of the vaccine. There were English cities where unvaccinated people did not get smallpox. Conversely, there were places where vaccinated people experienced smallpox epidemics. England launched its Anti-Vaccination League in 1870 and exposed statistical manipulation. For seven years the Royal Commission gathered evidence and repealed England's compulsory vaccination law in 1907. When hygiene, sanitation, and nutrition were adopted, the disease rate significantly declined. The anti-vaccine movement, with its alternative solutions, was vindicated. In 1919, England and Wales had a population of nearly 38 million people and only twenty-eight smallpox fatalities. Conversely, in that same year, the Philippines, a country with a population of ten million, who were all triple vaccinated against smallpox over the previous six years, had nearly 48,000 deaths from smallpox. Improved sanitation, and not vaccines, helped to eradicate this infectious disease. University research shows that the unproven theory behind vaccinations does not pass the test of scrutiny, nor can it compare to the powerful forces of a healthy body, as health cannot arise from poisoning the body. The smallpox vaccine contains the cowpox (vaccinia) virus and not the smallpox virus. Improved sanitation, and not vaccines, helped to eradicate this infectious disease. Doctors have documented many cases of disease and death caused by vaccines. The resulting litany of present-day vaccines are generally regarded as being scientifically tested, even though they are not. Doctors have documented many cases of disease and death caused by vaccines.

Turmeric is a potent anti-viral plant which interferes with the ability of an infected virus to continue infecting and binding to cells, as an infected virus must bind to a cell in order to infect it. A healthy immune system, exercising in quality fresh air, a healthy lifestyle, good quality water, sufficient sleep, a whole plant-food diet and a happy disposition while trusting in God, result in an alkaline bodily environment where infected viruses are unable to replicate because they only attack unhealthy tissue. Exosomes can also be mistaken for viruses. **A virus is not a living organism but is a well organised minuscule bacteriophage** which has a simple composition that is comprised of a core of genetic material of either RNA or DNA. It is surrounded by a protective coat of protein

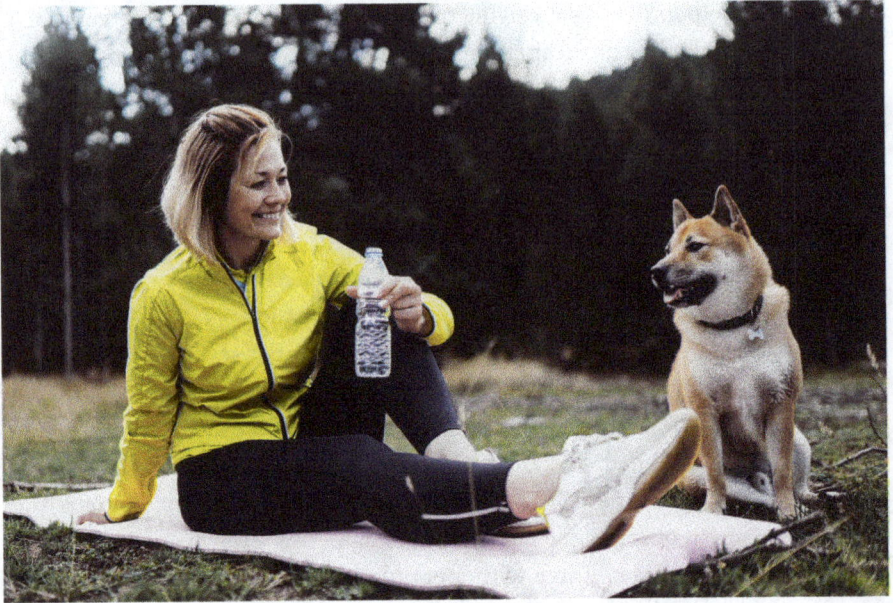

called a capsid. It cannot reproduce by itself and is only able to multiply inside living cells. Viruses are an integral component of every ecosystem. They can infect bacteria but do not necessarily destroy the bacteria. **Up to 45% of the genetic information in the DNA is viral information.** The body contains trillions of viruses and micro-organisms that live in the intestines, mucous membranes and skin. **Many viruses can change in response to alterations in their environment.** The presence of viruses or other organisms in the body does not mean that they will cause illnesses. Viruses are the smallest of all the microbes and generally much smaller than a bacteria, with the vast majority being submicroscopic and usually spanning in size from 5–400 nanometres (one nanometre is one-billionth of a metre). The smallest bacteria are approximately 400 nanometres. When an infectious virus particle, known as a virion, attaches itself to a specific susceptible host cell in which it will reproduce, the virion then infects the host cell by injecting its genetic material into it and implements the apparatus of that cell to generate new viruses. The release of these viruses occurs when the host cell breaks open.

"And that we may be delivered from unreasonable and wicked men: for all men have not faith. But the Lord is faithful, who shall stablish you, and keep you from evil" (2 Thessalonians 3:2, 3).

There are cancer-causing enzymes in vaccines, and vaccine ingredients do not instigate disease prevention but to the contrary, they cause the growth of tumours and other diseases. Today's vaccines are responsible for more deaths than the diseases that they are supposed to create immunity against. Injecting disease-causing agents into healthy bodies does not equate to disease immunity. Conversely, the only guaranteed immunity that is generated is for indemnified vaccine manufacturers against the potential devastation which they generate. There is a seemingly endless list of unethical, needless, and toxic ingredients to be found in vaccines that poison the body. The toxins inside vaccines are exponentially more toxic if the body is mineral and vitamin deficient. Vaccines are grown in questionable proteins and also contain many substances which, when injected directly into the bloodstream, can cause enormous harm to the body. These substances include heavy metals, MSG, live viruses, African green monkey kidney (vero) cells, human baby foreskins, formaldehyde, artificial sweeteners, glutaraldehyde, formalin, acetone, aluminum hydroxide, aluminum phosphate, sheep blood, aluminium salts, ammonium sulfate, bovine calf serum, amorphous aluminum hydroxyphosphate sulfate, alcohol, casein, chicken fibroblasts, D-fructose, genetically modified human DNA, egg proteins, hydrolyzed pig gelatin, guinea pig cell cultures, genetically mutated human blood cells, pig blood, human diploid cell cultures (MRC-5), human diploid cell cultures (WI-38), human serum albumin, rabbit brains, sorbitol, human-diploid fibroblast cell cultures (strain WI-38), horse blood, peanut oil (allergenic), canine kidney cell protein, canine kidney cell DNA, processed bovine gelatine, sodium bicarbonate, cow hearts, squalene, urea, thimerosal, WI-38 human diploid lung fibroblasts, yeast extract, human embryonic lung cell cultures, GM aborted fetus cell tissues, urea, neomycin, glyphosate, and much more. Many have died as a result of vaccinations, including newborns. Heavy metal contaminants have been found in pediatric vaccines and include aluminium, tungsten, iron, copper, nickel, chromium, lead, and stainless steel. When heavy metal contaminants cross the blood-brain barrier, this causes a secretion of inflammatory chemokines and cytokines, which can cause many adverse health issues. A vaccination puncture wound, to which the body needs to instigate an immediate acute inflammatory response to localize and eliminate the injurious agent in its effort to enable the body to heal, reveals why there is no lifetime immunity from vaccinations: it is because the proper immune system cells are not built. Vaccines also contain heavy metal nanoparticles, which not only cause a leaky gut but also cross the blood-brain barrier. These enter the brain as a result of inflammation which weakens this important barrier, thereby allowing foreign particles to pass through, which often results in neurological diseases. These nanoparticles can also travel from mother to fetus and cause miscarriage, malformation, and cancer of the fetus. Nanoparticles can also enter cells and interact with nuclear substances which damage the DNA, especially during cell reproduction. Cells can defend themselves against external attacks and even repair the DNA in some instances. However, if the attackers are nanoparticles, the cells are unable to commit apoptosis.

Researchers have reported that the aluminium and mercury contained in vaccines are highly neurotoxic and have resulted in a prevalence of serious adverse health issues such as autism, Alzheimer's disease, enhanced excitotoxicity of the brain, multiple brain disorders, kidney failure, disruption of energy metabolism, anorexia, immune system issues, respiratory illness, coagulation of proteins, gastrointestinal problems, anxiety disorder, abnormal regulation of gene function, food allergies, neurological damage, interference of gene expression, nervous system illness, obsessive-compulsive disorder, brain dysfunction, damage to cell membranes, and increased brain inflammation. Turmeric supports heavy metal detoxification of the body. This deadly, profitable practice of big pharma continues damaging and claiming many lives today, as not one vaccine has ever been proven to be safe or effective.[16] Fear of disease drives people to vaccinate against rationality and commonsense. Vaccines are now a vehicle for perpetuating diseases that would otherwise have been eradicated. The human race was created with an immune system which is designed to take care of the body if the body is properly taken care of, and turmeric has a profound positive effect on the body. Education before vaccination is a very wise strategy.

"Yea, the light of the wicked shall be put out, and the spark of his fire shall not shine" (Job 18:5).

Autism is known to be caused by vaccines, as evidenced by vaccine injury compensations, and can be reversed. Researchers have discovered that the mercury in vaccines depletes the vital antioxidant glutathione and blocks crucial neurodevelopmental pathways leading to neurodevelopmental disabilities, which have been correlated with much higher rates of autism. The body first metabolizes ethylmercury into methylmercury, which then becomes metabolized into inorganic mercury. Both methylmercury and inorganic mercury are toxic substances which are responsible for causing many serious health conditions and even death. The pathological processes of autism are characterized by mitochondrial

---

[16] See footnote 7.

dysfunction, oxidative stress, brain inflammation, and low antioxidant levels. Following a healthy lifestyle together with a healthy whole plant-food diet makes an enormous difference. Using as many healthy foods as often as possible including berries and especially citrus fruits, cilantro, turmeric, ginger, and sulphur-containing foods such as garlic, onions, and crucifers will be of great benefit. Sulphur-rich vegetables are extremely advantageous as the sulphur activates two crucial detoxifying pathways known as Phase I and Phase II enzymes, that help to flush toxins out of the body. Organic is the most healthful as research has concluded that glyphosate is a major culprit in the development of autism and causes many associated health issues, including a leaky gut. Vitamins A, B, E, folate, and glutathione are also needed by the body to assist with detoxifying. The master antioxidant glutathione is needed by every cell. Sufficient supplementation of vitamins B12, C, and D3 are also needed. A vitamin D deficiency is linked to autism. Omega-3 fatty acids, Himalayan crystal salt, and unrefined coconut oil are also important. The body needs plenty of beneficial gut probiotics (anti-biotics destroy probiotics) which do make a difference.

Autistic children often suffer from gastrointestinal problems with up to 90% having gut issues. Research has shown they have less diversity and reduced amounts of some types of gut bacteria. Research also demonstrates that there is a profound dynamic interaction between the brain, the gut and the immune system. Insufficient stomach acid is often a problem with autism and should be addressed, otherwise nutrient deficiencies can occur. Epsom salts baths also benefit the whole body. The removal of amalgam fillings and root canals will assist with the toxic load of heavy metals and toxins in the system and should be followed by heavy metal detoxification as well as general detoxifying, which can be undertaken with healthy foods and herbs. It will be extremely beneficial if animal products are gradually removed from the diet. It will also be greatly beneficial if refined oils, refined grains, refined salt, refined sugars, artificial sweeteners, MSG, toxic beverages, food additives, GMOs, and other neurotoxins are removed. Chiropractic adjustments may also be necessary.

"The face of the LORD is against them that do evil, to cut off the remembrance of them from the earth" (Psalm 34:16).

The human body is an exceptionally intricate and marvellously designed living structure. The nervous system controls all aspects of the body and is brought forth into existence in the embryo just seven hours after conception. The autonomic nervous system is part of the nervous system. It is a control system for the inside of the body that acts mostly unconsciously and regulates bodily functions such as the heart rate and blood vessels, sweating, digestion, urination, the pupils, respiratory rate, and more and is regulated within the brain by the hypothalamus. The autonomic nervous system has two main divisions: the parasympathetic and the sympathetic. Imbalances in the autonomic nervous system, such as not utilizing the parasympathetic nervous system as much as the sympathetic nervous system, can cause diseases. Human beings are designed to benefit by connecting with nature and having loving relationships with

> *The human body is an exceptionally intricate and marvellously designed living structure.*

others as well as sound nutrition and lifestyle practices. The sympathetic nervous system prepares the body for intense physical activity and is often referred to as the *fight-or-flight* response. It is faster-acting than the parasympathetic system, as it travels along very short, fast neurons. The parasympathetic nervous system is sometimes called the *rest, digest, and repair* system. It conserves energy by slowing the heart rate, increases gland and intestinal activity, and relaxes the sphincter muscles in the gastrointestinal tract. Only one of these two systems is active at any given time. Powerful turmeric helps to protect the nervous system.

"For ye are bought with a price: therefore glorify God in your body, and in your spirit, which are God's" (1 Corinthians 6:20).

Current statistics indicate that 98% of all diseases are controlled by the molecule NF-Kappa B (nuclear factor kappa-light-chain-enhancer of activated B cells), which is a powerful, significant cellular protein that promotes an abnormal inflammatory response in the body. Curcumin deactivates NF-Kappa B, and when it becomes inactive, skin cancer cells stop repairing themselves and die, and basal cell carcinomas literally dry up and fall off. An excess of NF-Kappa B can lead to a wide range of diseases, and studies show that as curcumin subdues NF-Kappa B, it is also capable of preventing a great many diseases that are afflicting the world today, including protection against acute liver damage. Researchers have concluded that, by inhibiting NF-kappa B activation, curcumin thereby inhibits the production of pro-inflammatory cytokines. Studies by cancer researchers have found that there is not a single cancer on which curcumin does not have a positive effect.

"Unto thee, O my strength, will I sing: for God is my defence, and the God of my mercy" (Psalm 59:17).

There are edible plants which can be used both topically and internally and turmeric is one of them. This flexibility gives turmeric an edge for skin cancer treatment. Organic is more healthful than non-organic and many herbs are irradiated, thereby destroying their potency. Curcumin is a safe and effective natural treatment for basal cell carcinoma and for other skin cancers. Curcumin creams are the most effective way to deliver curcumin directly to the skin. A good natural skin-care cream with added curcumin applied directly onto the basal cell carcinoma both in the morning and at night can help to facilitate healing. Curcumin prevents and halts the progression of basal cell carcinoma by turning on apoptosis, which is its intracellular death programme. A multicellular organism has cells which are members of a highly organized community. The amount of these cells is highly regulated and, if they are no longer required, they commit suicide by mobilizing apoptosis. Cancerous cells mobilize apoptosis and self-destruct because their DNA has been damaged.

"Now therefore stand and see this great thing, which the LORD will do before your eyes" (1 Samuel 12:16).

The skin weighs approximately twice as much as the brain and is a porous body covering that functions as a thermostat to help regulate the body temperature through the sweating process. It also has its own microbiome. The body's heat production, or thermoregulation, is a by-product of metabolism for which the hypothalamus is primarily responsible. The breakdown of food molecules causes energy, in the chemical bonds of food, to be released. This powers the body, and 75% of the energy from food is released as heat, which is conserved to maintain an adequate body temperature. If excess heat has been produced, some of it is allowed to radiate from the body through blood that has been directed to blood vessels close to the surface of the skin. For cooling, the hypothalamus can accelerate sweat production, which cools the body through evaporation on the skin's surface. If the body becomes too cold, the skin triggers shivering, and the blood vessels supplying warm blood to the skin become vasoconstricted. This restricts the flow of warm blood to the surface of the skin, which reduces heat loss. Several studies have shown that exposure to excess cold or heat requires a high bodily requirement for antioxidants. Powerful turmeric is very beneficial for the skin. Turmeric contains high amounts of antioxidants and inhibits the proteolytic enzyme elastase by up to 65%. This elastase enzyme reduces the ability of elastin from forming, which is needed for the skin. Connective tissue is comprised of the two proteins, elastin and collagen, which are needed to make the skin supple, firm, and smooth. Vitamin C promotes the formation of collagen. A paste made with turmeric and aloe vera gel is prized for its efficacy in treating many inflammatory skin conditions and blemishes. It can be applied topically to the skin to soothe pain and itching, burns, poison ivy, poison oak, chickenpox, red rashes, blisters, bites, external ulcers, shingles, psoriasis, dry and wet eczema, and scabies. The paste can then be covered with gauze or left open, depending on the location of the issue. Turmeric can also be used externally in poultices for pain. Many skin conditions are often caused by low stomach acid and leaky gut issues. Among these are vitiligo, urticaria (hives), psoriasis, eczema, and acne rosacea (or rosacea). A nutrient deficiency of vitamins A, B, C, EFAs and zinc can also cause skin problems as the skin is the window to the physiology of the body.

"Thou hast clothed me with skin and flesh, and hast fenced me with bones and sinews" (Job 10:11).

Smoking is an insidious weapon of mass destruction. It has been well established that over a quarter of all cancers are entirely caused by smoking tobacco, which is mostly GMO. The radioisotope Polonium-210 pollutant contained in cigarettes, which the industry has been aware of since the 1960s, is not only carcinogenic and a lethal poison but also an extremely addictive, highly radioactive substance. It causes cell damage and profoundly mutates, damages, and destroys the DNA. Tobacco smoke contains thousands of chemicals, with over seventy that are known to be cancer-causing. One of the harshest chemicals in tobacco smoke is nicotine. Other harmful chemicals include carbon monoxide, arsenic, lead, hydrogen cyanide, formaldehyde, polycyclic aromatic hydrocarbons, ammonia, benzene, and nitrosamines. The cigarette filter is a most effective delivery system for the poisons, which go directly to the pleasure centre of the brain and cause a greater addiction than heroin. Recent studies on e-cigarettes have disclosed that these devices can carry about 10 times more cancer risk than smoking cigarettes and have also been found to contain fungi. E-liquid substances deactivate protective lung cells. As with other addictions, high dose vitamin C helps with withdrawal symptoms from the damaging consequences of using these toxic substances.

"But the wicked shall perish, and the enemies of the LORD shall be as the fat of lambs: they shall consume; into smoke shall they consume away" (Psalm 37:20).

Tattooing originates from the ancient magical practices of the occult, as historically it was connected with ancient rites of bloodletting and scarification for the purpose of putting human beings, made in the image of God, in harmony with evil supernatural demonic forces. Society as a whole still views tattoos as a stigma. Tattoos (meaning to puncture the skin) are detrimental to the whole body as they often contain heavy metals such as mercury, lead, chromium, cobalt, iron oxide, nickel, beryllium, titanium, antimony, cadmium, copper, and arsenic. These give tattoos their permanence in the skin. Toxic tattoo ink ingredients induce genotoxicity and cytotoxicity and can accumulate in the lymph nodes, creating a life-long cancer risk. As well as cancer, they have also been linked to birth defects, allergies, and eczema. Other symptoms of tattoo infections include fever, redness and swelling, muscle aches and pains, prolonged or severe pain, diarrhoea, nausea, and vomiting. There is also the possibility of inflammation and infections to open wounds caused by the tattoo needles, which can also cause skin reactions, including scarring. Tattoo ink is mostly industrial grade and can be a major contributor to chronic illness, and a study found that adverse reactions to tattoos are relatively common. Most of those who have them develop an acute reaction to this invasive procedure, with a large percentage of those further developing chronic health issues including constant infections and swelling. The ink can also enter vital organs, with the darker colours causing the most damage. Laser tattoo removal surgery can take quite some time and be very expensive and very painful. Even if tattoos are removed from the skin, the organs can still be damaged as the ink can remain in the organs. According to the American Society of

> *Tattooing originates from the ancient magical practices of the occult, as historically it was connected with ancient rites of bloodletting and scarification for the purpose of putting human beings, made in the image of God, in harmony with evil supernatural demonic forces.*

Dermatological surgery, over 50% of everyone who has a tattoo would like it removed. *So thinking before inking is a very wise strategy!*

"Ye shall not make any cuttings in your flesh for the dead, nor print any marks upon you: I am the LORD" (Leviticus 19:28).

Body piercings also originate from the occult and are not harmless either, as they can cause many detrimental health issues including pain, scarring, disfigurement, fevers, chronic infections, prolonged bleeding, boils, allergies, blood-borne diseases, hepatitis, nerve damage, swellings, abscesses, and more. Statistically, one in four ends badly.

"And they shall be mine, saith the LORD of hosts, in that day when I make up my jewels; and I will spare them, as a man spareth his own son that serveth him" (Malachi 3:17).

Whatever is put onto the skin and nails penetrates to the underlying tissues where it is absorbed into the body. There are many harmful ingredients in everyday products such as nail polish, cosmetics, hair dyes, soaps, shampoos, toothpastes, antiperspirants, lotions, and more. It has been observed that there is a much higher increase in breast cancer, asthma, and severe allergic reactions for those who dye their hair on a regular basis. The majority of commercial nail polish contains harmful chemicals, which can be found in the body just hours after application and cause health issues. Applying artificial acrylic nails can cause exposure to formaldehyde and resins, which have been known to cause cancer. Over time they can result in nail loss due to the destruction of the nail matrix, as whatever is applied to the body will be absorbed into the body.

"There is a way which seemeth right unto a man, but the end thereof are the ways of death" (Proverbs 14:12).

Asbestosis, or mesothelioma (also called pulmonary fibrosis and interstitial pneumonitis), is a lung disease that develops when inhaled asbestos fibres cause scarring to the lungs, triggering inflammation, restriction of breathing, and also interferes with the ability of oxygen to enter the bloodstream. This serious health condition can be significantly ameliorated with turmeric and a healthy lifestyle and diet (organic if possible). Sufficient supplementation is also needed, including vitamins B12, C, D3, E, and Omega-3 fatty acids. Hyperbaric oxygen treatment can also be utilized to support the health of the body.

"Let every thing that hath breath praise the LORD. Praise ye the LORD" (Psalm 150:6).

Hyperbaric oxygen treatment can be beneficial for many different health conditions including cancer, strokes, and injuries. Oxygen is the most essential element that the body utilizes, and when the body is enclosed in a hyperbaric oxygen chamber, the pressure inside the chamber causes the 100% pure oxygen to infuse into bodily fluids at extremely high levels, which then seeps into the cells and saturates them, thereby promoting incredible healing and also increases stem cells. When the body is under this pressure, the blood vessels become a little constricted and start to generate tiny new blood vessels (angiogenesis), which helps the existing ones to heal, repair, and grow with each succeeding treatment, thereby promoting further healing. Angiogenesis is the growth of new blood vessels from existing vasculature (the distribution or arrangement of blood vessels in a body part or organ). All metabolically active tissue is within a few hundred micrometres of capillaries. In all tissues, capillaries are needed for the diffusion exchange of nutrients and metabolites (formed by and in the body) such as amino acids.

"One is so near to another, that no air can come between them" (Job 41:16).

In India and Pakistan, where curry and turmeric are a dietary staple, there is a much lower incidence of cancer than in other countries where turmeric is not regularly consumed. Turmeric fights cancer by neutralizing substances and conditions which can cause cancer. It acts directly to help the cells to retain their integrity if threatened by carcinogens, which are substances showing significant evidence of causing cancer or growth of cancer cells. If a tumour does grow, the curcumins can destroy it.

"Who forgiveth all thine iniquities; who healeth all thy diseases" (Psalm 103:3).

There are over 100 different forms of arthritis and related diseases. Turmeric is such a powerful anti-inflammatory herb that it has been shown to be beneficial in the pain, treatment, and reversal of arthritis (the suffix *itis* means inflammation), rheumatoid arthritis, bursitis, osteoarthritis, psoriatic arthritis, tendonitis, fibromyalgia, gout, and lupus. It is also congruous after surgery, injuries, trauma, and stiffness from both under activity and over-activity. Inflammation can be caused by an acidic condition of the body, which can be changed to a more

173

alkaline state by healthy changes in diet and lifestyle, including the consumption of adequate amounts of important nutrients, and especially sufficient high anti-oxidant Omega-3 and vitamin C, which can help to reverse these painful conditions, including rebuilding cartilage. Turmeric also supports the regeneration of articular cartilage. Chronic inflammation is damaging, but acute inflammation is the body's natural defence against viruses, bacteria, damaged cells, and more, as its purpose is to remove foreign or harmful invaders and heal itself. After surgery, turmeric and vitamin C are helpful for decreasing pain and inflammation and accelerating healing. Turmeric minimizes pain and inflammation related to any kind of exercise or strenuous activity. It also helps with exercise-induced oxidative stress by increasing blood antioxidant capacity. Turmeric de-activates the enzyme that is responsible for pain-generating hormones and has been proven to be three times more effective at alleviating pain than some popular drugs. Perhaps the most important anti-inflammatory mechanism of turmeric centres on its effects on the prostaglandins, which are a group of potent lipids created at sites of tissue damage or infection that are involved in dealing with illness and injury. They control processes such as inflammation, blood flow and the formation of blood clots. Studies indicate that the beneficial properties of turmeric also accelerate the wound healing process. Topical application shows increased cell proliferation at the wound site as well as increased tissue strength.

"And God shall wipe away all tears from their eyes; and there shall be no more death, neither sorrow, nor crying, neither shall there be any more pain: for the former things are passed away"
(Revelation 21:4).

Every organ and tissue is believed to contain a small sub-population of stem cells that have self-renewal capabilities and the ability to generate each mature cell type. From the initial stages of embryonic development and on into adulthood, the pool of stem cells is hierarchically organized according to the cells' differentiation capacities. Hence, one of the most propitious sources of beta cells may be pancreatic stem cells. Pancreatic regeneration has also been induced by other natural substances such as curcumin, which can down-regulate the T cell response that kills pancreatic beta cells. Curcumin also reduces blood glucose, and scientific literature indicates that not only does it possess anti-diabetic effects, but it also mitigates diabetes complications. The anti-diabetic activity of curcumin may be due to its potent ability to suppress oxidative stress as well as inflammation, as these play a significant role in the pathogenesis of diabetes.

Inflammation causes leptin, the master weight control hormone, to be less effective, thereby causing weight gain. Studies show that the amount of adipocytes (fat cells) stays constant in adulthood regardless of the size of an individual, even after substantial weight loss, thereby indicating that the number of adipocytes is laid down during childhood and adolescence. When weight is gained these adipocytes expand, and the fat contained in them leaks into the bloodstream, which can explain the link between diabetes and obesity (diabesity), as the fat is being utilized to protect the body from its own toxins. Scientists have discovered that body fat and not body weight is the key to evaluating obesity. Body mass index is a very poor indicator of health, and body composition is much more accurate. Hundreds of adiposity studies have been linked to many forms of cancer. An increase of just several kilograms in body weight can significantly increase the likelihood of cancers developing, and fat cells can stimulate the processes that regulate cancer cell growth. Brown fat is darker than white fat because it contains a high density of iron-containing mitochondria. These brown fat cells can divert substantial amounts of caloric energy into thermal energy. The primary function of the white fat cells is the storage of energy as adipose tissue for prospective use. Brown and white fat cells are completely different from each other, as they originate from an entirely diverse stem cell lineage. Curcumin is able to induce apoptosis in white fat cells and the browning of white fat cells. It also inhibits adipogenesis (the formation of fat or fatty tissue), thereby demonstrating promising implications for obesity treatment as it may permanently contribute to reducing unhealthy body fat storage.

"The liberal soul shall be made fat: and he that watereth shall be watered also himself" (Proverbs 11:25).

Diabetes is not only a preventable condition but is also reversible. Many studies have found that turmeric has strong anti-diabetic properties as it activates glucose uptake. Chronic inflammation, which can be devoid of symptoms, is similar to having a fire smouldering in the body. Inflammation causes insulin resistance, which is the main cause of type 2 diabetes. Diabetes injures blood vessels and inflammation is also the leading cause of diabetes complications. Type 2 diabetes is the most common form of diabetes in the world. It can be prevented and reversed by a whole plant-food diet together with a healthy lifestyle, including adequate exercise and good hydration levels. In this type of diabetes, the beta cells in the pancreas do produce insulin, but not enough may be produced or the body's cells are insulin resistant, meaning that they are resistant to the actions of insulin. It often occurs in adults who are overweight or obese and is due to an excess of animal fat inside the organs of the body. When animal fats prevent insulin from allowing glucose to enter muscle cells, this is insulin resistance. An acidic pH also causes insulin resistance. Fatty muscles predispose a fatty liver, which in turn leads to a fatty pancreas, and for every pound of fat, there is about a mile of blood vessels. Beta cells are killed by the excess build-up of unhealthy fat in the pancreas, after which insulin production starts to fail, resulting in high blood sugar levels. A whole plant-food diet with its high fibre content, including healthy non-animal fats, has been demonstrated to protect the beta cells of the pancreas, improve insulin sensitivity, and greatly assist in the prevention and reversal of this disease. Refined vegetable oils are detrimental to good health, and soybean oil is not only diabetogenic (causes diabetes) but also obesogenic (causes obesity).

The drug-based pattern of symptom suppression and disease management has fatal failings. A study revealed that oral anti-diabetic drugs and synthetic insulin can worsen the condition and actually increase the risk of death as they are both carcinogenic and cardiotoxic, and most big pharma insulin is mass-produced using GMOs. Big pharma clearly does not abide by the wise words of Hippocrates, "Do no harm." People are routinely informed that they will need to use drugs for the rest of their lives without being given a better option that is effective, natural, and harmless. Many people are realizing that superior natural healing methods, which resolve the root causes of diseases, offer a far superior method of addressing health issues than toxic drugs ever could. There are thousands of studies of many natural substances with therapeutic properties that can alleviate blood sugar disorders and their complications. Turmeric is a powerful plant that is an exceptionally valuable anti-diabetic agent and a therapeutic intervention for type 2 diabetes. It may also reverse pancreatic damage in insulin-dependent type 1 diabetes as the primary cause of this disorder is the deficiency or dysfunction of the beta cells, which are responsible for the production of insulin and which can be repaired together with the immune system. Turmeric, as well as avocados, black cumin, sulphoraphane (from crucifers), chard, vitamin D, and a healthy diet and lifestyle, can also assist in restoring health to a point where insulin replacement is no longer required for those with type 1 diabetes. Recent studies have shown that type 1 diabetes is not only connected to inflammation but also problems with a leaky brain and leaky gut. A leaky gut has fewer proteobacteria, which help to produce vitamin K, and also higher levels of Firmicutes, which is a bacteria group that includes streptococcus and bacilli. A healthy, whole plant-food diet containing adequate nutrients, including minerals and vitamins A, B12, C, D, E, and Omega-3, are vital for antioxidant enzymes, such as superoxide dismutase, catalase and glutathioneperoxidase, to work, and can squelch this inflammation. Cells are protected by a shield that is a rich combination of antioxidant enzymes, minerals, vitamins, and other components that work together.

"And this is the confidence that we have in Him, that, if we ask anything according to His will, He heareth us" (1 John 5:14).

Turmeric is especially recommended for cancers of the female reproductive system, specifically breast and uterine cancer. It also assists in pregnancy and birthing in India and is a mild and supportive uterine stimulant, meaning that there is a possibility of over-stimulation. It is essential to consult a healthcare practitioner before utilizing any herbs during pregnancy. Turmeric taken in the last two weeks of pregnancy helps to expedite an uncomplicated birth, while also increasing the health of the mother and child. It is also a pain reliever and is sometimes used in natural childbirth to decrease pain. It has also been used as an application to the cut umbilical cord after the placenta has been delivered following childbirth.

"For I will pour water upon him that is thirsty, and floods upon the dry ground: I will pour my spirit upon thy seed, and my blessing upon thine offspring" (Isaiah 44:3).

Researchers are examining curcumin as an immune stimulator that can boost different cells of the immune system, such as the B cells, T cells, natural killer cells, macrophages, and neutrophils. It also treats benign tumours and is even effective at low concentrations. A strong immune system is the best defence for defeating illnesses and infections, and curcumin demonstrates immune modulation activity in the immune system cells. Experiments with curcumin have shown that it can prevent tumours from forming as it acts against transcription factors, which are similar to a master switch that regulates all the genes needed for the formation of tumours. When they are turned off, the genes that are involved in the invasion and growth of cancer cells are shut down.

"And Jesus went about all Galilee, teaching in their synagogues, and preaching the gospel of the kingdom, and healing all manner of sickness and all manner of disease among the people" (Matthew 4:23).

Turmeric is one of the most potent weapons that can be used to extirpate different parasites from the body. Parasites are organisms which can live inside the body and cause numerous illnesses by harming the body in many different ways. In some instances, they can become fatal. There are over 100 different parasites that can infect and live inside the body, including bacteria, viruses, and worms. If left untreated, parasites can feed on the body's nutrients and produce toxic waste products, which can lead to the destruction of body tissues. Intestinal parasites thrive in an acidic digestive system and changing their environment from acidic to alkaline naturally kills and eliminates them. Turmeric, garlic, ginger, and lemon are excellent natural remedies which can destroy intestinal worms and limit the inflammation caused by their extensive tissue damage. Turmeric is not only able to be used externally but is also an internal antiseptic which contains antimicrobial properties, which help to kill intestinal worms. It can also help to alleviate abdominal pain, nausea, flatulence, and bloating, which are common symptoms of parasitic invasions. When the body is acidic, the likelihood of an exponential growth of parasites is higher, which decreases nutrients and beneficial intestinal flora. This results in a weakened immune system, which can lead to many diseases.

"Thy dead men shall live, together with my dead body shall they arise. Awake and sing, ye that dwell in dust: for thy dew is as the dew of herbs, and the earth shall cast out the dead"
(Isaiah 26:19).

Malaria is a terrible mosquito-borne infectious disease which kills many and occurs mostly in the tropics. It is transferred through the bite of a mosquito that has been infected with various types of parasitic micro-organisms. Turmeric destroys the parasites that cause malaria, and also fatal cerebral malaria. It has proven parasiticidal activity against many tropical parasites, with one of them being the most fatal malaria-causing Plasmodium falciparum species, which causes about 90% of deaths. Once infected, these parasites migrate to the liver where they reproduce. The immune and circulatory systems also become affected, with the symptoms starting to manifest about ten to fifteen days after the initial bite, as the parasites infect and multiply inside the red blood cells, which they then kill. Symptoms include fever, weakness, convulsions, headaches, vomiting, jaundice, and fatigue, with the most severe infection emanating from Plasmodium falciparum. In 25–40% of these incidences, the infection results in respiratory distress, shock, low blood sugar, spontaneous bleeding, encephalopathy, and even death. Turmeric causes cellular toxicity to parasites and produces molecules known as reactive oxygen species, which destroy the parasites and not the host. Turmeric also works on infected animals. The powerful anti-parasitic compounds in turmeric are geraniol, which blocks the development of Plasmodium falciparum parasites; quercetin, which likewise prevents Plasmodium falciparum parasites from developing; the terpene farnesol, which also arrests parasite development; and limonene, which repels mosquitoes. Garlic, ginger, lemon juice (which destroys malaria microbes), crucifers, berries, beetroot, and peppers are also anti-parasitic. Activated charcoal significantly assists in detoxification as it prevents the poisonous activity of many harmful micro-organisms by adsorbing the toxins and enzymes that they generate. Dried leaves from the Artemisia annua plant (also called sweet wormwood and sweet annie) have proven to be 100% effective at treating malaria and have been used by the Chinese for thousands of years. It is also called Qing Hao by the Chinese. Vitamin A and high dose vitamin C, including IV, are also protective. For the best results, turmeric should be taken with freshly ground black pepper.

"And when Jesus was come into Peter's house, He saw his wife's mother laid, and sick of a fever. And He touched her hand, and the fever left her: and she arose, and ministered unto them" (Matthew. 8:14, 15).

Tapeworms are flat, ribbon-shaped parasites that cannot live freely on their own and survive only in the gut of animals and humans. The tapeworm parasite literally feeds off of its host. The consumption of animal products can cause tapeworm infections, especially raw or undercooked meat or fish. An infection of these parasites can also be caused by contact with faeces or contaminated water. Depending on the species, these tapeworms can vary greatly in length. Echinococcus multilocularis is less than one centimetre long, whereas an adult Taenia saginata can be up to ten metres long. These are the longest parasites in the world and can live in their host for decades, typically unnoticed. Tapeworms have a crown of tiny hooks on the top of their head, which they use to attach themselves to the inside of the body of their host where they are able to assimilate nutrients by absorbing them through their skin.

"Thou shalt also be a crown of glory in the hand of the LORD, and a royal diadem in the hand of thy God" (Isaiah 62:3).

179

Hookworms can infect humans in countries with a warm humid climate and poor sanitation. Hookworm larvae are found in soil that has been contaminated with human faeces. Walking barefoot in contaminated soil can cause hookworms to penetrate into the skin, which can result in an itchy rash where the larvae have penetrated. This can then cause symptoms of fever, coughing, insatiable exhaustion, loss of appetite, abdominal pain, and diarrhoea. They bite into the intestinal wall and ravenously suck blood, and this blood loss can cause malnutrition, weight loss, anaemia (iron is critical for brain function), and fatigue for an unsuspecting host. They can lay about 30,000 eggs a day, and each worm usually lives from one to five years. Many hundreds of millions of people globally are infected by this parasite.

"In whom we have redemption through His blood, the forgiveness of sins, according to the riches of His grace" (Ephesians 1:7).

Roundworms are the largest and one of the most common parasitic worms that infect humans. Giant roundworms can grow to around half a metre long and 6 millimetres in diameter. They are capable of laying 200,000 eggs a day. Over a quarter of the world's population is infected with this parasite, which annually causes an estimated 20,000 deaths. Infection typically occurs from poor hygiene habits, and once inside the body they are difficult to remove because of their protective coating. Signs and symptoms of these infections include nausea, abdominal pain, diarrhoea, fatigue, and weight loss. Due to their size, they can chew through bodily tissues, completely block vital organs, including the intestines, and can be fatal. A loss of nutrients from the host leads to malnutrition and deficiencies, and their infestation causes many inflammatory and serious health conditions such as pancreatic infections, gallbladder and intestinal inflammation, kidney disease, appendicitis, peritonitis, cardiomyopathy, encephalopathy, and even blindness.

"And though after my skin worms destroy this body, yet in my flesh shall I see God" (Job 19:26).

The human brain is a fascinatingly complex organ. It weighs an average of nearly three pounds in an adult male and nearly 2.7 pounds in an adult female and should be approximately 80% water. It begins to function about ninety days after conception and is capable of rejuvenating and regenerating itself throughout life. It has a lymphatic system and also contains a highly specific semi-permeable

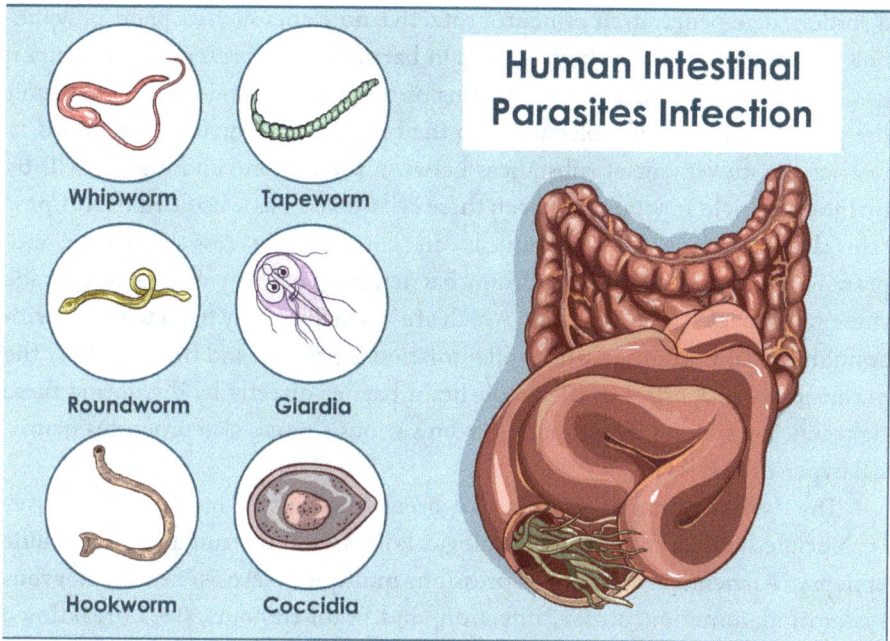

Human Intestinal Parasites Infection

Whipworm

Tapeworm

Roundworm

Giardia

Hookworm

Coccidia

blood-brain barrier. The blood-brain barrier was discovered in the late nineteenth century by a German physician named Paul Ehrlich. This dynamic and unique complex barrier separates the blood vessels of the brain from the central nervous system. The major functions of this highly specialized structural, transport, and biochemical barrier include the transport of nutrients and the protection of the brain from toxic substances. The blood-brain barrier is comprised of specialized brain microvascular endothelial cells that assist with regulating the passage of blood-borne molecules in and out of the brain. It is a diffusion barrier that impedes the influx of many substances from the blood to the brain, and its selective permeability effectively prevents the entry of most micro-organisms and molecules and protects the brain from infections. This barrier preserves ionic stability within the brain micro-environment, plays a pivotal role in brain health and is often compromised in disease. The selective delivery of small molecules such as amino acids, sugars, vitamins, and trace elements are transported across the blood-brain barrier with carrier-mediated transport. Whereas, large biomolecules such as lipoproteins, protein, and peptide hormones are transported across the blood-brain barrier by receptor-mediated transport. Dysfunctions in the transport of nutrients at this crucial barrier causes neurological diseases and disorders. The penetration of neuroprotective nutrients such as plant polyphenols and alkaloids across the blood-brain barrier have a protective effect upon it. Complex intercellular tight junctions of these special endothelial cells limit the passive diffusion of molecules into the brain, as the barrier's function is to restrict the movement of substances between the cerebral endothelial cells by maintaining tight junctions between these cells. It also has specific transport proteins that determine which substances can transcellularly cross this barrier, and, prior to passage across this important barrier, enzymes may change or degrade these substances. These junctions, which are normally firmly fixed together with zonulin, are compromised when inflammation is present, and this can affect the permeability properties of the blood-brain barrier directly by disrupting these tight junctions. Brain inflammation from various sources also promotes neuronal hyper-excitability.

The dysfunctional disruption and breakdown of the blood-brain barrier is associated with a variety of neurological diseases and trauma. These include epilepsy, Alzheimer's disease, depression, multiple sclerosis, central nervous system inflammation, stroke, infection, and brain tumours. This breakdown of the blood-brain barrier permits blood-to-brain extravasation of molecules that would normally be excluded. Extravasation is a process whereby cells and molecules are able to squeeze between loosened gaps in a cell wall barrier. According to a study, traumatic brain injury can also damage the gut, which is likely to cause even more brain damage.[17] Strokes are conditions that occur when blood vessels, which provide blood to the brain, are blocked by blood clots or when a blood vessel bursts in the brain. These are hemorrhagic and ischaemic strokes. Hemorrhagic stroke occurs when a weakened blood vessel ruptures, such as an aneurysm or an arteriovenous malformation. Ischaemic strokes are much more common and occur as a result of an obstruction, such as a blood clot that forms within a blood vessel supplying blood to the brain. The blood-brain barrier is an extremely specialized structure of the fully differentiated neurovascular system, and is present in all brain regions, except in those regulating the autonomic nervous system and the endocrine glands. It also forms a route of communication between the circulating blood and the underlying brain tissues.

Intriguingly, the blood-brain barrier has its own system for waste elimination and is called the glymphatic system. The glymphatic system is a macroscopic

[17] "A Review of Traumatic Brain Injury and the Gut Microbiome," June 2018, Vol. 8:6, p. 113, https://1ref.us/1p2 (accessed June 6, 2021).

waste clearance system which promotes efficient elimination from the central nervous system. It can also function to help distribute other compounds including lipids, glucose, and amino acids. The glymphatic system enters the brain by piggy-backing blood vessels in the brain and functions mainly during sleep but mostly disengages during wakefulness. It pumps cerebral spinal fluid through the tissues of the brain and flushes the brain's waste back into the circulatory system for elimination by the liver. Endothelial cells remodel and extend the network of blood vessels, which repair and cause tissue growth, and have an amazing capacity to adjust their arrangement and amount to suit adjacent requirements. They also create an adaptable life-support system and extend, by cell migration, into almost every area of the body. Nitric oxide is manufactured in the endothelium, which is the inner lining of the blood vessels. The endothelium is the most important organ in the entire cardiovascular system and converts the amino acid L-arginine into nitric oxide, which is critical for well-being. It is a multi-functional organ, which is involved in immunological, metabolic, and cardiovascular processes. Endothelial cells line all the blood vessels of the body from the large coronary arteries of the heart to the tiny capillaries that transfer oxygen and nutrients from the bloodstream to the tissues, which all depend on a blood supply. The endothelium also lies attached to the interior of the heart chambers. There are approximately six trillion endothelial cells in the body, which line about 60,000 miles of blood vessels in a single layer. Curcumin increases nitric oxide bioavailability, which enables the endothelium to fully dilate. Nitric oxide produces more oxygen to the muscles and thereby provides more energy. Consuming animal products and processed foods kill endothelial cells, but a whole plant-food diet reverses this process.

"Every word of God is pure: He is a shield unto them that put their trust in Him" (Proverbs 30:5).

Wherever there is blood vessel inflammation, damaged tissue cells release inflammatory chemical signals that activate the endothelial cells of nearby capillaries. Within the capillaries, these activated endothelial cells display selectin (cell surface lectin) adhesion molecules, which attract and slow down moving neutrophils (a type of white blood cells), causing them to roll along the endothelium. These neutrophils encounter chemicals that activate integrins, which are adhesion receptors on their surfaces that tightly attach to adhesion receptor molecules on the endothelial cells. This causes the neutrophils to stick to the endothelial cells and stop rolling. The inflammatory mediators released by the injured tissue changes the environment. Mast cells release histamine, which causes vasodilation and loosens the tight zonulin junctions between the endothelial cells, thereby allowing fluid and leucocytes (white blood cells) to leave the capillaries and enter the infected tissues. During the process of extravasation, the neutrophils change shape dramatically, enabling them to squeeze between the loosened endothelial cell wall into the interstitial tissue fluid. Neutrophils and other types of phagocytes, such as macrophages, are attracted to substances at the injured site that have been released by bacteria and products of tissue breakdown, and which attack, ingest, and destroy invading bacteria at the site of inflammation. The primary antioxidant vitamin C fights inflammation, as does turmeric, and promotes the formation of epithelial and endothelial barriers with tight junctions throughout the body. An abundance of other antioxidant vitamins A, E, and healthy Omega-3 fatty acids, which can be found in hemp seeds, chia seeds, nuts, and flax seeds and other natural sources can also be both protective from inflammation and can therapeutically lower inflammation when taken on a regular basis. Both Omega-3 and Omega-6 have anti-inflammatory properties but can become pro-inflammatory if they are consumed in the incorrect ratio, as generally more Omega-3 are required.

"And it shall be said in that day, Lo, this is our God; we have waited for Him, and He will save us: this is the LORD; we have waited for Him, we will be glad and rejoice in His salvation"
(Isaiah 25:9).

Endothelial dysfunction, which is caused by the natural healing process of inflammation, is considered to be a principal cause of scar tissue development, but turmeric can help to ameliorate this issue and can thereby prevent, reduce, or reverse endothelial dysfunction, thus reducing mortality and morbidity associated with cardiovascular disease and other diseased states. Turmeric dilates the arteries, thereby inducing the ability of the endothelium to fully dilate. The vascular endothelium also releases anti-atherosclerotic molecules, including nitric oxide. To ameliorate the underlying cause of cardiovascular disease, antioxidants such as vitamin C and nitric oxide bioavailability can protect against endothelial dysfunction. Many heart diseases are associated with fibrosis, and cardiac fibrosis is the scarring of the cardiac tissue which leads to the thickening of this tissue. This thickening of cardiac tissue leads to a reduction of the heart chambers, which can cause arrhythmia. A study has shown that curcumin exerts anti-fibrotic action in cardiac fibrosis and also attenuates the occurrence of cardiac fibrosis as a result of continuous stress on blood vessel walls.

"The LORD is my strength and my shield; my heart trusted in Him, and I am helped: therefore my heart greatly rejoiceth; and with my song will I praise Him" (Psalm 28:7).

Heart disease is a general term for conditions which indirectly or directly affect the heart or blood vessels and is one of the leading causes of death globally. The heart is a unique organ and is in constant communication with the brain. The heart's magnetic energy is 5,000 times more powerful than the brain. A heart attack, or myocardial infarction, occurs when a blood clot blocks the blood flow to the heart. Turmeric supports the heart in many ways. A study found that its administration reduced the frequency of a heart attack after a coronary artery bypass as myocardial infarction associated with coronary artery bypass grafting has a poor outcome. Turmeric also helps with cardiac repair and function after a heart attack as it facilitates and regulates the repair of heart muscle cells, even after surgery. Research shows that turmeric's benefits decrease pro-inflammatory cytokines during cardiopulmonary bypass surgery and also decreases the occurrence of cardiac cell death. Arrhythmia is an abnormal electrical condition of the heart rhythm, which is often caused by a lack of nutrients. A recent study concluded that painkillers are linked to an increased risk of atrial fibrillation.[18] Turmeric's anti-inflammatory action can benefit and also help to prevent arrhythmia.[19] Arrhythmia can also be caused by an infection, such as a UTI. In 1937 it was discovered that low magnesium levels, and not the consumption of too much saturated fat, was the leading cause of many aspects of heart disease. Turmeric acts on various enzymes and angiotensin receptors, which regulate cardiovascular functions. Hundreds of studies have shown that turmeric protects the heart and blood vessels as it combats various metabolic conditions that could serve as risk factors for the development of heart diseases. Risk factors leading to heart disease involve a lack of exercise, an unhealthy diet with insufficient antioxidants, obesity, the use of alcohol, tobacco, and stress-related factors. The toxic effects of deadly chemotherapy drugs weaken heart function. Conversely, turmeric is cardioprotective as it

---

[18] "Non-steroidal anti-inflammatory drug use and risk of atrial fibrillation or flutter," *BMJ*, July 4, 2011, https://1ref.us/1p3 (accessed June 6, 2021).

[19] "The effects of curcumin on the prevention of atrial and ventricular arrhythmias and heart failure in patients with unstable angina," *AJP*, 2019, Vol. 9:1, https://1ref.us/1p4 (accessed June 6, 2021).

protects the heart from heart attacks, clot formation and drug-induced toxicity. It also promotes the normalizing of pulse pressure and expedites the healing of damage caused by diabetes and smoking.

"Be of good courage, and He shall strengthen your heart, all ye that hope in the LORD" (Psalm 31:24).

Depression can be a life-changing issue from which a great many diseases emanate. The biggest cause of depression and anxiety is a traumatic life event. Usually, depression is caused by emotional suppression and the limbic system is the emotional centre. The frontal lobe is responsible for the conscience, the judgment, the intellect, the will, and reasoning. If life is navigated by the limbic system and is not filtered through the frontal lobe this means that emotions are in place and not the reasoning powers. The frontal lobe begins to shut down if a hopeless situation is perceived because depression results when suppression of feelings occur as the frontal lobe has been compromised. Poor nutrition is also a cause of depression and inflammation and the primary cause of chronic illnesses. Anti-inflammatory turmeric has been shown to be effective as a natural treatment for depression and can halt this disorder more effectively than toxic dangerous antidepressant drugs without the negative and harmful side effects. Turmeric is extremely beneficial when used therapeutically for this health issue, whilst also boosting the neurotransmitters dopamine and serotonin. Serotonin is a feel-good hormone that is produced by the gut. However, serotonin levels that are too high have been linked to a range of health issues, including autism and schizophrenia. It has been discovered that components of the immune system, which mediate inflammation, may be intimately involved in depression. Inflammation is usually understood to be the primary response of the body to physical injury or infection. There is now substantial evidence that psychological stress can also trigger significant increases in the inflammatory response, which can then elicit profound changes in behaviour and initiate depressive symptoms. Long-term sleep deprivation can lead to a neurotoxin buildup in the brain, which not only impairs memory but prolongs

> *Heart disease is a general term for conditions which indirectly or directly affect the heart or blood vessels and is one of the leading causes of death globally.*

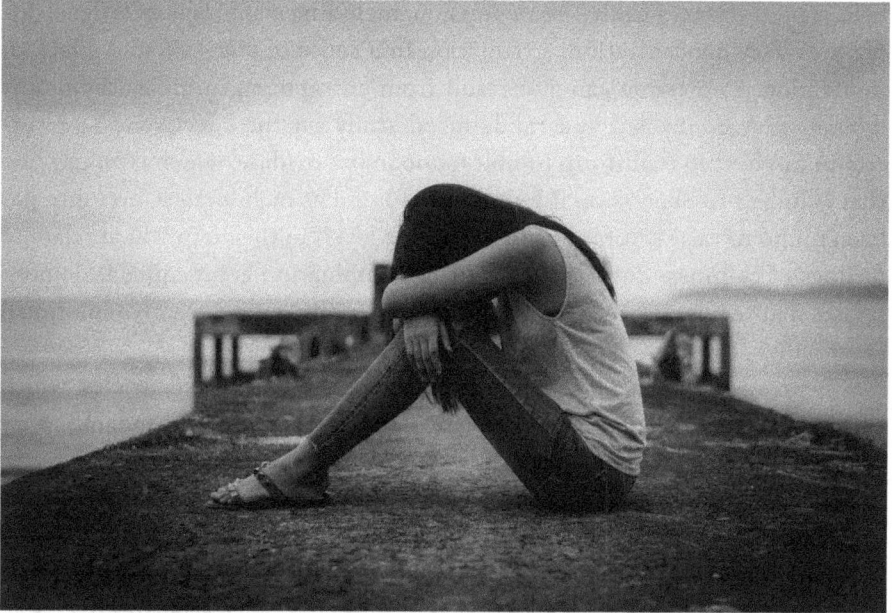

insomnia. Those whose body clocks are thrown off by night light exposure and whose melatonin levels are suppressed are more prone to depression, which can also be a precursor to Alzheimer's disease and cancer. Probiotics destroy toxic chemicals in the gut, and a study showed evidence that probiotics, particularly Bifidobacterium longum, Lactobacillus helveticus, and other Lactobacilli strains, significantly reduce negative thoughts that are associated with anxiety, depression, and stress, and stress causes a loss of these beneficial bacteria, according to an enormous number of studies. A study revealed that consuming 500 milligrams of standardized, bioavailable curcumin twice daily showed tangible brain benefits and was also effective against major depressive disorders. In addition to being fat-soluble, curcumin is also resistant to water solubility, which is why absorption is enhanced by ingesting it with healthy fats, such as unrefined coconut oil, avocados, nuts, and olives.

A healthy lifestyle, together with a whole plant-food diet, including foods high in polyphenols, will also improve brain function. According to a study, polyphenols that are prevalent in plant foods are effective at improving psychiatric disorders, the mood, cognitive functioning, and the synaptic plasticity of the brain, in addition to reducing oxidative stress. There can be many reasons for depression, and a new study demonstrates that inflammation can induce behavioural changes similar to depression, including symptoms of fatigue, difficulties with concentration, a reduction in a sense of pleasure, and a lack of motivation. Depression can also result from entrapment in unhealthy family dynamics. A controlled and randomized study on the effectiveness of curcumin discovered that it can inhibit monoamine oxidase, which is an enzyme that is linked to depression if found in the brain at high levels. Curcumin has been found to raise serotonin and dopamine levels in the brain which relate to feelings of calmness and well-being. This combination is potent as it demonstrates that regular use of curcumin can significantly reduce negative emotional symptoms.

Depression can also be the result of different nutrient deficiencies, which can include the essential, highly effective antioxidant and anti-inflammatory Omega-3 fatty acids. Foods high in Omega-3 fatty acids, including flax seeds, hemp seeds, and chia seeds, can be easily incorporated into the diet and are quite effective against this disorder. The Omega-3 fatty acids DHA and EPA can perform as anti-depressants and are essential polyunsaturated fatty acids that work together synergistically. EPA assists, from a physiological perspective, as an anti-inflammatory agent. DHA assists in normal growth and development and helps with the cell membrane structure. Minerals (especially iron for energy) and vitamins, including all of the B-vitamins, adequate essential vitamin C taken frequently, vitamin D3, and folate are also important for this condition. A vitamin D deficiency is linked to depression and schizophrenia. Low levels of the amino acid tryptophan can also often lead to depression, as can low blood sugar levels. Tryptophan is an important component of a healthy diet and ensures that balanced levels of the essential serotonin neurotransmitter are present. Niacin (vitamin B3) has been proven to be safe and highly effective and has been successfully used for decades to treat schizophrenia, alcoholism, depression, anxiety, and other mental disorders. High niacin containing foods include cashews, peanuts, avocados, guavas, mangos, bananas, nectarines, passion fruit, potatoes, mushrooms, acorn squash, green peas, asparagus, tomatoes, whole wheat, brown rice, and lentils. There are generally two types of depression: atypical and typical. Atypical depression is associated with an increase in appetite, weight gain, and excessive sleeping or sleepiness. Typical depression can often be associated with a loss of appetite, weight loss, and difficulty with sleeping. To de-intensify symptoms, big pharma drugs typically impair and disable various normal brain processes, thereby limiting the ability of the brain, which often shrinks in the process. Studies on saffron have shown that its two active components, safranal and crocin, also have anti-depressant effects. Dutch researchers studied 30,000 men and discovered that low cholesterol levels showed increased rates of depression.

"A merry heart doeth good like a medicine: but a broken spirit drieth the bones" (Proverbs 17:22).

The way that people feel and think has a major effect on the physiology of their body. Physical pain and the distress that comes from social rejection have both been traced to the same region of the brain. It is persistent, negative thoughts that cause changes in the brain, including a change in serotonin levels. The effect is psychosomatic (physical symptoms that occur for psychological reasons). The moment that a thought comes into the mind, neuropeptides, which are powerful hormones, are produced in the brain and the thought is changed into biochemicals, which instantly changes the biochemistry of the body. Thoughts can also change protein production and the receptor sites on a cell. A shock or any negative thoughts and emotions that are retained can cause lesions in the brain and become a poison to the body, which in turn can lead to cancer and other diseases. The solution is to take control of negative patterns of thinking. When unresolved issues become resolved, cancer is generally healed. Gastrointestinal inflammation in particular, can play a crucial role in the development of depression and is often associated with immune diseases, type 2 diabetes, neurodegenerative diseases, cardiovascular diseases, and cancer. The study of these connections is known as psychoneuroimmunology. Being in a state of happiness releases the protein BDNF (Brain-Derived Neurotrophic Factor) to protect the brain from stress. BDNF is a type of growth hormone that functions in the brain. This has a reparative and protective element for memory neurons. Happy people have better immune function, a lower heart rate, and better stress levels, as happiness works on the cellular level.

"For as he thinketh in his heart, so is he" (Proverbs 23:7).

Brain neurons are capable of forming new connections. However, in particular areas of the brain, they can also multiply. One of the main proponents of this process is BDNF. Minerals are involved in the activation of BDNF and among the most promising are magnesium and zinc. Many common brain disorders have been linked to decreased levels of this hormone, but curcumin can increase brain levels of BDNF, and in doing so, it may be effective at delaying or even reversing many brain diseases and decreases in brain function. Sage also helps to protect brain cell health by maintaining higher levels of BDNF. BDNF is a strong anti-inflammatory, thereby helping to protect the brain from free radical damage and oxidative stress while blocking and repairing damage to brain cells. Interestingly, neurons are not only found in the brain but also in the heart and the gut.

"But even the very hairs of your head are all numbered. Fear not therefore: ye are of more value than many sparrows"
(Luke 12:7).

The phenomenal brain is comprised of some of the highest energy-demanding tissues in the body. It burns about 25% of the body's oxygen and also controls and co-ordinates every bodily function. There are about 100,000 miles of blood vessels in the brain and about 100 billion neurons, with anywhere from 1,000–10,000 synapses for each neuron. Synapses are small gaps at the end of neurons and are connecting points between the neurons which allow neural communication. Synaptogenesis is the formation of new brain synapses. Synapses are also found throughout the body. It has been said that there are more synapses in the human brain than there are stars in the galaxy. A neuron is an electrically excitable cell that processes and transmits information by electro-chemical signalling. The brain has plasticity, and its structure is changed and reshaped by experiences and stimulus, and neuronal synapse nerves regrow, depending on the stimulus that they receive. Consistent stimulus causes consistent firing of the neurons, which produces consistent chemicals, and the plasticity of the brain forms to the thought process and the body responds through neural firings to the input. Neurons that fire together wire together. Every new thought creates a new neuronal pathway and every emotional experience creates a chemical. By continually thinking the same thoughts, the brain is not expanding but shrinking. Continually memorizing the emotions of past events not only creates the same circumstances in the mind but also reinforces the same chemical pathways and neuronal connections. Dependence on these chemical pathways produces a chemical addiction, as emotions are chemicals. Thoughts cause neurons to connect and fire, which produces chemicals that stimulate particular emotional pathways and triggers a bodily response, which creates feelings. Scientists have discovered that selenium protects brain neurons from depression and cell death. Those who are depressed have shrunken brains, less grey matter, and a smaller hippocampus. However, exercise improves memory and increases the size of the hippocampus. By becoming self-aware of thought processes, a brain change can occur.

"A merry heart maketh a cheerful countenance: but by sorrow of the heart the spirit is broken" (Proverbs 15:13).

A study of curcumin reveals a mechanism by which this extensively studied phyto-compound may alleviate cognitive disorders. Long-chain essential fatty acid DHA is the most prevalent Omega-3 fatty acid in the brain tissues, and its deficiency is linked to several neurocognitive disorders. Essential fatty acids are messengers that must be obtained from dietary sources for optimal health as they cannot be synthesized by the body. These fatty acids are involved in the immune system and the functioning and synthesis of brain neurotransmitters. A DHA deficiency is quite common and can have a wide range of adverse consequences on the optimal functioning of the brain. The human brain is around 70% fat, and Omega-3 DHA represents about 30% of brain matter. Omega-3 tends to reduce cancer cell growth, while highly processed Omega-6 has been found to cause cancer growth. DHA synthesis occurs primarily in the liver and curcumin increases DHA synthesis. Researchers have discovered that because curcumin enhances DHA biosynthesis, the result is an elevated brain DHA content. These findings have important implications for health and the prevention of cognitive diseases, as DHA is essential for brain function. Curcumin-induced DHA levels may be an indirect result of reduced oxidative stress because of the anti-inflammatory properties of curcumin.

"Thou wilt keep him in perfect peace, whose mind is stayed on thee: because he trusteth in thee" (Isaiah 26:3).

For about 100 years it was believed that a damaged brain could not regenerate. It is now accepted by medical science that the brain does regenerate and is pliable and resilient—this is known as neuroplasticity. Neurogenesis is the production of new neurons and glial cells which make new connections when they are stimulated by learning new skills. Conversely, antibiotics stop the growth of new neurons. The brain, which voraciously consumes oxygen and glucose, also needs sound nutrition and plenty of physical and mental exercise for optimal functioning, enabling it to regenerate throughout life. Turmeric is a remyelinating compound, as it repairs the protective myelin nerve sheath, having proven nerve-regenerative effects. Studies have found that the fat-soluble, aromatic substance turmerone or ar-turmerone within turmeric may support regeneration in neurologic diseases. Researchers evaluated the effects of this turmeric-derived compound on neural stem cells, the subgroup of brain cells capable of continuous self-renewal required for brain repair. When brain cells were exposed to ar-turmerone, the number and complexity of neural stem cells increased through enhanced proliferation. These newly formed neural stem cells also increased the number of fully differentiated neuronal cells, indicating that a healing effect was taking place. Ar-turmerone is not only the principle flavouring compound of turmeric but is also another of the potent volatile oils found in turmeric root.

"And be renewed in the spirit of your mind" (Ephesians 4:23).

Curcumin modulates various neurotransmitter levels in the brain and is a powerful inhibitor of reactive astrocyte expression, thus preventing cell death. Astrocytes are specialized glial cells that outnumber neurons more than five-fold. Curcumin can also provide an effective therapeutic strategy to reverse cerebrovascular dysfunction, which includes stroke, cerebral amyloid angiopathy, and cognitive decline. When penetrating the blood-brain barrier, curcumin demonstrates neuroprotective functioning in epilepsy, which is caused by inflammation of the brain. In a study, a water extract of black Nigella sativa seeds was also found to significantly reduce seizure activity in epileptic children. Adequate vitamin C can also be utilized for this issue as it is a potent anti-inflammatory. Curcumin also protects from Parkinson's disease and other related neuropsychiatric and neurodegenerative disorders through its supplies of additional protection to the brain cells with its anti-inflammatory and antioxidant properties.

"That ye may with one mind and one mouth glorify God, even the Father of our Lord Jesus Christ" (Romans 15:6).

When the sense of smell begins to deteriorate, it is an indication that there may be a problem in the nervous system, and this is linked to a higher risk of Parkinson's disease, which is caused by inflammation that damages cells in the nervous system and is essentially the malfunction and death of vital brain nerve cells. Parkinson's disease is a neurodegenerative disease whose symptoms are characterized by a reduction of dopamine and its related norepinephrine. Dopamine is a neurotransmitter that sends signals between various parts of the brain. Dopamine-producing nerve cells in the substantia nigra of the brain are responsible for relaying messages that design and control body movement. These nerve cells are more susceptible to damage and death when a nutrient-deficient diet is consumed, including much-needed folate, DHA, and vitamins B12 and D. Heavy metals and toxins are also a problem. As Parkinson's disease progresses, the dopamine neurons are damaged in the substantia nigra part of the brain. This decreases the availability of dopamine as the substantia nigra is one of its largest suppliers. When 80% of dopamine is lost, symptoms such as slowness of movement, tremors, stiffness, and balance problems occur. As turmeric is anti-inflammatory, it will help with this condition. Other anti-oxidants are also beneficial. The brain and gut are created before birth from the same type of tissue, and during the development of the fetus, one part develops into the enteric nervous system and the other part develops into the central nervous system. These two systems are connected via the vagus nerve, which is the longest of twelve cranial nerves that exits from the medulla oblongata of the brain and runs from the brainstem to the abdomen. It contains sensory and motor fibres and has the widest distribution in the body because it passes, by way of multiple organs, through the neck and thorax before reaching the abdomen. Studies of Parkinson's disease patients have discovered that their motor conditions correlate with problems with the vagus nerve, which has about 90% of its neural fibres transmitting information from the gut to the brain. When there is insufficient dopamine to provide smooth nerve impulses between the parts of the brain that control motor movement, motor control and coordination start to deteriorate. Exercise also helps with this condition.

"Jesus said unto him, Thou shalt love the Lord thy God with all thy heart, and with all thy soul, and with all thy mind"
(Matthew 22:37).

In the early 1900s, Parkinson's disease began to be linked with unhealthy microbiome conditions including nausea, constipation, GI inflammation, and heartburn. Research found that Parkinson's disease patients had significantly more pathogenic (disease-causing) Enterobacteriaceae, which cause a myriad of diseases throughout the digestive tract and the rest of the body. If the pathogenic bacteria overtake the probiotics, this often results in a bacterial overgrowth in the small intestine. More of the healthy probiotic bacteria are needed in these cases as pathogenic bacteria fight for territory in the gut and are the enemies of probiotics. The gut flora needs nourishing with a healthy whole plant-food diet which can include probiotic foods. Research has discovered that probiotic bacteria can increase the levels of the important neurotransmitters dopamine and serotonin. The greatest concentration of serotonin is not found in the brain but in the gut, as 95% of serotonin is produced in the gut and 50% of dopamine is found in the gut. High concentrations of curcumin remain in the GI tract following ingestion and this significantly boosts gut microbes.

"But he that shall endure unto the end, the same shall be saved" (Matthew 24:13).

Most cases of Parkinson's disease are caused by a whiplash effect to the back of the neck if the medulla oblongata, the pons (meaning bridge), and the mid-brain are involved, as damage to this region can cause a deficiency in the production of dopamine. A good corrective chiropractor can mitigate this problem and can also check the nervous system for any other issues. Free-radical damage to the fatty tissue of the brain, because of an antioxidant deficiency, can also be a cause, as can insufficient brain cholesterol, since almost 100% of the myelin is cholesterol.

"They that sow in tears shall reap in joy" (Psalm 126:5).

According to researchers, Alzheimer's disease begins with brain changes thirty years or more before the commencement of symptoms. Alzheimer's disease is now known as type 3 diabetes, and research has proven that diabesity (diabetes and obesity) plays a pivotal role in implementing a cascade of brain damage as there is a strong correlation between dementia and obesity. Mounting evidence from research indicates that Alzheimer's disease is intricately connected to insulin resistance that adversely impacts the blood vessels in the brain. Even mildly elevated blood sugar is associated with an elevated risk of dementia. Vaccines contain aluminium and Alzheimer's disease victims have very high brain levels of this potent inflammatory neurotoxin. Alzheimer's disease occurs when toxins accrue in the brain and produce inflammation and oxidative stress. This can result in an accumulation of the amyloid-B protein fragment, which forms plaques between the neurons in the brain that disrupt brain function. Amyloid is a protein that occurs naturally throughout the body, but this protein inappropriately divides in Alzheimer's disease, thereby creating a form of amyloid which is toxic to brain neurons. Inflammation directly fuels amyloid plaque build-up. In a healthy brain, the amyloid-B are broken down and eliminated. However, in Alzheimer's disease, these fragments accumulate, forming hard, insoluble plaques between the neurons. The compounds in anti-inflammatory turmeric may strike at the origin of the pathological cause of Alzheimer's disease by preventing amyloid-B protein formation. Turmeric boosts amyloid plaque clearance, and a study on those with Alzheimer's found that taking less than one gram of turmeric daily for three months resulted in remarkable improvements.

When curcumin crosses the blood-brain barrier it binds to amyloid-B, and once bound the amyloid-B are unable to clump together to form plaques.

Curcumin also boosts immune and macrophage activity to normal levels, which facilitates the clearance of the chemically sticky amyloid-beta that gradually forms into amyloid plaques. The most injurious form of beta-amyloid may be aggregations of a few pieces rather than the plaques themselves. These small clumps may prevent cell-to-cell signalling at the synapses. In those who are healthy, immune cells called macrophages, which engulf and destroy suspected pathogens and abnormal cells, efficiently clear amyloid-beta, while macrophage activity is suppressed in those with Alzheimer's disease. Regular use of turmeric has been found to reduce the occurrence of Alzheimer's disease and

> *According to researchers, Alzheimer's disease begins with brain changes thirty years or more before the commencement of symptoms.*

is potent in its therapy as it produces remarkable recovery in those with this disease. The antioxidant melatonin has also been identified to inhibit the formation and progression of amyloid-B. Epidemiological studies show that in elderly Indian populations where turmeric is commonly consumed, levels of neurological diseases such as Alzheimer's are minimal. Curcumin also has metal-chelating properties and has a higher binding affinity for iron and copper rather than zinc, which may contribute to its protective effect in Alzheimer's disease, as iron-mediated damage may also play a pathological role.

As an effective chelating agent, curcumin not only neutralizes the toxicity of aluminium, mercury, and lead in the body but also pesticides and herbicides. Pesticides and herbicides accumulate and are stored for a long time in the fatty tissues of the brain. Curcuminoids are neurorestorative and may regress physiological damage by restoring distorted neurites and disuniting existing plaques. Whole turmeric root restores the injured brain, and recent research has exposed how it may contribute to the regeneration of the damaged brain. The brain also produces a soluble type of amyloid plaque that is protective for dendrites and neurons. A healthy lifestyle and diet, integrating a whole plant-food diet with adequate amounts of vitamins A, B12, C, D, E, Omega-3, turmeric, and medium-chain unrefined coconut oil instead of unhealthy refined oils and fats, is paramount in the prevention and reversal of Alzheimer's disease. The brain's primary fuel source is glucose, and reduced glucose metabolism is a defining characteristic of Alzheimer's disease. Another alternative fuel source are ketones, which are metabolized by the brain faster than glucose; they increase the efficiency of the mitochondria, provide more energy, and are available as usable energy when stored fat is broken down. Keytones are formed when there is a carbohydrate deficiency, as glucose is produced when carbohydrates are digested or metabolized. Medium-chain triglycerides are essential for the production of ketones, and unrefined coconut oil contains 65% of these healthy triglycerides which boosts cognitive function and supplements a glucose deficiency in the brain.

"For God hath not given us the spirit of fear; but of power, and of love, and of a sound mind" (2 Timothy 1:7).

Alzheimer's disease is a multi-factorial condition which is primarily caused by chronic inflammation. Anything that causes inflammation in the brain can produce amyloid plaques including a lack of sleep, infectious diseases, stress, aluminium, mercury, cadmium, lead, pesticides, herbicides, excitotoxins, fungicides, and emotional or physical trauma. Aluminium and mercury, which work synergistically as a toxin, can enter the body through dental fillings, the water supply, and vaccinations. As these heavy metals accumulate in the astrocytes and microglial cells of the brain they become the motivation for destructive Alzheimer's disease. Silica removes toxic aluminium from the body by binding to it, which the kidneys then filter from the blood. Silica is made of silicon and oxygen and is the most abundant element in the earth's crust as it comprises 59% of its total composition. Good sources include whole grains, green beans, leafy greens, artichokes, asparagus, cucumbers, melons, bananas, mangos, dandelion, horsetail, rose hips, nettle leaf, and oat straw. Unfortunately, it has a low bioavailability and the majority of it is in a form called orthosilicic acid, which is located in the liver, kidneys, aorta, bones, and tendons. Amyloid plaques suppress the mitochondria, which is a part of the cell that generates chemical energy in the form of the chemical adenosine triphosphate (ATP). It is also the first part of the brain that is affected by Alzheimer's disease. Curcumin stimulates the energy production of the mitochondria and also stimulates the production of more mitochondria. The brain contains its own immune system (neuroimmune system), and the microglia, which are resident immune cells of the central nervous system, become activated when the brain becomes inflamed under an inflammatory attack. Curcumin reduces microglial activation and amyloid plaque deposits. Exercise increases the production of anti-inflammatory compounds and also reduces microglial activation. When the microglia are activated, they release chemicals which damage the connections of the dendrites, synapses, and brain neurons. The microglia become provoked to implement their activities for inflammation but are not fully activated until they become exposed to toxins. Glial cells are similar to immune cells of the brain. When they become activated it leads to neuroinflammation or inflammation of the brain cells. When this occurs they then produce instant intense inflammation and enter into a full destruction process by releasing toxic inflammatory compounds and damaging excitotoxins, which then becomes Alzheimer's disease. Spinach dramatically decreases a declining brain by reducing immunoexcitotoxicity, microglial stimulation, and activation. Obesity and the consumption of a diet high in damaging oils and fats over a long period of time can lead to brain inflammation and dementia. Obesity is one of the biggest influences that leads to preventable chronic diseases. Those who are obese and have cancer are typically in far worse danger than their leaner counterparts as cancer stem cells have the ability to bury themselves in adipose fatty tissue. The most unhealthy fats are the oxidized Omega-6 fats, which, in the brain, have been demonstrated to trigger immunoexcitotoxicity. Adipocytes in the abdomen contain special immune cells called macrophages, which produce elevated levels of the inflammatory chemicals chemokines and cytokines, in those who are obese. These disperse in the bloodstream and rapidly activate inflammation in the brain. The inflammation in the brain calms down when these excess fat cells no longer exist. Curcumin powerfully inhibits excitotoxicity, stimulates energy production in the brain, and reduces microglial activation and brain inflammation. The carotenoid astaxanthin is also a powerful brain protector.

"And be not conformed to this world: but be ye transformed by the renewing of your mind, that ye may prove what is that good, and acceptable, and perfect, will of God" (Romans 12:2).

Inspirational new research from Harvard proposes that beta-amyloid buildup in the brain may not be abnormal but may perform as a natural probiotic that safeguards the brain from infections of which Alzheimer's disease might be a side effect when the brain tries to fight infectious diseases. Beta-amyloid proteins appear to be antimicrobial peptides that perform a beneficial role in the brain and are part of the inborn immune response. Beta-amyloid traps and kills bacteria, infectious proteins, fungus, and viruses that cross the blood-brain barrier. The resulting plaque accumulation that is seen in Alzheimer's disease is the result of this process. When these plaques have been tested, each one contained a single bacterium at its centre. The antioxidant capability of curcumin demonstrates anti-inflammatory properties. Inflammation caused by viruses and also by direct viral action results in neuronal damage which leads to progressive synaptic dysfunction, neuronal loss, and finally Alzheimer's disease. Fortunately, turmeric is anti-inflammatory. Neurons are highly specialized nerve cells and the basic building blocks of the nervous system. They are designed to transmit information, both electrical and chemical, throughout the body. Scientists have discovered that brain cells do regenerate, and some of this regeneration occurs in the hippocampus, a region which is devastated by Alzheimer's disease.

"Let this mind be in you, which was also in Christ Jesus"
(Philippians 2:5).

Whilst most molecules are prevented from crossing the incredible blood-brain barrier, curcumin is proficient at traversing this barrier, not only acting efficiently against cancerous cells but also targeting brain cancer stem cells. Studies have shown that in the rare and usually fatal highly aggressive brain tumour glioblastoma, curcumin activates particular cell signalling routes that destroy the advancement of the glioblastoma cells, shutting down the signal that safeguards the glioblastoma cells, which in turn effectively allows apoptosis. Glioma stem cells are present in glioblastoma tumours, and curcumin is much superior at homing in on this distinct subpopulation of chemoresistant and radioresistant cells in a way that conventional treatments cannot. The anti-inflammatory effects of curcumin can also provide relief from intracranial pressure in the brain due to the development of a tumour. Curcumin halts glioblastoma and has been proven to decrease brain tumours with no evidence of toxicity or adverse effects on healthy cells, demonstrating that curcumin is fully capable of selectively targeting cancer stem cells at the centre of cancer malignancy. Recently published studies contribute compelling evidence that curcumin can be a viable option in prohibiting and treating this deadly brain disease. All cells, including cancer cells, need blood for their growth, as without it they would perish. Curcumin performs as an angiogenesis inhibitor, meaning that it prevents the growth of any new blood vessels around the metastasized cells, thereby impeding the blood supply to a tumour. This privation of blood inhibits the proliferation of cancer cells and also quickly destroys the mutated cells so that they do not metastasize throughout the body.

"And Jesus looking upon them saith, With men it is impossible, but not with God: for with God all things are possible"
(Mark 10:27).

Spinal cord injury often has irreversibly devastating effects. A promising new study states that curcumin may provide victims of spinal cord injury with a more effective and safer approach than conventional treatments, which primarily rely on surgery and corticosteroids, a class of anti-inflammatory drugs that are notorious for their adverse health effects. Turmeric is able to stimulate the regeneration of injured neurological tissues through neural stem cells. Damaged axons are due to a primary injury that begins after a physical impact. Axons are nerve fibres which are long slender neuronal projections that conduct electrical impulses away from neurons. The outpouring of the inflammatory events following an impact causes a large amount of axons to be lost, resulting in secondary injury sensorimotor losses. There are both primary and secondary inflammatory processes in spinal cord injuries that are believed to be responsible for the often-permanent damage caused by these injuries. The spinal cord contains stem cells that are capable of regenerating damaged tissues. Curcumin may help to assuage both the primary and secondary dimensions of inflammation-mediated spinal cord injuries by behaving as a powerful anti-inflammatory pleiotropic (a gene which affects more than one characteristic of the phenotype). Inflammation is the primary driver in damaged tissues. Curcumin triggers the proliferation of neural progenitor cells, which can assist the root cause of impairment caused by a spinal cord injury and heal the spinal cord. Turmeric is not only neuroprotective, neurorestorative, and a natural analgesic, but it also mitigates damage, stimulates accelerated healing, and can generate recovery and improvement of function.

"Delight thyself also in the LORD; and He shall give thee the desires of thine heart" (Psalm 37:4).

Turmeric may be the most important plant in the world at reducing the risk of harm from many diseases, infectious exposures, electromagnetic radiation, cognitive disfunction, stress-induced adverse physiological changes, and modern-day chemicals including toxic dangerous cancer-causing DNA destroying preservatives. Sodium benzoate is a preservative, a cheap mould inhibitor, and a solvent which is found in many foods and beverages and steals essential nutrients from the body whilst also depriving the mitochondria of oxygen. The potent carcinogen benzene is formed when sodium benzoate is combined with vitamins E or C. Bisphenol A (BPA), a chemical that is used in a wide range of plastics, has also been found in high concentrations within the human body. It is linked to over fifty adverse health effects as it is neurotoxic, carcinogenic, cardiotoxic, a well-known potent endocrine disruptor, and also disrupts human hormones. Exposure to thermal printer receipts has also been proven to contaminate the body with toxic BPA. A new study indicates that there is a natural way to mitigate the adverse effects of exposure to this chemical. Curcumin is able to reverse the BPA induced activation of oncogenic pathways within cells exposed to this chemical. Additives that are used in place of BPA and are sold as BPA-free can potentially be just as harmful.

"For, behold, I create new heavens and a new earth: and the former shall not be remembered, nor come into mind" (Isaiah 65:17).

Curcumin attenuates the neurotoxicity induced by the forced medication of the unprocessed highly toxic industrial waste that is known as fluoride (fluorosilicic acid), which is added to the water supply and dental products in some countries. It should not be confused with the natural fluoride that is found in the soil. Scientific research has proven that fluorosilicic acid is a drug, an insecticide, a chemical compound that destroys bone mass, including spinal discs, and an endocrine disruptor which can affect blood sugar levels, the bones, the brain, and the pineal and thyroid glands. It has also been proven to lower IQ levels and nearly doubles the risk of hypothyroidism. Once fluoride crosses the blood-brain barrier it causes degeneration of the neocortex, the cerebellum, and the hippocampus. When fluoride comes into contact with aluminium it is able to cross the blood-brain barrier in the form of aluminium fluoride, which studies have linked with the development of Alzheimer's disease. Fluorosilicic acid was used during World War II to keep concentration camp victims placid and dumbed down and it still works the same way today. There have been many studies linking this dangerous poison to brain damage and a wide variety of other health problems. It has been established that toxic fluoride exposure contributes to the calcification of the pineal gland, a small endocrine gland in the brain that is best known for its role in producing the hormone melatonin from serotonin, and its calcification is associated with quite a number of diseases. Prozac® (fluoxetine) is approximately 30% fluoride by weight and marketed as an anti-depressant, and a major side effect of using or withdrawing from it is suicidal depression. Curcumin is a protective agent against fluoride's various adverse health effects, including an increased rate in tumours and various cancers, including bone cancer. Curcumin also appears to raise endogenous glutathione production in the brain, which is a primary antioxidant defence system. Anti-inflammatory tamarind is not only iron and vitamin C rich but has been found to remove dangerous fluoride deposits from the bones. Iodine can also effectively remove this contaminant. According to the Congressional Record of 21st July, 1976, Dr. Dean Burk, Ph.D., chief chemist of the National Cancer Institute, made the following statement: "Fluoride causes more human cancer death, and causes it faster than any other chemical."

"The LORD shall preserve thee from all evil: He shall preserve thy soul" (Psalm 121:7).

Approximately one third of the world's population are infected with Mycobacterium tuberculosis, which is the bacterium present in tuberculosis. It mostly affects the lungs and can also damage the kidneys, spine, and brain. Macrophages are a special type of white blood cell which are implicated in the immune response. They eliminate foreign materials including cancer cells, cellular waste, and bacteria. Curcumin is able to improve the macrophages' ability to both kill and eliminate TB bacteria, as it has been found to be a potent apoptosis inducer, an effective mechanism used by macrophages to kill intracellular Mycobacterium tuberculosis. This process depends upon the prevention of the cellular molecule NF-Kappa B, which is deactivated by curcumin. Scientists found that by stimulating a key part of the immune system, curcumin is able to successfully remove Mycobacterium tuberculosis from infected cells. Curcumin also increases autophagy in infected cells. In autophagy, cells encapsulate, destroy, and recycle various elements inside the cells.

According to researchers at National Jewish Health, curcumin enhances cellular defense against tuberculosis. In cell culture studies, curcumin enhanced the death of infected cells and also the destruction of the bacteria inside the infected cells. A lead study author at the Denver Veterans Affairs Medical Center stated that their study has provided basic evidence that curcumin protects against Mycobacterium tuberculosis infection in human cells.

"By the word of the LORD were the heavens made; and all the host of them by the breath of His mouth" (Psalm 33:6).

Turmeric can be powerful in many health conditions simultaneously and improve conditions that are completely resistant to conventional treatments. It not only inhibits cancer cell growth but also metastasis (the development of secondary malignant growths at a distance from a primary cancer site). Epidemiological studies have linked the frequent use of turmeric to lower rates of various cancers.

Experiments have demonstrated that curcumin can prevent tumours from form-ing and exerts its biological activities through epigenetic modulation. The science of epigenetics proves unequivocally that cancer is not a genetic disease. This phe-nomenon has powerful effects with wide-ranging implications and can alter gene expression by changing the environment of the cells. When retinoblastoma (a rare malignant tumour of the retina that affects young children) was exposed to curcumin, it altered the expression of over 2,000 genes. Genes that have mutated into cancer-promoting genes can be re-modified and changed again simply by altering the environment of the cell with diet and lifestyle modifications. To maximize health benefits, this health-giving brilliant orange plant root can be cut up, grated, crushed in a garlic press, and added to almost anything. Other ways to boost the absorption of curcumin is to consume turmeric as a whole food or powdered with other foods. The natural oils contained in whole turmeric can enhance the bioavailability of curcumin by about seven-fold. When con-sumed with healthy fats, such as unrefined coconut oil, curcumin can be directly absorbed into the bloodstream through the lymphatic system and bypass the liver.

"The LORD is nigh unto all them that call upon Him, to all that call upon Him in truth" (Psalm 145:18).

European herbalists of the past believed that God gave clues as to which plants are most beneficial for specific body parts and ailments by their shape and colour. Paracelsus (1491–1541) stated: "Nature marks each growth ... according to its curative benefit." He called this the *doctrine of signatures*, a concept that God placed His seal upon plants to indicate their medicinal uses. Thus, the yellow colour of turmeric emulates the sallow complexion of those who have jaundice or chronic hepatitis, which are liver problems that turmeric effectively treats. What people consume and the quantity of bile they produce determines how effectively the food they eat is digested and how efficiently their liver cleanses the blood. Turmeric assuages liver disease and facilitates its detoxification by increasing the secretion and movement of bile, which is utilized to digest fats, eliminate toxins, and may prevent all forms of liver disease. It is the favourite herb of the liver as it helps to boost the liver's detoxification process by assisting enzymes that actively flush out dietary carcinogens. When the liver works more proficiently, the blood will be purer and have a more positive influence on the genetic blueprint of the cells. If toxins are not efficiently disposed of by the liver and they enter the envi-ronment of the cell, the outcome will affect the expression of the gene as the cell environment modifies the genetic blueprint. Turmeric not only protects the liver from toxins and pathogens but it is also known to destroy toxins in the liver and to rebuild the liver after a toxic attack. It also helps to remove stagnant blood while stimulating the formation of new blood tissues. Its many actions on the liver suggest that it may also assist in balancing hormone levels. According to preliminary experimental research, turmeric appears to delay liver damage that can eventually lead to cirrhosis. Preclinical studies demonstrate that it also kills liver cancer cells and tumours and has the potential to protect, regenerate, and reverse damage in the diabetic liver. Turmeric and curcumin also protect the liver against a wide range of chemical and drug exposures. To activate and rebuild the liver, about five grams of turmeric can be mixed with a glass of water and taken morning and evening for a month. In essence, turmeric helps to keep the liver healthy so that it can detoxify the body.

Curcumin also has the ability to quell potential damage from hepatitis. Documentation shows that it also slows cirrhosis, which is a chronic liver disease where the liver has become significantly scarred and is marked by inflammation, a fibrous thickening of tissues, cell degeneration, and is typically a result of alcoholism. It targets multiple steps in the inflammatory pathway at the molecular level. Scientists have confirmed that curcumin protects the liver and gallbladder by acting as an anti-inflammatory agent. It also helps to create the master anti-oxidant glutathione, which detoxifies the liver. No diseases, and especially degenerative diseases, including cancer, can survive for longer than a few weeks in the presence of a healthy liver. Having a healthy liver is extremely crucial for those with cancer in terms of their health and for recovery, and an unhealthy gut flora can undermine natural liver detoxification. Selenium is also important for the health of the liver, partially due to its ability to enhance glutathione levels. Glutathione is a potent antioxidant that protects the lungs

> *No diseases, and especially degenerative diseases, including cancer, can survive for longer than a few weeks in the presence of a healthy liver. Having a healthy liver is extremely crucial for those with cancer in terms of their health and for recovery, and an unhealthy gut flora can undermine natural liver detoxification.*

and blood, and its depletion can result in damage to the lung tissue. Fortunately, exercise increases glutathione levels. Antioxidant and chelating agents are generally employed for the treatment of heavy metals poisoning, and curcumin plays a protective role against liver injury induced by heavy metals. In clinical and preclinical studies, it has demonstrated therapeutic efficacy and anti-hepatotoxic effects against environmental or occupational toxins. Curcumin reduces the hepatotoxicity induced by arsenic, cadmium, chromium, copper, lead, and mercury. It maintains the antioxidant enzyme status of the liver and protects against mitochondrial dysfunction. The preventive effect of curcumin on the noxious effects induced by heavy metals has been attributed to its scavenging and chelating properties.

"Then spake Jesus again unto them, saying, I am the light of the world: he that followeth me shall not walk in darkness, but shall have the light of life" (John 8:12).

Turmeric is seldom contra-indicated but in the case of weak kidneys, it may increase the risk of kidney stones due to its soluble oxalate content. Those suffering from poor gut health are particularly susceptible to oxalates. Nevertheless, the citric acid in lemons can not only help to eliminate calcium deposits from kidney stones but also gallstones and pancreatic stones. Lemon juice can eliminate the occurrence of stones by forming urinary citrate, which prevents the formation of crystals. Turmeric performs as a natural blood thinner by preventing platelet aggregation in the body and can increase the risk of bleeding in those with bleeding disorders. Cayenne pepper can effectively halt bleeding disorders. Curcumin has the potential to trigger gallbladder pain in those with gallstones and therefore is contraindicated for those with biliary tract obstruction due to its powerful ability to induce gallbladder contractions. However, as a preventative, it can effectively induce the gallbladder to empty and thereby reduce the risk of gallstone formation and gallbladder cancer. Bitter foods are important as they trigger the gallbladder to release bile and the pancreas to secrete digestive enzymes.

"The righteous cry, and the LORD heareth, and delivereth them out of all their troubles" (Psalm 34:17).

For sores and wounds, turmeric acts quickly to help stop bleeding and because of its anti-bacterial qualities, it also helps to prevent infections. Turmeric essential oil is efficacious as an external antibacterial to prevent infections in wounds.

Turmeric can be applied to cuts and pressure may also be applied to the area to stop bleeding if necessary. Added cayenne pepper can also assist to stop bleeding, and it does not sting. Of course, serious wounds will require immediate medical attention. Turmeric also purifies and nourishes the blood and skin and external applications can stop pain and swelling and assist in healing wounds rapidly.

"Then Peter said, Silver and gold have I none; but such as I have give I thee: In the name of Jesus Christ of Nazareth rise up and walk" (Acts 3:6).

Turmeric can be used to treat ant bites and also bee, wasp, and scorpion stings, as well as poisonous snake-bites. Topical turmeric extract effectively reduces the severity of symptoms directly at a snake bite area, as it contains compounds that can neutralize the venom, thereby diminishing its poisonous effects. Application at the wound site also helps to control haemorrhaging, swelling, and tissue death. Curcuminoids have been shown to almost completely inactivate cobra venom, and the ar-turmerone in turmeric counteracts venom from both pit vipers and rattlesnakes. Research indicates that the potent antioxidant protein compound turmerin in turmeric can prevent organ damage from cobra venom and neutralize its lethal effects by 90%. Conventional antivenom drugs typically do not resolve these local symptoms.

"And the LORD God said unto the serpent, Because thou hast done this, thou art cursed above all cattle, and above every beast of the field; upon thy belly shalt thou go, and dust shalt thou eat all the days of thy life" (Genesis 3:14).

According to the Bible, the serpent was cursed to eat dust after tempting God's creation to disobey. In the roof of a snake's mouth, there is an organ called the *Jacobson's organ*, which, together with its nose, gives a snake its sense of smell. It samples particles of dust by picking them up on the end of its darting, forked tongue. The serpent has a pair of sensory organs in its mouth which recognizes the dust and immediately uses its mouth to clean its tongue so that the process can be repeated. Therefore, serpents do purposely lick dust and eat it.

"They shall lick the dust like a serpent, they shall move out of their holes like worms of the earth: they shall be afraid of the LORD our God, and shall fear because of thee" (Micah 7:17).

Research indicates that diets which include turmeric or curcumin stabilize and protect biomolecules in the body at the molecular level, which is demonstrated by its anti-oxidant, anti-mutagenic, anti-inflammatory, and anti-carcinogenic actions. These substances may be effective by protecting the body directly by shielding the biomolecules, or indirectly by stimulating the natural detoxification and defence mechanisms and assisting the body to heal and preserve itself naturally.

"Our soul waiteth for the LORD: He is our help and our shield"
(Psalm 33:20).

Curcumin helps to destroy cancer by its ability to inhibit the enzyme topoisomerase, which is required for the replication of cancer cells. Topoisomerase works within the nucleus of the cell, where it first adheres to supercoiled DNA and then catalyses the passage of one DNA helix through another by utilizing a transient double-stranded division. This process splits the DNA and thereby allows cell replication to occur. Preventing topoisomerase prohibits replication, which stops the proliferation of cancer cells.

"For thou hast been a shelter for me, and a strong tower from the enemy" (Psalm 61:3).

It is known that oxygen-deprived cells can develop into cancer cells simply as a matter of survival. Cancer cells produce new blood vessels (angiogenesis) that supply oxygen and more glucose to these cells to enable them to proliferate. Curcumin can prevent the formation of these new blood vessels which support tumour cells, thereby preventing existing cancer cells from ever proliferating into solid tumours. It denatures and decomposes existing blood vessels that nurture tumour cells, and has the ability to change the environment of a tumour or cancer cells to the point where cancer cells either die or become inactive.

"Commit thy way unto the LORD; trust also in Him; and He shall bring it to pass" (Psalm 37:5).

Curcumin is one of the most studied natural COX-2 inhibitors, which blocks the enzyme cyclooxygenase-2. This is beneficial because the COX-2 enzyme helps to make carcinogens more active in the body and allows cancerous cells to survive by growing new blood vessels. Curcumin completely blocks the formation of cancer-causing enzymes and decreases the likelihood of cancerous cell formations. Other food antioxidant COX-2 inhibitors include sweet cherries, red grapes, bee propolis, chamomile, rhubarb, cardamom, celery seeds, marjoram, lavender, sage, currants, chives, cabbage, ginger, rosemary, thyme, nuts, Omega-3 fatty acids, and various other fruits and vegetables.

"Plead my cause, O LORD, with them that strive with me: fight against them that fight against me" (Psalm 35:1).

Another effective quality of turmeric is its anti-fungal properties. Candida albicans is a form of yeast (fungus) which is a naturally occurring micro-organism in the mouth, reproductive organs, and intestines. It is the most common human pathogen. A healthy body is a host to a delicate balance of friendly micro-flora and yeasts, and a very small amount of it should reside in these bodily organs to aid with digestion and nutrient absorption. The mucous membranes throughout the body are lined with a protective bacteria, and if this becomes compromised through the effects of medications and poor lifestyle choices then the underlying bodily tissues will be attacked by opportunistic organisms such as fungus and yeast. Candida flourishes when there are insufficient beneficial bacteria in the gut, and when it is left unchecked, it can cause a wide variety of symptoms due to the release of numerous toxins that are secreted as bi-products. This can cause a leaky gut by breaking down the intestinal barrier and entering the bloodstream. The brain is one of the most sensitive organs and is, therefore, most affected by mycotoxins, which are the toxic by-products of Candida. Effective treatment of Candida overgrowth reverses the symptoms of Candida, including the psychological ones. Another by-product of Candida is the potent cell mutating acetaldehyde neurotoxin, which causes symptoms similar to those that occur with alcohol consumption. Acetaldehyde has the ability to alter the structure of proteins, and not only causes brain damage but also liver damage, pancreas degeneration, damage to the immune system, direct muscle tissue damage, nutritional deficiencies, peripheral nerve damage, and the reduced capability of the stomach lining to produce stomach acid. Fungal and other parasitical infections cause enormous amounts of toxic substances to overwhelm the body, causing cellular damage throughout. The infection also feeds on dead and decaying cells, which in turn leads to more dead and decaying cells. Candida is kept in check by Lactobacillus bacteria, which cannot work effectively if there is a system imbalance. Current Candida research has discovered that Candida colonization delays the healing of inflammatory lesions and inflammation promotes the colonization of Candida, which can create a vicious cycle of Candida causing inflammation and the colonization of the gut with Candida.

The majority of inflammatory diseases originate in the gut, which can progress into systemic inflammation. The gut is made of an incredibly large and intricate semi-permeable lining with a surface area that could cover the dimensions of two full-size tennis courts if stretched out flat. Its degree of permeability fluctuates in response to a variety of chemically-mediated conditions. Repeated gut damage causes the microvilli to become dysfunctional, which leads to an inability to process and utilize vital enzymes and nutrients. Digestion then becomes impaired, and with further exposure to these toxins, the body responds with various symptoms of inflammation, allergies, and much more serious and debilitating diseases such as cancer, as the immune system drives the inflammatory process in diseases. An anti-inflammatory diet and lifestyle with adequate anti-oxidants effectively overcomes inflammatory processes. Unrefined coconut oil also fights deadly yeast infections.

"Being confident of this very thing, that He which hath begun a good work in you will perform it until the day of Jesus Christ" (Philippians 1:6).

Another major use of turmeric is for support of the respiratory system. The word asthma derives from the Greek word for panting, and this malady is due to a problem with the nervous system and the smooth muscle control of the lungs. The allergic response in asthma is generated when immune system T-lymphocytes release specific substances that cause inflammation. According to research, turmeric can block the release of these inflammation-causing phenomenon. As an antioxidant, it protects the lungs from pollution and toxins and also assists with the oxygen transfer from the lungs to the blood. Turmeric also helps to dilate blood vessels, thereby allowing for better breathing capabilities by restoring normal breathing patterns. It also relaxes muscle spasms and relieves asthmatic inflammation that causes swelling in the lungs and breathing problems, as does ginger. Researchers have found that vitamin D3 is also helpful for asthmatic conditions as it reduces the frequency and severity of asthma attacks. Black seed oil from Nigella sativa seeds has also been proven to alleviate asthma symptoms. It has been stated by a well-known drug manufacturer that asthma medications actually increase the risk of death.[20]

---

[20] Peggy Peck, "FDA Documents Say Drugs Increase Risk of Asthma-Related Death," *MedPage Today*, December 5, 2008, https://1ref.us/1p5 (accessed June 6, 2021).

"The Spirit of God hath made me, and the breath of the Almighty hath given me life" (Job 33:4).

Combining turmeric, spices, onions, garlic, cruciferous vegetables, coconut cream, and other healthful ingredients together into a flavourful curry can be an effective, beneficial therapy, not only to help prevent prostate cancer but also to help inhibit the spread of established prostate and other cancers. The flavonoid quercetin is the beneficial antioxidant in onions, and research shows that the combination of onions and turmeric reduces both the size and number of pre-cancerous lesions in the intestinal tract. Quercetin also has the ability to target cancer stem cells and is contained in grapes, cruciferous vegetables, green leafy vegetables, ginger, garlic, tomatoes, peppers, berries, cherries, citrus fruits, and apples.

"O taste and see that the LORD is good: blessed is the man that trusteth in Him" (Psalm 34:8).

Turmeric has obviously stood the test of time. It has been highly revered for centuries and is still today one of the most significant plants for the prevention and treatments of serious diseases as well as an aid in the general ailments of life. Whether suffering from an acute or chronic health issue, or as preventative maintenance in the bumps and bruises and aches and pains of life, turmeric is an affordable plant that can be utilized by anyone on an everyday basis.

"And my soul shall be joyful in the LORD: it shall rejoice in His salvation" (Psalm 35:9).

Due to its tremendous array of powerful health benefits and its efficacy, safety, and versatility, turmeric is one of the most important plants in the world. It reduces unhealthy levels of inflammation, protects against heavy metal toxicity, safeguards against acute liver damage and radiation-induced destruction, destroys multi-drug resistant cancers and cancer stem cells, which are arguably at the root of all cancers and which drive its growth. It also prevents and reverses Alzheimer's disease and associated pathologies, diabetes, heart disease, depression, Parkinson's disease, TB, Candida, and parasites as well as a plethora of other health issues. Turmeric is also an important food additive as a preventative or reversal strategy for pets that suffer from ailments and diseases, and especially those that cause pain.

"I will open rivers in high places, and fountains in the midst of the valleys: I will make the wilderness a pool of water, and the dry land springs of water" (Isaiah 41:18).

God-given turmeric and curcumin extract have been extensively studied for their ability to kill cancer stem cells. The information that corroborates its uses is so abundant that it is disheartening that so many of those who are in need of safe, effective, and affordable treatments are not being supplied with information about it.

"He will swallow up death in victory; and the Lord GOD will wipe away tears from off all faces; and the rebuke of His people shall He take away from off all the earth: for the LORD hath spoken" (Isaiah 25:8).

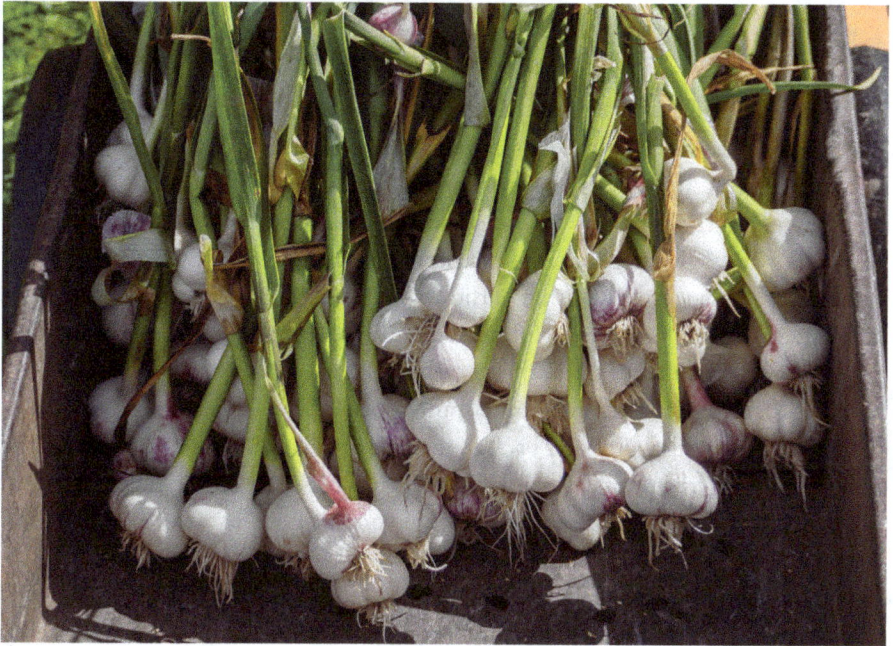

Chapter 4

Garlic

"THE DOCTOR OF THE FUTURE WILL GIVE NO DRUGS, BUT WILL EDUCATE THEIR PATIENTS IN THE CARE OF THE HUMAN BODY, IN A PROPER DIET, AND IN THE CAUSE AND PREVENTION OF DISEASE."

Garlic, or Allium sativum, was originally indigenous to central Asia and is believed to be descended from Allium longicuspis, a wild strain of Asian garlic. Garlic is a member of the lily (Liliaceae) family and is a cousin to onions, chives, leeks, and shallots.

Allium vegetables are the richest sources of powerful beneficial organo-sulphur compounds. The word garlic means *to exhale* and comes from the old Anglo-Saxon word *gārlēac* which is derived from *gār-leek*. The prefix *gār* stems from the word spear because the shape of the cloves resembles a spearhead. Elephant garlic has larger cloves and is more closely related to the leek, and therefore does not offer the full potent health benefits of regular garlic.

Pungent garlic is one of the oldest documented and cultivated plants in the world that has been used for the maintenance of health and the treatment of diseases. It has been proven that garlic was one of the first plants to have been cultivated by man. This powerful beloved little bulb has been used throughout history by many cultures for both its medicinal and culinary properties.

Garlic has been used since time immemorial. The reputation of garlic as a powerful medicinal plant dates back thousands of years and has been used for the prevention and treatment of many diseases. It has been found in every medical book of every culture since antiquity and is one of nature's most potent foods. Ancient, well-documented medical texts from all the major civilizations including that of the Sumerians, Egyptians Chinese, Indians, Assyrians, Babylonians, Greeks, and Romans all prescribed medical applications for garlic. Over twenty uses of garlic were listed for a variety of disorders, including hepatic degradative diseases and protection against toxins and infections. Garlic was also used later for parasites and respiratory ailments. There are at least four ancient cultures that grew garlic and referred to it well over 4,000 years ago. These are the Sumerians (Sumerian cuneiform clay tablets mention garlic), the Egyptians, the Chinese, and the Indians.

"Heal me, O LORD, and I shall be healed; save me, and I shall be saved: for thou art my praise" (Jeremiah 17:14).

It is thought that garlic was first cultivated by the Sumerians on the shores of the Mediterranean Sea. At the beginning of recorded history, in the ancient, recorded Sumerian story of the *Epic of Gilgamesh*, there is the first extra-biblical mention of Noah and the great flood. The Sumerians lived before the Egyptians and did not build pyramids, as did the Egyptians, but instead they built ziggurats, which were huge structures constructed of brick and comparable in size to that of the Egyptian pyramids, although, in appearance, they resembled step pyramids. These were not tombs, but rather were pagan temples, which are similar to pyramid temples in the Americas. One of these structures was the Etemenanki ziggurat which was also known as the biblical Tower of Babel. Over 2,000 years BC, the Sumerians were actively utilizing the healing properties of garlic, and it is believed that they brought garlic to China, where it was later spread to Korea and Japan. There is also clear historical evidence for its use by the Babylonians, where it was grown in the ancient gardens of Babylon. It was one of the most used remedies in ancient China and Japan and was prescribed to aid digestion, respiration, diarrhoea, worm infestation, and was also used as a food preservative. The Tibetans also possess ancient recipes to cure stomachache with garlic.

"But Noah found grace in the eyes of the LORD" (Genesis 6:8).

Therapeutic garlic has been found in ancient Egyptian pyramids and Greek temples. Archaeologists have discovered paintings of garlic in Egyptian tombs and the Great Pyramid of Cheops. The ancient Egyptians cultivated garlic and it played an important role in their culture. It was not only placed in the tombs of the pharaohs but was also used to pay and feed the labourers and slaves working on the great pyramids. Herodotus, the Greek historian, claimed that the workers who built the pyramids were fed garlic to maintain and increase strength and work capacity. A garlic crop failure, due to the flooding of the River Nile, caused one of the only two recorded Egyptian slave revolts. The bulb was so popular with those who worked on the great pyramids that garlic shortages caused work stoppages. Egyptian priests worshipped garlic but actively avoided cooking and eating the fragrant cloves. It has been used since ancient times to treat wounds, infections, tumours, intestinal parasites, and more. Well-preserved garlic cloves and clay models of garlic bulbs were found in the tomb of King Tutankhamun, who ruled from 1334 BC–1325 BC. The Egyptian crypts have some of the oldest visible inscriptions for the existence of garlic, which the Egyptians ate to not only help increase their strength and productivity but also their stamina and endurance. There is also a Biblical reference to garlic being used in ancient Egypt:

"We remember the fish, which we did eat in Egypt freely; the cucumbers, and the melons, and the leeks, and the onions, and the garlick" (Numbers 11:5).

Garlic has been associated with healing processes in India from antiquity. The first available written records show that it was used for many therapeutic purposes including arthritis, heart disease, fatigue, digestive diseases, parasites, and leprosy. The healers of ancient India prescribed garlic for leprosy, which was a practice that continued for thousands of years, and modern research supports the ability of garlic to treat leprosy. In India, leprosy became known as *peelgarlic* because lepers spent a great deal of time peeling and eating the health-inducing cloves. Leprosy is contagious and very difficult to treat conventionally. It is induced by an organism called Mycobacterium leprae, which is very similar to Mycobacterium tuberculosis, which causes tuberculosis. Garlic has been used successfully to combat this terrible disease when all other forms of conventional therapy have failed.

"And it came to pass, when He was in a certain city, behold a man full of leprosy: who seeing Jesus fell on his face, and besought Him, saying Lord, if thou wilt, thou canst make me clean. And He put forth His hand, and touched him, saying, I will: be thou clean. And immediately the leprosy departed from him" (Luke 5:12, 13).

During archaeological excavations in the Knossos palace on the Greek island of Crete, garlic bulbs were discovered dating from 1850–1400 BC. The Codex Ebers (named after George Ebers who discovered it in 1872), is an authoritative very ancient medical papyrus from around 1500 BC and is thought to be the oldest medical reference in western civilization. It mentions various medicinal plants, and amongst these is the much-appreciated garlic. It prescribed garlic for the treatment of circulatory ailments, general malaise, abnormal growths, and infestations with parasites and insects. Civilizations and cultures that never came in contact with each other came to many of the same conclusions about the role of garlic for the treatment of diseases. Garlic was introduced into various regions throughout the world by migrating tribes and explorers. Ashurbanipal, who reigned from 668–627 BC as the last great Tsar of Assyria, hid clay plates on which various pieces of evidence of the life, rituals, and customs of the Assyrian world were recorded. Amongst the 10,000 volumes of this clay library were volumes devoted to medicinal plants, and garlic was given a special place in the first Assyrian book of medicinal plants.

"But in the first year of Cyrus the king of Babylon the same king Cyrus made a decree to build this house of God" (Ezra 5:13).

The Greek physician Hippocrates, revered as *the father of medicine*, was born around 460 BC on the island of Kos, off of the southwest coast of Asia Minor, which is present-day Turkey. He prescribed garlic to treat a variety of health conditions and recommended that his patients eat large amounts of crushed garlic to cure their cancer. He also used garlic as part of his therapeutic armamentarium, promoting its use for pulmonary disorders, as a cleansing or purgative agent and for abdominal growths. The Greek philosopher and scientist Aristotle (384–322 BC) recommended garlic as a preventative of rabies lyssavirus.

"A merry heart doeth good like a medicine: but a broken spirit drieth the bones" (Proverbs 17:22).

In the vast and influential Roman Empire, garlic and onion were used as remedies, spices, and food for the survival of the poor. Aulus Cornelius Celsus (25 BC–AD 50), used garlic to cure fever and tuberculosis. He was a Roman encyclopaedist who was known for his extant medical work *De Medicina*, which is a primary source on diet, surgery, pharmacy, and related fields. It is one of the best sources concerning medical knowledge in the Roman world. Pliny the Elder (AD 23–79), a Roman scientist and physician from the first century, considered garlic to be a universal remedy, and he wrote that the Egyptians took an oath by mentioning garlic and onion because they were considered to be two miraculous, holy plants. This strength-enhancing quality was honoured by the ancient Romans and Greeks, whose athletes consumed it before sporting events and whose soldiers ate it before going to war. The Greeks also prescribed it for leprosy. In ancient Rome, the chief physician to Nero's army, Pedanius Dioscorides, who wrote a celebrated treatise on herbs, also recommended garlic to clean the arteries, even though the circulation of the blood was not discovered until hundreds of years later. Garlic was also recommended for gastrointestinal tract disorders, a treatment for animal bites, and for the alleviation of joint disease and seizures. Galen (AD 121–200), the renowned physician and medical writer among the Romans and later among other nations, spoke of garlic as the most popular folk remedy which cured many diseases. He also used it for colic and the regulation of digestion.

"To all that are in Rome, beloved of God, called to be saints: Grace to you and peace from God our Father, and the Lord Jesus Christ" (Romans 1:7).

During the Middle Ages, in the Arabic school of medicine, garlic was a specially valued remedy and Arabic physicians contributed to the expansion of using garlic as a remedy. In ancient Europe, it was used without restrictions, particularly in Italy, while the French added it to many of their dishes. Garlic was brought into Great Britain from the coasts of the Mediterranean Sea. Wild garlic grew and was cultivated in church courtyards in England for centuries. Ostensibly, the cultivation of garlic commenced in England before the sixteenth century.

"O taste and see that the LORD is good: blessed is the man that trusteth in Him" (Psalm 34:8).

Garlic even eradicates the deadly bacillus Yersinia pestis, which was identified by Swiss bacteriologist Alexandre Yersin in 1894 as the cause of the Bubonic Plague or *Black Death*, which is now known to be a bacterial infection. Those afflicted developed buboes, after which the bubonic plague was named, and these were agonizing egg-sized lymph-node swellings. This is an extremely virulent bacterium that is transmitted through the bite of fleas that feed on infected rodents and has emerged repeatedly to cause subsequent plagues. It was identified as the causative agent of the plague of the Emperor Justinian in the sixth century AD. In AD 540, mice bearing the disease from lower Egypt arrived at the harbour town of Pelusium, from which the disease spread to Alexandria and on to Justinian's capital of Constantinople in AD 542 before spreading throughout his empire. By AD 590, about half of the population of Europe, amounting to around 100 million victims, had died from this dreaded disease. During the Middle Ages, another plague in Europe resulted in the deaths of a further 25 million casualties. During the same period, French priests used garlic to protect themselves from the Bubonic Plague. Garlic was brought to Great Britain from the Mediterranean in 1548. In 1720 a thousand inhabitants of Marseille were saved from the spread of an epidemic of the plague as a result of using garlic. Subsequently, it has had numerous other encounters including a pandemic that occurred in China and India in the last half of the nineteenth century.

"For He had healed many; insomuch that they pressed upon Him for to touch Him, as many as had plagues" (Mark 3:10).

This amazing, delicious, aromatic plant is time-tested, highly accessible, very potent and affordable, and has also been used for its efficacy in other epidemics, including typhus, dysentery, and cholera. Whenever an epidemic has emerged, garlic has been the first curative and preventative remedy. During World War I, European soldiers prevented infections by putting garlic directly onto their wounds, and it was also used in military hospitals to help prevent the spread of gangrene by wrapping infected limbs in garlic-soaked bandages, which saved many an infected limb from amputation. It was also used during World War II. Rubbing garlic on an infected staphylococcus area will stop infections in their tracks.

"Yea, though I walk through the valley of the shadow of death, I will fear no evil: for thou art with me; thy rod and thy staff they comfort me" (Psalm 23:4).

There are approximately 300 varieties of garlic grown worldwide, and it is one of the most intensively studied herbs in natural medicine today. Garlic plays a significant role in preventing or treating well over 160 health conditions and contains a wide range of phytocompounds that have at least 150 recognizable physiological responses. Over 1,800 scientific studies detail the chemical complexity and multifaceted roles of garlic in the prevention and treatment of disease.

"The LORD is good, a strong hold in the day of trouble; and He knoweth them that trust in Him" (Nahum 1:7).

This most nutritious, pungent bulb has more than 400 chemical compounds, including over eighty different sulphur compounds, one of which is sulphuric acid. Garlic is a rich source of calcium, copper, chromium, iodine (valuable for the thyroid), manganese, phosphorous, quercetin, selenium, sulphur-containing amino acids, and zinc. It contains a good source of the primary antioxidant vitamin C, and also vitamin A, vitamin B1, vitamin B2, iron, magnesium, potassium and an excellent source of vitamin B6, which helps to prevent heart disease by lowering homocysteine levels. It also contains oligosaccharides, fibre, polyphenols, arginine, and vitamin-like flavonoids, plus eight essential amino acids and nine non-essential ones. Many of these micronutrients contribute to the immunity of the body.

"This is the LORD'S doing; it is marvellous in our eyes" (Psalm 118:23).

Powerful garlic is efficacious for virtually any disease and infection and rapidly diffuses throughout the system. It has many health-promoting properties. It is anti-ageing, anti-allergenic, anti-angiogenic, antiarrhythmic, anti-arthritic, anti-asthmatic, anti-atherogenic, anti-bacterial, anti-carcinogenic, anti-coagulant, antidiabetic, antifungal, anti-infective, anti-inflammatory, anti-ischaemic, antiprotozoal, anti-malarial, anti-microbial, antimycotic, anti-parasitic, antiphlogistic (prevents or relieves inflammation), antiseptic, antithrombotic, antiviral, anxiolytic, apoptotic, cytotoxic (to cancer stem cells), detoxifying, epigenetic, immune-protective, neuroprotective, and neurorestorative. It is also an analgesic, an antibiotic, an antioxidant, an anti-ulcer, an expectorant, a diuretic, a stimulant, a vasodilator, and a vermifuge. A Washington University study found that garlic is 100 times stronger than the best of the antibiotics that big pharma has to offer.

"Oh that men would praise the LORD for His goodness, and for His wonderful works to the children of men!" (Psalm 107:15).

Garlic has been known to kill many cancers, including glioblastoma (brain cancer), acute lymphoblastic leukaemia, acute myeloid leukaemia, basal cell carcinoma, breast cancer, cervical cancer, chronic lymphocytic leukaemia, colon cancer, endometrial cancer, gastric cancer, leukaemia, liver cancer, lymphoma, melanoma, osteosarcoma, and pancreatic cancer.

"For our conversation is in heaven; from whence also we look for the Saviour, the Lord Jesus Christ: Who shall change our vile body, that it may be fashioned like unto His glorious body, according to the working whereby He is able even to subdue all things unto Himself" (Philippians 3:20, 21).

The powerful therapeutic action of garlic is beneficial for many health issues including cholera, leprosy, plague, viral hepatitis, colds, coughs, flu, seizures, athlete's foot, arrhythmia, insomnia, epilepsy, endothelial and epithelial dysfunction, hemorrhoids, liver disease, sinusitis, ulcers, varicose veins, pancreas issues, candidiasis, pituitary issues, liver problems, measles, mumps, adrenal issues, thyroid problems, diphtheria, ringworm, rheumatic bacteria, cardiovascular disease, typhoid fever, scarlet fever, urinary tract infections, bacterial dysentery, cholera, whooping cough, diabetes, asthma, chickenpox, anthrax, viruses, infections, gangrene, meningitis, mononucleosis, botulism, rabies, diarrhoea, tuberculosis, herpes simplex 1 and 2, tetanus, herpes zoster, macular degeneration, cataracts, sinus issues, circulatory problems, digestive disorders, and sore throats.

"And the LORD will take away from thee all sickness, and will put none of the evil diseases of Egypt, which thou knowest, upon thee; but will lay them upon all them that hate thee" (Deuteronomy 7:15).

The beneficial effects of garlic are numerous. It helps to reduce the adverse effects of radiotherapy and chemotherapy. It is a preventative, including a preventative for strokes, heart attacks, dementia, Alzheimer's disease, arterial calcification, and the growth of Mycobacterium tuberculosis. It is a body heater, a blood thinner, and a preservative. It is also efficacious for infections of the mouth, throat, upper respiratory tract, stomach, gastrointestinal, genitourinary and skin. It prevents and heals arthritis, kidney, and muscle problems. It aids in the prevention of inflammation, including vascular inflammation. As a bile stimulator, it enhances digestion. It promotes respiratory health by removing excess mucus and facilitates the recovery from respiratory ailments such as bronchitis and asthma. It also promotes sweating, strengthens the immune system, stimulates urine flow, retards tumour growth, builds strong bones, kills and expels parasites, including pinworms, heals bloating and cramps, assists with immunity, protects the circulatory system, destroys Streptococcus and Staphylococcus infections, regulates blood sugar, boosts the metabolism, serves as a poison antidote, blocks carcinogens, removes warts and corns, promotes weight control, helps with abnormal hair loss, alleviates allergies, eliminates toxins, slows the rapid division of cancer cells, enhances DNA repair, kills gram-positive and gram-negative bacteria, heals herpes (when a garlic clove is cut in half and applied to the afflicted area), and destroys harmful bacteria whilst increasing good intestinal flora (fresh and raw is best). Exposed peeled garlic kills viruses and bacteria in the air. Garlic is one of the best foods for detoxification as it stimulates the liver to produce detoxification enzymes. Garlic and cilantro both chelate heavy metals from the body. Garlic has also been scientifically proven to be a much more powerful pro-biotic (meaning *for life*) than any toxic chemical anti-biotic (meaning *against life*), as its antimicrobial properties act against pathogenic gut bacteria whilst sparing beneficial gut bacteria. A study has established that antibiotics that are strong enough to kill gut bacteria also stop the growth of new brain cells in the hippocampus. Research has shown that crushed garlic can help to prevent infection by the bacterium Pseudomonas aeruginosa in burn patients.

"Then He called His twelve disciples together, and gave them power and authority over all devils, and to cure diseases"
(Luke 9:1).

Chemotherapy is not a therapy or even a medicine but is a toxic poison to every living cell. It increases the number of tumour cells circulating in the blood and spreads them to previously unaffected areas of the body, speeding cell death, and creating conditions for the development of future cancers. It causes mitochondrial destruction and the mitochondria is the powerhouse of the cell. These debilitating effects cause oxidative stress, weakness, fatigue, muscle wasting, and

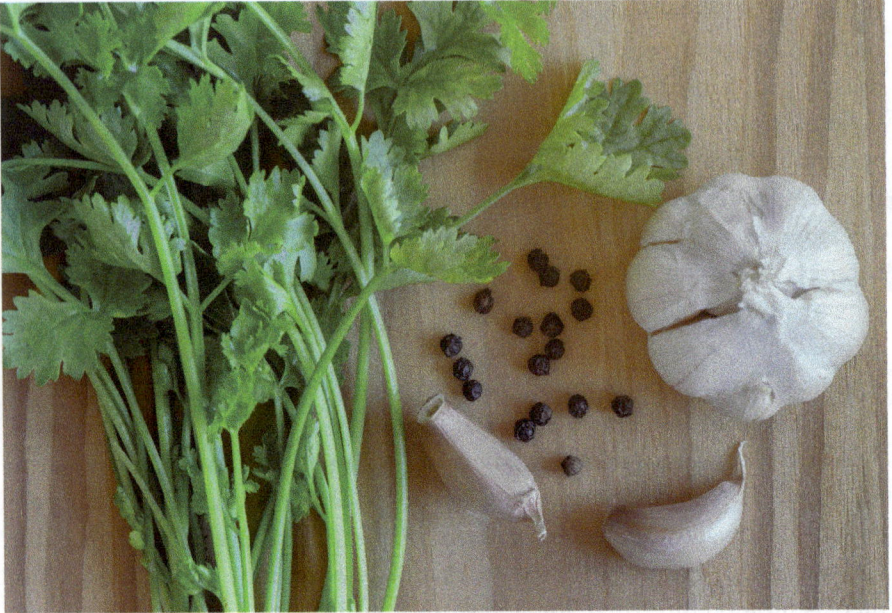

also initiates chronic disease conditions. The reason why so many people die with conventional cytotoxic (toxic to living cells) cancer drugs is that, while damaging healthy cells, these dangerous poisons also trigger them to secrete a protein that sustains tumour growth and is resistant to further protocols. Conversely, the allyl-sulphur compound in garlic preferentially suppresses neoplastic (any abnormal new growth of tissue or tumour) over non-neoplastic cells. Properties within this powerful little bulb produce reactive oxygen species in cancer cells, activating multiple death cascades, and blocking pathways of tumour proliferation. The oil contained in garlic can suppress haematological disorders induced by radiotherapy and chemotherapy. Nefarious chemicals, as proffered by big pharma as the only solution to a sick body, do great harm to the entire system while failing to deal with the root cause of the problem, which is the cancer stem cells. This obscenely sick, chemical medication industry preys upon endless victims with so-called incurable diseases to generate vast corporate profits whilst offering no cures for anything. Commonly subscribed chemotherapy drugs can inflict serious brain damage, resulting in constant brain fog, poor concentration, memory loss, dementia, impaired vision, seizures, and more. Chemotherapy also extensively damages the cells that make myelin, which is the material that insulates the nerve cells and allows them to effectively send signals to each other.

"The face of the LORD is against them that do evil, to cut off the remembrance of them from the earth" (Psalm 34:16).

The medicinal efficacy of garlic is measured by its allicin content. Allicin was discovered in 1944 by the Italian chemist Chester John Cavallito. Allicin is a chemical compound which is sourced from raw garlic and imparts much of the pungent characteristics of garlic. As the primary ingredient responsible for its broad spectrum of anti-bacterial activity, it is an effective weapon against some of the most dangerous bacteria and kills or incapacitates over seventy infectious forms of bacteria. Even in a dilution of 1:85,000–1:250,000, allicin shows anti-bacterial activity against certain gram-positive and gram-negative bacteria.

"Behold, God is mighty, and despiseth not any: He is mighty in strength and wisdom" (Job 36:5).

This amazing little bulb is a rich source of a wide variety of powerful organo-sulphur compounds, which are responsible for its pungent odour and which undergo further chemical modifications when the garlic clove is cut, minced, chopped, or crushed. The chemistry of garlic is exceptionally complex. Fresh garlic contains the enzymes alliinase and alliin, which are contained in different compartments of the garlic. Alliinase is a glycoprotein that catalyses the conversion of alliin (derived from the amino acid cysteine) to powerful allicin. This unique structure is designed as a defence mechanism against microbial pathogens which attack the garlic cloves. The garlic cloves also react the same way to produce powerful allicin when garlic is being prepared for consumption. When the membranes of these compartments are destroyed, within ten seconds the alliinase is released and the alliin is converted into allicin, which is a compound that gives off hydrogen sulphide. This hydrogen sulphide helps to relax the blood vessels and is also responsible for the cancer-fighting properties of garlic. Crushed garlic releases the most allicin because more of its cells are damaged. It is through this natural chemical reaction that allicin is able to fight cancer. Just like Jesus Christ, some plants do not release their full power until they are battered, bruised, and pierced.

"But He was wounded for our transgressions, He was bruised for our iniquities: the chastisement of our peace was upon Him; and with His stripes we are healed" (Isaiah 53:5).

This defence system of the garlic clove is only activated in a very small location for a short period of time, whereas the rest of the alliinase and alliin remain preserved in their respective compartments and are available for subsequent microbial or human attacks. A large amount of generated allicin could be destructive to the remaining plant tissues and enzymes, so the very limited, short-lived manufacture of allicin that is confined to the area where the attack occurs, minimizes self-damage to the plant. Allicin blocks the activity of a peptide called angiotensin II, which helps the blood vessels to contract, thereby forcing the blood to pass through a narrower space. Therefore, allicin helps to prevent undesirable contractions of the blood vessels.

"My defence is of God, which saveth the upright in heart"
(Psalm 7:10).

Allowing the prepared garlic time to rest for at least fifteen minutes before utilizing it will result in the release of its significant health-promoting component allicin. Changing its temperature through immediate cooking without resting, or its pH through the immediate addition of an acidic substance, such as lemon juice, without resting, will lessen its powerful allicin content. Ingredients with a pH below 3.5 can also deactivate the enzymatic process. Consuming garlic and other members of the allium family on a regular basis has obvious benefits for cancer prevention and also helps to build the immune defences, including macrophage, T cell, and natural killer cell activity.

"Look unto me, and be ye saved, all the ends of the earth: for I am God, and there is none else" (Isaiah 45:22).

The allicin in garlic is a very strong and effective natural defence against bacteria, viruses, fungi, and intestinal amoeba without the toxic side effects. It is also a broad-spectrum antimicrobial which is capable of fighting a wide range of infections. By eradicating these pathogens it can help to fight against cancer in several indirect ways. The antibiotic activity of one milligram of allicin is equal to the antibiotic activity of fifteen units of penicillin. Cysteine proteinase enzymes are among the main culprits that cause infections, as they provide infectious organisms such as bacteria, fungi, and viruses with the means to damage and invade tissues. Researchers discovered that very diluted allicin solutions of just one part in 125,000 inhibited the growth of fourteen of fifteen species of bacteria including Streptococcus, Shigella, Staphylococcus, and Vibrio cholerae, which causes cholera. A slightly stronger concentration of allicin was effective against all of the fifteen species.

"The LORD shall fight for you, and ye shall hold your peace" (Exodus 14:14).

Garlic imparts its most healthful properties when eaten in its fresh, raw state, and in this raw state, it acts as a powerful antioxidant by reversing the damage inflicted on cells by cancer-causing free radicals. Research has demonstrated that minimal low-temperature cooking of three minutes or less of this crushed or minced delicious aromatic herb is more beneficial for health than prolonged or high-temperature cooking. If roasting whole garlic, anti-cancer activity is partially retained if the top of the bulb is cut off prior to heating. Commercial garlic formulas often remove the powerful pungent principle allicin and are not as effective as fresh garlic as they cannot be used by the red blood cells in the same way and do not provide the same level of efficacy.

"The voice of the LORD is powerful; the voice of the LORD is full of majesty" (Psalm 29:4).

The powerful and vital trace mineral selenium in garlic can become a significant part of the antioxidant defence system of the body, including supporting immune system function, and selenium, together with the iodine in garlic, is beneficial for the thyroid. As a co-factor of the most important internally produced anti-oxidant enzyme glutathione peroxidase, selenium also works with vitamin E in some vital antioxidant systems. Garlic is an excellent source of the trace mineral manganese, which also operates as a co-factor in some other significant antioxidant defence enzymes, such as superoxide dismutase. Selenium is extremely important for many health issues including eye health, Crohn's disease, and cystic fibrosis. Garlic is not only a good source of selenium; additionally, it may also be a more reliable source and helps to fight tumour growth as selenium kills cancer stem cells. Scientists refer to garlic as a seleniferous plant, as it can uptake selenium from the soil even when soil concentrations do not favour this.

> *Garlic imparts its most healthful properties when eaten in its fresh, raw state, and in this raw state, it acts as a powerful antioxidant by reversing the damage inflicted on cells by cancer-causing free radicals.*

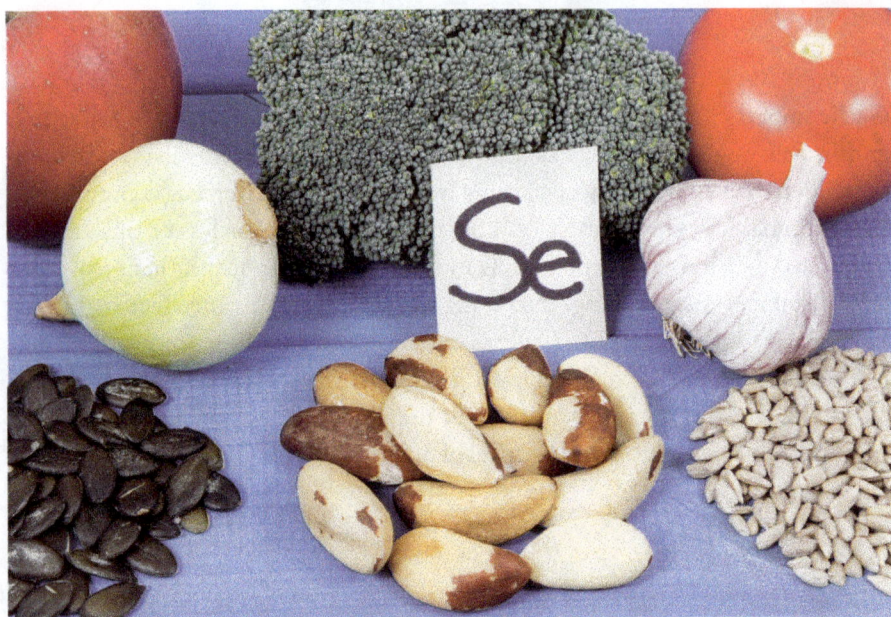

There is an abundance of other whole plant foods that contain selenium including onions, Brazil nuts, sunflower seeds, sesame seeds, flax seeds, whole wheat and whole rye grains, crimini, shiitake, and white button mushrooms, broccoli, spinach, cabbage, pinto beans, lima beans, brown rice, and chia seeds. Selenium is vital for heart health and a deficiency can cause cardiomyopathy. Arrhythmia is an electrical problem in the heart that disrupts the normal heartbeat rhythm. Magnesium and selenium, in particular, have an antiarrhythmic effect on the heart, and a significant deficiency of these nutrients may cause arrhythmia. Adults need between 200 to 300 micrograms of selenium per day, depending on their particular needs (it is best to keep below 400 mcg. a day). Selenium is important for DNA production, thyroid gland function, and reproduction and also protects the body from damage caused by free radicals. As selenium is an anti-inflammatory it not only reduces cancer risks but also fights bacterial and viral infections, assists the body to detoxify, and many other health issues.

"I will walk before the LORD in the land of the living"
(Psalm 116:9).

Garlic supports cardiovascular protection by squelching inflammation and preventing blood vessels from becoming blocked. Clogged blood vessels can occur because of inflammation in the vessel wall. Cholesterol is deposited at these sites in an effort to cover the damage and is not the cause of the problem, as is commonly assumed. A build-up of lactic acid in the heart cells can also cause heart attacks. Vitamin E improves the metabolism of heart cells and can be found in green leafy vegetables, nuts, avocados, papaya, olives, and seeds. Vitamin E reduces platelet aggregation, thereby preventing blood clots. It is naturally designed to prevent fats from becoming rancid and creating toxic free radicals. It also stimulates the formation of new small blood vessels in the heart. Garlic prevents and keeps the platelets from becoming too sticky, and thereby lowers the risk of them clumping together to form internal blood clots that can trigger heart attacks and strokes. Garlic is a good source of iron and low iron causes red blood cells to stick together, which increases the likelihood of blood clots. Being a blood thinner and adaptogenic, garlic allows clotting when needed, even while thinning the blood, and has been repeatedly shown to have anti-clotting properties and thus prevents blood clots, or thrombosis, from forming inside the blood vessels, thereby reducing the risk of cardiovascular disease. It also prevents the oxidation of important lipids that leads to cellular destruction. The polysulphides of garlic dilate the blood vessels and help to boost blood flow. A great quantity of research indicates the widely recognized importance of the role of garlic in preventing and treating many cardiovascular diseases and cancers, the two primary causes of death in developed countries. Medical scientists have sufficient evidence of the potency of garlic to counteract cancers and heart disease.

"Be of good courage, and He shall strengthen your heart, all ye that hope in the LORD" (Psalm 31:24).

Garlic has a curative effect for many pathogenic diseases. By consuming it daily, the body is provided with prophylactic (preventative) protection against pathogens. It kills a broad spectrum of harmful bacteria whilst keeping the friendly intestinal bacteria intact. Research shows that garlic is efficacious for even the very worst types of infections and several garlic phytochemicals contain virus-killing activity against common respiratory viruses. Patients suffering from cryptococcal meningitis, which is usually fatal, were successfully treated and recovered after several weeks of garlic therapy.

"O spare me, that I may recover strength, before I go hence, and be no more" (Psalm 39:13).

As an amazing carrier of oxygen, garlic contains a significant amount of sulphur, which is one of the best oxygen-carrying minerals as sulphur carries the oxygen in the body directly to an infected area. The important sulphur compounds contained in garlic penetrate the red blood cells and are converted to hydrogen sulphide, which not only dilates the blood vessels but also helps to boost the blood flow. The distinctive beneficial characteristics of garlic are mainly attributed to the presence of volatile sulphur-containing compounds, which constitute almost 1% of its dry weight. These compounds are ajoene, allicin, alliin, allyl mercaptan, allylmethyl disulphide, allylmethyl tetrasulphide, allylmethyl trisulphide, diallyl sulphide, diallyl disulphide, diallyl sulphide, diallyl tetrasulphide, diallyl trisulphide, dimethyl trisulphide, L-glutamyl-S-alkyl-l-cysteine, methyl allyl thiosulphinate, 1-propenyl allyl thiosulphinate, S-allyl cysteine, S-allyl mercaptocysteine, 2-vinyl-4-H-1,3-dithiin, 3-vinyl-4-H-1,2-dithin, and 1,2-vinyldithiin, which is one of the unique sulphur substances in garlic that has long been recognized as being anti-inflammatory.

"Sing unto the LORD; for He hath done excellent things: this is known in all the earth" (Isaiah 12:5).

Researchers have confirmed that specific micromolecule organo-sulphur compounds, which are present in garlic, prevent and kill glioblastoma cells (an aggressive form of brain tumour) without disturbing healthy cells, and have demonstrated efficacy in eradicating these brain cancer cells. Glioblastoma is the most prevalent and the most invasive primary malignant type of cancer, while also being the fastest growing lethal brain cancer tumour among all primary brain tumours which are common to adults. This type of tumour originates from the glial cells of the brain and accounts for 20% of all intracranial tumours and 52% of all the brain tissue tumours. Garlic contains sulphone-hydroxyl ions, which are active compounds that can penetrate the blood-brain barrier and enter the brain tissues. Garlic's protective compounds diallyl sulphide, diallyl disulphide, and diallyl trisulphide are easily able to penetrate the blood-brain barrier to induce cancer cell apoptosis and prevent future cell growth as it possesses anti-tumourigenesis effects. According to a published study, these compounds can enter glioblastoma cells and interfere with their metabolism. Ginger and turmeric are also an effective treatment for this type of health issue, and taking ginger, turmeric and garlic together delivers a powerful natural defence system.

"The LORD is my rock, and my fortress, and my deliverer; my God, my strength, in whom I will trust; my buckler, and the horn of my salvation, and my high tower" (Psalm 18:2).

Cancer cells have a high metabolism and require a great deal of energy for rapid growth. They also utilize mechanisms which allow them to evade apoptosis, thereby enabling them to grow. However, garlic not only boosts the immune system but several compounds other than garlic's antibiotic allicin, sulphur, and selenium, contribute to cancer cell apoptosis and one of them is diallyl trisulphide. Apoptosis is the body's normal way of eliminating abnormal or unneeded cells. Cancer stem cells have a pro-survival strategy which promotes their growth and metastasis. These cells are not regulated by normal cell functions but promote inflammation and are able to self-renew. However, they are adversely affected by phytochemicals in the diet which manipulate the pathways of communication between the cancer stem cells and the corresponding cancer cells. Garlic contains the flavonoid quercetin, which kills cancer stem cells and can contribute to preventing damaged cells from becoming cancerous as it has anti-inflammatory effects that encourage cancer prevention. Garlic, onions, and their family members not only contain flavonoids, but also phenols. Red and yellow onions are richer in these antioxidants than white onions, with red onions being particularly rich in quercetin and anthocyanins (which are also abundant in berries). Quercetin is also contained in blueberries, pears, elderberries, romaine lettuce, spinach, kale, red apples, and cranberries. Shallots are especially high in antioxidant polyphenols, which is a generic term for several thousand plant molecules that are the most abundant antioxidants.

"The last enemy that shall be destroyed is death" (1 Corinthians 15:26).

Many cancers are thought to be caused by DNA damage, which could be the result of exposure to environmental toxins. Over sixty years ago, several statistical studies indicated that cancer occurred the least in countries where garlic and onions were regularly consumed. Garlic, like onions, also helps to eliminate waste materials and dangerous free radicals from the body. Even a small amount of this pungent little bulb has the ability to activate liver enzymes that help the body to flush out toxins. The high amounts of allicin and selenium found in garlic are two natural constituents that aid in cleansing the liver.

"That He might sanctify and cleanse it with the washing of water by the word" (Ephesians 5:26).

As one of nature's most broad-spectrum antibacterial agents, garlic has been studied, not only for its ability to fight viral and bacterial infections, but also for its ability to fight infections from other microbes, including worms, fungi, and yeasts. It counteracts the growth of many forms of bacteria and fungi that cause diseases. The ajoene property of garlic not only has powerful anti-leukaemic action but has also been successfully used to help prevent infections with the Candida albicans yeast. Garlic is an antifungal, and research studies have clearly shown its effectiveness against the Candida pathogen as its anti-candidal activity inhibits both the function and growth of Candida albicans. A wide range of scientific literature supports the use of garlic as a proven antifungal and is an easy and simple addition to a Candida treatment plan. Ajoene is formed when allicin combines with the enzyme alliinase and is a key compound in garlic and a proven antifungal. It has been shown to be effective against many fungal strains. As garlic improves immune system functioning, yeast and garlic cannot co-exist. When detoxifying too quickly the body can suffer a Herxheimer reaction, which is a detoxification response that is generally known as die-off symptoms. This response occurs if too many harmful toxins are released into the blood and tissues faster than the body can eliminate them. The body can then become overloaded with toxic waste, which can cause suffering from adverse reaction symptoms. This is usually taken as a positive sign that a beneficial response is happening and the body is cleansing itself, when in fact the opposite is true as creating too many die-off toxins too soon can cause strong debilitating symptoms, which cause a negative reaction that literally poisons the body with an overload of toxic substances. Detoxifying is best performed at a pace that gently assists the body to unload its toxic burden. Unrefined organic coconut oil is an antifungal to which Candida cannot adapt, and it is especially beneficial in establishing a positive environment to ensure the survival of beneficial gut bacteria.

"Behold, I will bring it health and cure, and I will cure them, and will reveal unto them the abundance of peace and truth" (Jerimiah 33:6).

Many scientists are already convinced that garlic contains compounds that are a potential remedy against cancer, and have achieved good therapeutic results. Garlic prevents free radicals from being generated, and it also supports protective mechanisms of the body that destroy free radicals. The unique set of sulphur-containing compounds in garlic helps to protect against oxidative stress and unwanted inflammation. Six powerful phenylpropanoids, which are a diverse family of organic compounds that are synthesized by plants from the amino acid phenylalanine, have been isolated from garlic peel.

"Thou wilt shew me the path of life: in thy presence is fulness of joy; at thy right hand there are pleasures for evermore" (Psalm 16:11).

The antidiabetic effect of garlic has been well documented, even in ancient medical literature. The active ingredients in garlic have been extensively studied for their anti-diabetic efficacy, and it has proven to be effective at reducing insulin resistance. It influences insulin activity instead of directly lowering blood sugar. Garlic is known to regulate blood sugar levels and to increase the amount of insulin released. A published study discovered that not only is garlic highly effective at increasing the insulin content of the body but it also improves glucose tolerance. Allicin competes with insulin for insulin-inactivating sites in the liver, which results in insulin activation and consequently free insulin is increased. Another study showed that garlic has the potential to protect the heart from diabetes-induced cardiomyopathy.

"For thou hast delivered my soul from death, mine eyes from tears, and my feet from falling" (Psalm 116:8).

The sulphur-containing compounds in garlic can help the inflammatory aspects of obesity. Fat cells cannot grow 100% unless they are able to move from a preliminary stage called preadipocytes to a more mature stage called adipocytes. One of the sulphur compounds in garlic halts this progress. Garlic eliminates fat from the cells as well as being a powerful detoxifier, an effective diuretic, and a metabolism booster.

"Therefore shall the Lord, the Lord of hosts, send among His fat ones leanness; and under His glory He shall kindle a burning like the burning of a fire" (Isaiah 10:16).

Garlic contains germanium, which is an anti-cancer agent and an ultra-trace mineral that was discovered by Clemens Alexander Winkler in 1886. Germanium protects against amyloidosis, which occurs when an abnormal amyloid protein accumulates in organs and tissues. It is a serious health issue that can cause life-threatening organ failure. Germanium also induces interferon-gamma levels, which boost the immune system and increase the activity of the macrophages and natural killer cells, which are a part of the defence system of the body. Interferons are glycoproteins that prevent the growth and proliferation of viruses.

"For the LORD is our defence; and the Holy One of Israel is our king" (Psalm 89:18).

Significant research and clinical studies have shown that garlic is a remarkable defence against cancer as it enhances the effectiveness of natural killer cells in the destruction of tumours and cancer cells based on its immune-modulating activity. Natural killer cells are the most powerful infection-fighting cells in the white blood cell arsenal. They kill viruses, fungus, and bacteria and secrete hydrogen peroxide, which kills cancer cells and anaerobic tetanus. It is well known that garlic strengthens the immune system, which is vitally important for fighting cancer. Its anti-carcinogenic properties can heal breast cancer, kidney cancer, lung cancer, pancreatic cancer, oesophageal cancer, prostate cancer, stomach cancer, and brain tumours. It is also able to restrict the blood supply to cancerous tumours.

"Seek the LORD and His strength, seek His face continually" (1 Chronicles 16:11).

The supposed HIV is said to cause an infection which may lead to the development of AIDS, which is a vague range of symptoms that are constantly being changed by the powers that be. Garlic has successfully been used to treat these issues. Very toxic carcinogenic and mutagenic drugs have been prescribed for these varying symptoms, leading to the demise of those who do not realize that good nutrition and lifestyle practices can reverse many unfortunate symptoms. Millions of people have been given positive fraudulent HIV tests and told that they were going to die from AIDS but they died from the effects of the poisonous drugs. Various trials have shown that garlic is effective against common infectious agents, including Cryptococcus (fungus), Cryptosporidium (protozoan parasite), herpes (virus), pneumocystis (fungus), and Mycobacteria, and can obstruct the spread of infectious agents. Garlic enhances the actions of several cell types in the arsenal of the immune system which are important in combating infections. These are phagocytes, which engulf invading germs; lymphocytes, which produce antibodies that kill specific microbes; cytotoxic T-cells, which attach themselves to microbes into which they secrete poisons and natural killer cells which are activated by the diallyl trisulphide in garlic.

"For God sent not His Son into the world to condemn the world; but that the world through Him might be saved" (John 3:17).

The brain is the only organ that is known to have its own security system—a network of blood vessels that allows the entry of essential nutrients whilst blocking other substances. Blood vessels of the brain are lined with endothelial cells that are wedged so tightly together that they create an almost impermeable boundary between the brain and the bloodstream. Scientists have discovered that minuscule, fat-soluble substances and many hormones are capable of slipping through these endothelial cells that comprise the blood-brain barrier, while larger molecules, such as insulin and glucose, need to be transported across with transporter proteins. These proteins, which are located in the blood vessel walls of the brain, selectively transport the desired molecules into the brain from the blood. The cells, which are in constant communication with each other on each side of the blood-brain barrier, know when and which molecules to allow through. They are highly specialized to allow precise control over the substances that enter and leave the brain. Unfortunately, inflammation can weaken the blood-brain barrier, which is why anti-inflammatory antioxidants should be consumed on a regular basis as part of an anti-inflammatory lifestyle.

> *Millions of people have been given positive fraudulent HIV tests and told that they were going to die from AIDS but they died from the effects of the poisonous drugs.*

"But thou, O LORD, art a shield for me; my glory, and the lifter up of mine head" (Psalm 3:3).

Garlic dilates the blood vessels, as does exercise, and is rich in well studied sulphur-containing molecules called polysulphides (two or more sulphur atoms bonded together as a group in a compound). Virtually all of these have been demonstrated to function as antioxidants, and many provide anti-inflammatory benefits. Once inside the red blood cells, these molecules can be further converted by the red blood cells into the gas hydrogen sulphide, which is described as a gasotransmitter. This gas not only helps the blood vessels to expand by triggering the dilation of the blood vessels but is also in the same category as nitric oxide. When the muscles are supplied with blood, the lining of the arteries releases nitric oxide into the blood, which relaxes the blood vessel walls, thus causing vasodilation which allows more blood to flow through. This expansion of blood vessels also reduces cognitive decline and improves brain functioning because it dramatically enhances blood flow to the brain and also functions as a secondary neurotransmitter between the neurons. The powerful nitric oxide vasodilator is a gaseous signalling molecule that the body produces. It enables the body to function more efficiently by assisting the cells to communicate with each other by transmitting signals throughout the entire body, which causes nutrients, oxygen, and red blood cells to arrive at their destination tissues and cells much faster. Nitric oxide also improves the quality of sleep, aids digestion, reduces inflammation, increases strength and endurance, aids the immune system by fighting bacteria and protecting against tumours, increases the sense of smell, and assists with behaviour and memory by transmitting information between neurons.

"Therefore my heart is glad, and my glory rejoiceth: my flesh also shall rest in hope" (Psalm 16:9).

Although garlic does not contain a large amount of nitrates, it does enhance their production by boosting the enzyme nitric oxide synthase. Nitrate is a nitric acid salt and is found naturally in grains, fruits, and vegetables. The highest nitrate content of fruit is in strawberries, followed by currants, gooseberries, cherries, and raspberries. Vegetables that are high in nitrates include spinach, celery, beetroot, green beans, cabbage, parsley, carrots, radishes, lettuce, and collard greens. Nitrate is converted into nitrite in the body almost immediately by bacteria on the tongue. Nitrite eventually becomes nitric oxide in the blood and also displays anti-platelet properties in addition to helping to prevent inappropriate blood clotting.

"In whom we have redemption through His blood, even the forgiveness of sins" (Colossians 1:14).

Garlic has powerful anti-cancer properties, and its allyl sulphides have an essential role in its cancer prevention benefits. These compounds activate a molecule called nuclear factor-erythroid (Nrf2), an antioxidant response element signalling pathway, which controls gene expression. It is a significant mechanism in the cellular defence against oxidative stress in the main compartment of the cells, which then moves into the cell nucleus where it triggers a wide variety of metabolic activities. Occasionally, these events can prepare the cells to engage in a strong survival response that is needed under conditions of oxidative stress. Under different situations, the same events can prepare the cell to engage in apoptosis. Garlic's allyl sulphide ability to activate Nrf2 suggests that garlic is able to help modify these critical cell responses and prevent potential cancerous cells from forming.

"Verily, verily, I say unto you, he that believeth on me hath everlasting life" (John 6:47).

Sulphides, which are available in garlic in large amounts, stop the growth of tumours and inhibit carcinogens. Garlic is among the most important foods that are ingested as a potential weapon against many types of cancer. Regular consumption of raw or minimally heated garlic decreases the risk of stomach and colorectal cancer by around 50%. Epidemiological studies from six different countries have consistently shown that garlic consumption is associated with a decreased risk of gastrointestinal cancer.

"No weapon that is formed against thee shall prosper; and every tongue that shall rise against thee in judgment thou shalt condemn. This is the heritage of the servants of the LORD, and their righteousness is of me, saith the LORD" (Isaiah 54:17).

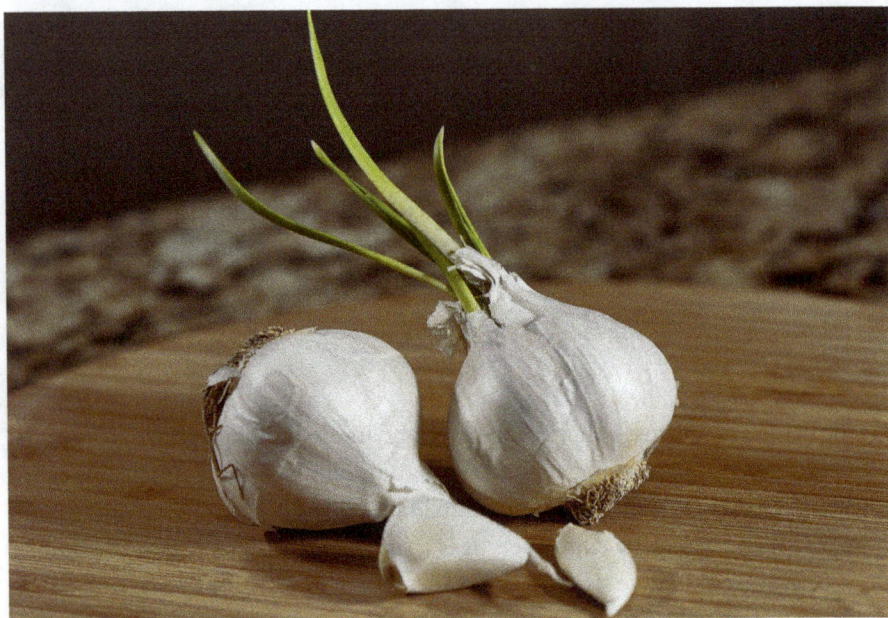

Sprouted garlic has more antioxidant activity than unsprouted garlic. Plants are very susceptible to attacks from viruses, bacteria, and insects during sprouting, causing them to produce a variety of chemicals called phytoalexins to defend themselves. Most of these are toxic to micro-organisms and insects but beneficial to human health. Extracts from garlic that have been sprouted for five days have a higher antioxidant activity than extracts from raw, unsprouted garlic. Sprouting may be a viable method to increase the antioxidant potential of garlic. It enhances raw garlic's proven immune-boosting, anti-inflammatory, and cardiovascular health protection and its ability to kill cancer cells. Researchers have suggested that diallyl sulphide, a compound released when garlic bulbs sprout into cloves, may be at the root of garlic's preventative potential. This active diallyl sulphide compound is known to inactivate potent carcinogens and is able to break through the tough membranes of bacteria better and faster than ineffective injurious antibiotic drugs.

"The LORD will give strength unto His people; the LORD will bless His people with peace" (Psalm 29:11).

Research has shown that garlic may be able to improve the body's metabolism of iron. When iron is stored in the cells, one of the most important pathways for it to be moved out of the cell and returned into circulation involves the protein ferroportin. This protein darts across the cell membrane, providing a bridge that facilitates the stored iron to cross over and leave the cell and become available wherever it is needed. Garlic may have the ability to increase the body's production of ferroportin and help to keep iron in circulation as needed.

"I will go before thee, and make the crooked places straight: I will break in pieces the gates of brass, and cut in sunder the bars of iron" (Isaiah 45:2).

Garlic has also been used successfully to detoxify lead from both children and adults and is a much safer natural detoxifier of this toxic metal. It has efficacy in naturally reducing tissue and blood lead concentrations in mild to moderate lead poisoning. Lead poisoning can be acute or chronic. Exposure to lead results in harm to the skeletal, gastrointestinal, reproductive, renal, cardiovascular, and nervous systems of the body. If left untreated, lead poisoning can damage the kidneys and central nervous system, which can lead to many serious adverse outcomes, and even death. It has been shown to be particularly harmful to infants and children, whose developing nervous systems are much more susceptible to lead toxicity than those of adults. Children who had been exposed to this heavy metal were found to have decreased brain volume in adulthood.

"Thou didst blow with thy wind, the sea covered them: they sank as lead in the mighty waters" (Exodus 15:10).

Deadly anthrax is most susceptible to garlic, which is a broad-spectrum probiotic that has been successfully used as a disease preventative from time immemorial. When tested, garlic was found to be a more potent probiotic than ampicillin, cephalexin, doxycycline, penicillin, and streptomycin, which are some of the very same drugs used in the treatment of anthrax. It was found to be effective against nine strains of E. coli, Staphylococcus, and other harmful microbes. The anthrax bacterium's toxicity emanates from its capability to kill macrophage cells, which are large white blood cells that are an integral part of the immune system. Macrophage cells locate microscopic foreign bodies and use the process of phagocytosis (engulf or ingest particles or cells) to eliminate them.

"And the Lord shall deliver me from every evil work, and will preserve me unto His heavenly kingdom: to whom be glory for ever and ever. Amen" (2 Timothy 4:18).

A traditional Chinese healing method for tuberculosis involves placing a thick compress of crushed, raw garlic onto a cloth on the back of those who are afflicted and then covering the garlic with a clean damp towel. A laundry iron is then used to heat the compress, which forces the garlic fumes through the skin into the chest cavity, where the bacteria are killed that are responsible for the ailment. Its pungency can also provide relief for those who suffer from chronic bronchitis or other lung disorders because of its airway clearing capabilities.

"And the LORD God formed man of the dust of the ground, and breathed into his nostrils the breath of life; and man became a living soul" (Genesis 2:7).

The odour of garlic tends to linger after it has been consumed. This is due to the fact that garlic releases the enzyme allyl methyl sulphide (which has a strong odour) when consumed, and can remain in the body for up to twenty-four hours. The resulting gas emanating from this enzyme becomes absorbed into the blood where it is transferred to the lungs for exhalation. It can also be excreted through the pores of the skin. Lemon juice neutralizes the allyl methyl sulphide enzyme, which helps to dissipates the odour.

"By the word of the LORD were the heavens made; and all the host of them by the breath of His mouth" (Psalm 33:6).

Garlic is a good source of prebiotics, which are non-digestible plant fibres that help beneficial probiotic gut bacteria to grow and flourish in the digestive system and also act as food for probiotics as fibre is the food source of prebiotics. Recommendations for the amount of prebiotics for general digestive health range from about five to eight grams per day. Three large garlic cloves provide about two grams of prebiotics (garlic contains 17.5% fibre by weight). Foods that are high in fibre, such as fruits, vegetables, grains, legumes, nuts, and seeds are also high in prebiotics. When healthy quantities of prebiotics feed the probiotics it causes these live gut bacteria to function more efficiently and produce a healthier gut environment. Stimulation of gastric juice secretion and the restoration of intestinal flora combined with the resulting prevention of gastrointestinal auto-intoxication helps to remove some causes of cancer. The antimicrobial properties of garlic act against pathogenic gut bacteria with relative sparing of the beneficial and friendly gut bacteria.

"For our heart shall rejoice in Him, because we have trusted in His holy name" (Psalm 33:21).

Outstanding garlic has a long history of killing parasites, and it also controls secondary fungal infections. Its antioxidant properties protect against oxidation, which is caused by the toxins produced by parasites. Garlic is able to target parasitic infestations, which have many symptoms, and even though it has powerful effects it does not negatively affect the beneficial gut flora and bacteria in the digestive system but gently stimulates elimination while also detoxifying. Allicin and ajoene are the active components in garlic which contribute to its ability to kill various parasites, including hookworms, pinworms, and amoebas—even one-cell varieties. To ward off all types of parasites from dogs and to eliminate the parasite Giardia from them, garlic is recommended, as it is a vermifuge (anti-parasitic). The recommended daily dose for dogs weighing ten to fifteen pounds is half a clove, fifteen to forty pounds is one clove, forty to seventy pounds is two cloves, seventy to ninety pounds is two and a half cloves, and one hundred and more pounds is three cloves. An effective anti-parasitic regime for both humans and canines alike would be to consume garlic, ginger, and turmeric on a regular basis. Garlic is also useful for dogs as a pest repellant.

> *God-given garlic is necessary for everyday life and has been used for medicinal treatments of many different ailments from ancient civilizations until now, and its intake should be as frequent as possible as it has tremendous health benefits.*

"Ask, and it shall be given you; seek, and ye shall find; knock, and it shall be opened unto you: For every one that asketh receiveth; and he that seeketh findeth; and to him that knocketh it shall be opened" (Matthew 7:7, 8).

God-given garlic is necessary for everyday life and has been used for medicinal treatments of many different ailments from ancient civilizations until now, and its intake should be as frequent as possible as it has tremendous health benefits. It is a powerful, safe, time-tested, affordable, and easily accessible natural healing agent that is extremely beneficial for numerous applications. Consequently, it appears logical to use this delicious, pungent bulb in as many ways as possible for prevention as well as healing.

"Behold, He cometh with clouds; and every eye shall see Him, and they also which pierced Him: and all kindreds of the earth shall wail because of Him. Even so, Amen" (Revelation 1:7).

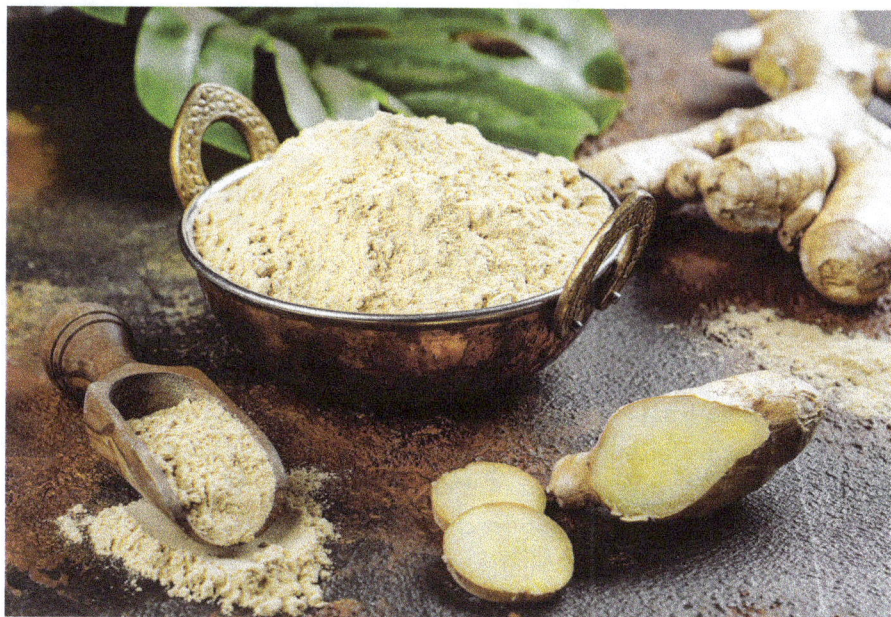

Chapter 5

Ginger

"REAL MEDICINE COMES FROM THE EARTH, NOT A LABORATORY."

Ginger (Zingiber officinale) was used as a flavouring long before history was formally recorded. It was of great medicinal and economic importance in ancient history and is among the truly great natural healing plants of the world. The properties of ginger make it one of the most unique and potent disease-fighting plants God ever created—not only for our benefit, but also for the benefit of animals and has many applications.

The origin of the word ginger is from the Old English word *gingifer*. This was readopted and became the Middle English word *gingivere*, which is from the Old French word *gingivre*. From Sanskrit comes the word *srngaveram*, which means *horn root,* because of its appearance. In Latin, it was called *zinziberi,* and in Greek, it was called *ziggiberis.*

This powerful, aromatic, pungent, and spicy flowering herbaceous perennial belongs to the same fragrant family of Zingiberaceae plants that produce an enormous amount of highly scented oils such as cardamom, turmeric, zedoary (white turmeric), and galangal, which have been used for centuries. The unique flavour and fragrance of ginger emanate from its natural oils, of which gingerol is outstanding.

Ginger is both a herb and a food, as is turmeric and garlic. It has been used as a safe medicine for millennia by a wide range of world cultures and features many of the same properties as its near relative, turmeric. The ancient Egyptians cultivated ginger and used it in their cooking to keep epidemics at bay. Ancient literature describes its impact from Asia, the Middle East, and Europe and it has been prized by many different cultures for thousands of years. There are approximately 1,600 varieties of ginger, and from its first use until the present, it is the most widely cultivated plant in the world. Most of the world's ginger is produced by India, followed by China and Nepal. The ginger plants grown in India show the largest numbers of genetic variations, indicating that the plant has grown for a longer period of time in that region. Though originating in Southeast Asia, it has a long history of being cultivated in other countries and was considered a tonic for every ailment by the early Indians and ancient Chinese. The Chinese records chronicled the enormous wealth that was associated with growing ginger, which has been a trading commodity longer than most other herbs. This delicious aromatic herb has influenced early history since the time of ancient China. The Chinese have been using it as a medicine for about 4,000 years, and references to its use are found in Chinese pharmacopoeias. Wars were fought and whole dynasties rose and fell with the objective of seizing it, and the trading of such plants was the basis of the world's economy for many centuries. Confucius wrote of ginger as being a digestive aid as far back as 500 BC and of never being without it when he ate. There is also recent evidence that ginger was traded in Greece in 300 BC. It could be found in commerce in Europe long before the days of Jesus Christ and has been the herb of choice for thousands of years.

In the famous De Materia Medica of AD 77, Pedanius Dioscorides the Greek (AD 40–90) recorded that ginger "warms and softens the stomach" and recommended its use as a stomachic, to help a sluggish system, and as a stimulant of digestion. He was a pharmacologist, physician, and botanist as well as the author of *De Materia Medica,* a five-volume pharmacopoeia of herbal medicine and related medicinal substances that was widely read for more than 1,500 years. Ginger was exported from India to ancient Rome at an early date and was used extensively by the Romans and Greeks who used it both medicinally and as a spice in cooking. The Romans used ginger in ophthalmics for advanced cataracts, for which a ginger preparation was made and applied to the eyes several times a day. When the Roman Empire fell, ginger almost disappeared, but the Arabs took control of the spice trade and ginger became a costly herb, as did many spices. The Greeks and Romans obtained the herb from Arab traders, and it was one of the first far-eastern herbs to arrive in Europe, where it was re-discovered and became popular again. By the first century, Arab traders had taken ginger to the Mediterranean regions.

Fifth-century Chinese mariners used the vitamin C from fresh ginger to ward off scurvy many hundreds of years before British surgeon Dr. James Lind discovered that limes could prevent scurvy on long voyages. It was also used by Welsh physicians in AD 507, and by the eleventh century, ginger was well known in England. St. Hildegarde, a twelfth-century German healer, recommended it as a stimulant and tonic and used its effectiveness for eye diseases. Explorers such as Marco Polo (1254–1324) and Vasco da Gama (1460s–1524) carefully documented the cultivation of ginger. During the thirteenth and fourteenth centuries, Arabs travelled to Zanzibar and Africa where they planted the rhizomes, thereby spreading its cultivation. In the fourteenth century, a half-kilogram of ginger was equal in value to one whole live sheep. In the fifteenth century, ginger plants were transported on ships to Africa and the Caribbean island of Jamaica, where it became popular and could be easily cultivated as it blooms in the wild. In the sixteenth century, Henry VIII suggested it as a remedy for the plague. Today ginger is grown freely throughout the humid tropics and sub-tropics.

Ginger is a flavoursome herb that is valued for its strong and lively flavour. It has been revered throughout the ages for its numerous health benefits while also being warming with a slightly sweet, distinctive, peppery flavour and a spicy, zesty aroma. It is produced from the rhizome (underground stem), or tubers, of the plant and is available in white, red, and yellow varieties. The rhizome is the horizontal stem from which the firm, striated, textured roots grow, and is the portion of ginger that is generally consumed. These rhizomes are known as *hands* as they often consist of several finger-like protuberances that can resemble gnarled arthritic hands, an affliction that ginger can help to alleviate as it is anti-arthritic. These *hands* are covered with a pale brownish skin which may

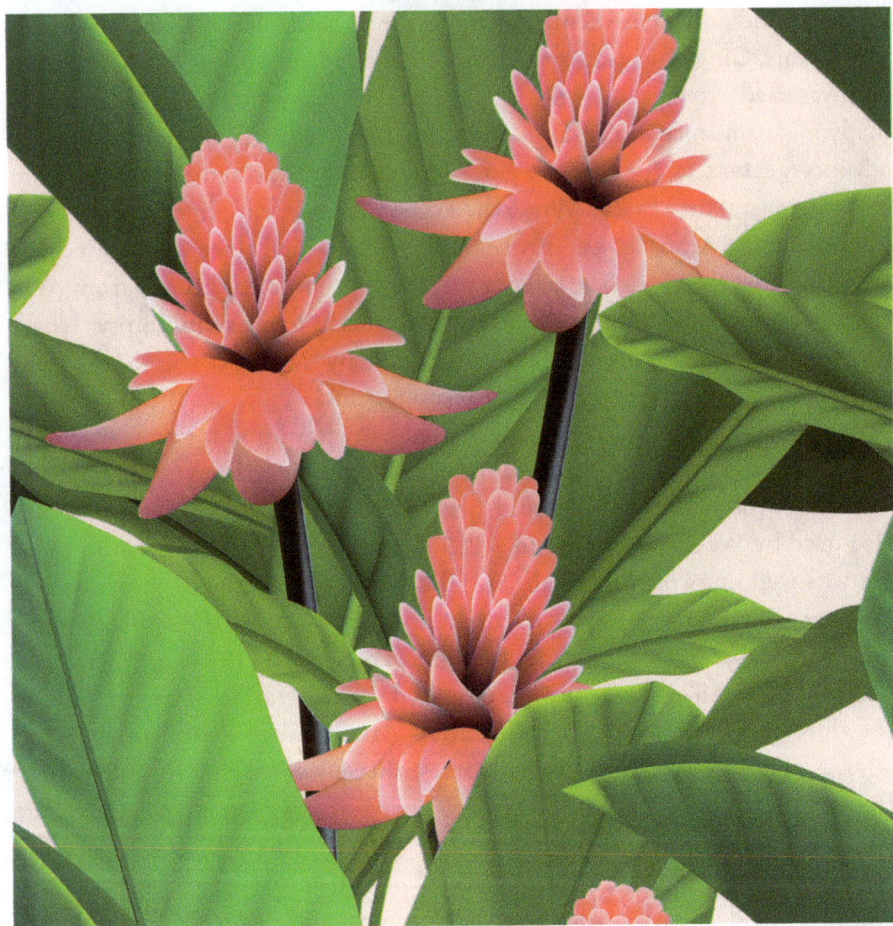

either be thin or thick, depending upon whether the plant was harvested when it was young or mature. The leafy stems grow to about a metre in height and the plants are propagated by planting rootstalk cuttings.

"Be ye strong therefore, and let not your hands be weak: for your work shall be rewarded" (2 Chronicles 15:7).

This multifaceted, aromatic plant has many medicinal uses. The fresh or dried rhizome is used in oral or topical preparations to treat a variety of ailments, while the essential oil is applied topically as an analgesic. Ginger has been referred to as a synergistic herb as it enhances other herbs by rendering them more effective. It is well researched and many of its traditional uses have been confirmed. In the scientific literature, there are over 2,100 published studies on its medicinal properties. Its powerful health benefits are astounding and have been extensively studied for over 170 different health conditions as well as over fifty different beneficial physiological effects. It has an extremely high level of phytochemicals and antioxidants and more than 400 components in fresh and dried ginger have been identified. This high concentration of active substances makes it one of the most versatile, evidence-based remedies in the world. Ginger contains potent proteolytic enzymes which facilitate the breakdown of rogue proteins in the bloodstream and soft tissues of the body. These enzymes are several hundred times more potent than the papain enzyme contained in papaya. It also has broad-spectrum antiviral, antiparasitic, and antibacterial properties, which are just a few of its forty-plus distinct pharmacological actions.

"Many, O LORD my God, are thy wonderful works which thou hast done, and thy thoughts which are to us-ward: they cannot be reckoned up in order unto thee: if I would declare and speak of them, they are more than can be numbered" (Psalm 40:5).

Powerful ginger has proven amazing medicinal properties with a wide range of molecular mechanisms working simultaneously. The main constituents in ginger rhizomes are 50%–70% carbohydrates, which are present as starches. Oleoresin provides 4%–7.5% of the pungent principles of various bioactive compounds, including gingerol homologues, shogaol homologues, zingerone, gingerdione, vallinoids, and paradols (which are active ingredients to reduce pain), plus volatile oils. Volatile oils are present in 1%–3% concentrations and mostly consist of zingiberene, beta-bisabolene, and sesquiterpenes, which include zingiberenol and zingiberol. The concentration of lipids in ginger is 3%–8% and includes the free fatty acids: capric acid, lauric acid, linoleic acid, linolenic acid, myristic acid, oleic acid, palmitic acid, and also lecithins. Numerous monoterpenes are also present, as are amino acids, phytosterols, raw fibre, protein, vitamins, minerals, and ash. At least thirty-one gingerol-related compounds have been identified from the extracts of fresh ginger rhizomes. Gingerols possess a hot taste, and shogaols are approximately twice as hot. The primary active ingredients in ginger are terpenes, which are substances that inhibit the reproduction of cancer cells, preventing their spread and leading to their death, of which gingerols and the ginger oil oleo-resin belong. It also contains zingibain, which dissolves parasites and their eggs. Studies show that zingibain has been shown to kill the anisakid worm, which is a parasite sometimes carried in raw fish such as sushi.

"This also cometh forth from the LORD of hosts, which is wonderful in counsel, and excellent in working" (Isaiah 28:29).

In addition to containing a variety of volatile essential oils, ginger also contains vitamin B3, vitamin B6, vitamin C, calcium, choline, folate, iron, lipids, magnesium, phosphorus, potassium, quercetin, starch, sulphur, resins, and zinc. It also contains numerous beneficial anti-inflammatory and antioxidant compounds such as beta-carotene, curcumin, capsaicin, caffeic acid, and salicylate.

"He loveth righteousness and judgment: the earth is full of the goodness of the LORD" (Psalm 33:5).

Ginger has many powerful therapeutic qualities which are anti-ageing, anti-allergenic, anti-arthritic, anti-asthmatic, anti-atherogenic, antibacterial, anti-carcinogenic, anti-clotting, anti-diabetic, anti-diarrhoeal, anti-emetic, antifungal, anti-hyperglycemic, anti-infective, anti-inflammatory, anti-ischaemic, anti-malarial, anti-metastatic, antimicrobial (including salmonella), anti-nausea, anti-parasitic, antiphlogistic (prevents or relieves inflammation), anti-proliferative, antipyretic, antiseptic, antispasmodic, antithrombotic, anti-toxic, anti-tumourigenic, antitussive, anti-ulcer, antiviral, anxiolytic, apoptotic, cytotoxic (to cancer stem cells) and detoxifying. It is also an analgesic, antibiotic, anti-coagulant, antidepressant, antihistamine, antioxidant, appetite stimulant, energy enhancer, and intestinal spasmolytic (a substance which relaxes and soothes the intestinal tract). It is a blood-thinner, bowel and kidney cleanser, cardiotonic, carminative, circulatory stimulant, diaphoretic, digestive, diuretic, heart stimulant, hormone balancer, mild laxative, pain reliever, peripheral blood vessel relaxer, stomachic, sudorific, tonic, and vermifuge. It is immune-protective, immuno-modulatory, lymph-cleansing, neuroprotective, neurorestorative, and radioprotective. It is also an epigenetic and expectorant.

"Oh that men would praise the LORD for His goodness, and for His wonderful works to the children of men!" (Psalm 107:21).

Being a powerful anti-inflammatory, ginger assuages chronic inflammation, an underlying cause of diseases, but not the root cause. Studies have demonstrated that it has been highly effective at preventing and healing a wide variety of diseases and health issues over the centuries, including many cancers such as glioblastoma (brain cancer), colds, coughs, congestion, flu, fevers, chillblains, constipation, toothache, ulcers, bursitis, allergies, heartburn, heart disease, arthritis,

Candida, tendonitis, food poisoning, dysentery, meningitis, rheumatism, asthma, bronchitis, osteoarthritis, DNA damage, cholera, macular degeneration, cataracts, diarrhoea, nausea, dizziness, travel and morning sickness, vomiting, rabies, tetanus, leprosy, obesity, diabetes, depression, pain, dysmenorrhea, sciatica, bursitis, pyrosis (heartburn), epilepsy, malaria, inflammation, endothelial and epithelial dysfunction, flatulence, dyspepsia, angina, colic, migraine, Alzheimer's and Parkinson's disease, diverticulitis, Salmonella, haemorrhage, irritable bowel, food poisoning, stroke and aneurysm protection, poor circulation, urinary problems, liver and kidney problems, menstrual issues and menopause, chills, stomachache and digestive issues, immune diseases, sore throats, spinal and joint pain, muscle spasms, cramps, viral infections, nervousness, minor burns, repetitive strain injury, and radiation. As an anti-fungal, it has already been established that ginger has powerful qualities that fight against Candida growth. But it may be contraindicated for those who have gallbladder problems as it may provoke a flare-up due to its powerful action.

"Now when the sun was setting, all they that had any sick with divers (various) diseases brought them unto Him; and He laid His hands on every one of them, and healed them" (Luke 4:40).

Ginger is accessible, time-tested, affordable, powerfully potent, and is abundantly superior to dangerous life-destroying pharmaceutical drugs at defeating cancer. Gingerols and shogaols are bioactive anti-inflammatory compounds that are found in abundance in ginger. A study conducted at the Rajiv Gandhi Centre for Biotechnology in India declared that 6-shagaol is 10,000 times more powerful than conventional chemotherapy at killing cancer stem cells. Powerful 6-shagoal induces apoptosis in leukaemia cells. While cancer stem cells are subject to the destructive effects of 6-shagaol it is harmless to non-cancerous cells, thereby displaying selective cytotoxicity and preventing the formation of tumours. A tumour requires new blood vessel development (angiogenesis), and the most important factor associated with the induction and maintenance of new vasculature in tumours is the vascular endothelial growth factor (VEGF). A study demonstrated that 6-shagaol inhibits angiogenesis-dependent tumours and is produced during the heating and drying of ginger roots. Another major component of ginger is 6-gingerol. Gingerols are the principal pungent compounds that are present in ginger rhizomes. Gingerols induce apoptosis in gastric cancer cells and leukaemia cells. Ginger is a powerful plant that selectively targets the root cause of tumour malignancy, which is the complex immunity of the cancer stem cell-based tumours. These destructive effects of ginger act only on cancer stem cells but do not harm non-cancerous cells. This is the crucial difference between ginger and the extremely lethal traditional cancer protocols that do not exhibit this kind of selective cytotoxicity and therefore do great harm to the body. As with other stem cells, cancer stem cells possess the ability to differentiate into various cell types. They differentiate into the various malignant cells that comprise a tumour colony and only comprise 0.2% to 1% of the cellular composition of a tumour. They also split off to form new tumour colonies. Cancer stem cells are capable of self-renewal and continuous differentiation. If these stem cells are not destroyed, they will create even more cancer cells that can metastasize.

Although cancer stem cells comprise a minute part of a tumour, they can regenerate the original tumour. Cancer stem cells can migrate through the blood vessels and spread cancer to secondary locations. Ginger has the effective ability to outperform many dangerous and toxic cancer drugs, which have not only been shown to be severely and completely ineffective at permanently shrinking tumours, but they actually cause tumours to grow larger and cause a quicker demise of the body. More specifically, the tumours have been found to be very aggressive, and they return bigger and stronger than their original size. There are no drugs in clinical use that specifically target the cancer stem cell population within a tumour. Cancer stem cells pose a serious obstacle to traditional toxic cancer protocols, as they are responsible for a poor prognosis and tumour relapse. Therefore any harmless natural substance that displays promise towards the destruction of cancer stem cells is a highly desirable step towards cancer treatment and should be part of a protocol to eradicate them. Conventional rapacious methods actually increase the populations of cancer stem cells, and if the cancer stem cell population is not destroyed, the tumours will regrow with a heightened vengeance and metastatic invasiveness, resulting in the survival of the cancer. These premium-priced, pernicious drugs are little more than a death sentence for many people. The medicinal properties of ginger far surpass the most advanced pharmaceutical inventions and have also been proven to provide significant benefits against radiation-induced lethality if taken before radiation is encountered.

> *Ginger is accessible, time-tested, affordable, powerfully potent, and is abundantly superior to dangerous life-destroying pharmaceutical drugs at defeating cancer.*

"The LORD preserveth all them that love Him: but all the wicked will He destroy" (Psalm 145:20).

Ginger also inhibits cell invasion, adhesion, motility, and activities of cancer cells. It contains bioactive natural compounds, which have proven epigenetic benefits and have a positive effect on cancers. Simple non-irradiated and non-GM ginger root powder can cause cancer cells to commit apoptosis, and research has found that it kills a range of cancer cells including skin cancer, colon cancer, rectal cancer, breast cancer, stomach cancer, prostate cancer, pancreatic cancer, lung cancer, liver cancer, melanoma, and other skin cancers. In laboratory studies, ginger extracts have shown potent activity against any type of cancer cells, including leukaemia, kidney cancer, skin cancer, lung cancer, and pancreatic cancer cells. It also suppresses the metastasis of lung cancer, prostate cancer, pancreatic cancer, liver cancer, breast cancer, colon cancer, and leukaemia. Cancer metastasis is responsible for 90% of all cancer deaths.

"Then they cried unto the LORD in their trouble, and He saved them out of their distresses" (Psalm 107:13).

Next to turmeric, powerful ginger is one of the world's most potent disease-fighting plants. It is also one of the best analgesics in the world and reduces pain-causing prostaglandin levels in the body, as it mitigates acute and chronic pain, including muscular. Phytonutrient gingerols are one of the primary active constituents in fresh root ginger, giving it its distinctive pungent flavour. Its spicy aroma is mainly due to the presence of vanillyl ketones. Gingerols are slightly reduced in dried ginger, which can be used for all the same applications that fresh ginger is utilized for. Research has shown that these substances can prevent joint inflammation and have exhibited reductions in pain and improvements in movement. Historically, anti-inflammatory ginger was one of the most respected herbs to use for joint health, and it is indicated for arthritis, osteoarthritis, and rheumatoid arthritis when taken on a regular basis. Ginger is a powerful tool for fighting these painful health issues because of its heat-stimulating characteristics. Researchers discovered that those with arthritis and osteoarthritis experienced a significant decrease in pain levels when ginger compresses were applied to an affected area, as it has the ability to decrease inflammation and reduce pain due to its powerful anti-inflammatory activity. When using ginger, 75% of arthritis patients and 100% of patients with muscular discomfort experienced relief from pain and swelling. A hot bath with slices of ginger is soothing for aching muscles. Ginger increases peripheral circulation and brings blood to the surface of the body. It is thereby an effective remedy for chilblains and is used clinically for cold hands and feet. Chilblains are areas of painful inflammation of small blood vessels in the skin that occur in response to repeated exposure to cold but not freezing air.

"Our help is in the name of the LORD, who made heaven and earth" (Psalm 124:8).

The medicinal properties of ginger are powerful and well known for their ability to shrink tumours, including mammary tumours. Researchers have ascertained that ginger inhibits the proliferation of breast cancer cells and causes apoptosis of breast carcinoma cells. They have also discovered that the 6-shogaol in ginger is superior at targeting breast cancer stem cells in several different ways. These include altering the cell cycle to increase the cancer cell death rate, inhibiting tumour formation and directly inducing apoptosis and cytotoxicity (poisoning) to cancer stem cells. It also inhibits breast cancer spheroids (lumps) from forming. Studies have shown that gingerols have breast cancer-fighting abilities including anti-metastasis.

"And He said to the woman, Thy faith hath saved thee; go in peace" (Luke 7:50).

Nausea has a great deal to do with nerve centres, receptors, and nerve endings. Motion sickness has everything to do with sensory perception and is usually an imbalance between the input from the visual and vestibular (inner ear) systems. It is often caused by dehydration, due to the inner ear not being lubricated with enough fluid and becoming viscous. It is thought that ginger works to desensitize the nerves that create the nauseous feeling. Ginger has a long history of consistently proving its effectiveness at reducing nausea and dizziness, and evidence suggests that it is most effective against vomiting, vertigo, travel sickness, and morning sickness. Its anti-vomiting action has been shown to be very useful at reducing the nausea and vomiting of pregnancy, even in its most severe form—hyperemesis gravidum, a condition that usually requires hospitalization. Unlike dangerous anti-vomiting drugs, which can cause severe birth defects, ginger is extremely safe, and only a small dose is required. It has a definite action on the nerves and can also prevent nausea following surgery.

"For, behold, I create new heavens and a new earth: and the former shall not be remembered, nor come into mind" (Isaiah 65:17).

Treasured for its warming and pain-relieving properties, ginger can significantly reduce dysmenorrhea, that is, discomfort throughout the menstrual cycle. Ginger may also help to control heavy menstrual bleeding. A healthy diet and lifestyle can significantly ameliorate these conditions. Research suggests that because ginger is an anti-inflammatory it can inhibit the body's excessive production of prostaglandins, which are a class of pro-inflammatory chemicals that are involved in triggering smooth muscle contractions to enable the uterus to shed its lining. Inflammation causes menstrual pain and ginger contains anti-inflammatory magnesium. Magnesium-rich foods include dark leafy greens, nuts, seeds, beans, whole grains, avocados, bananas, pumpkin seeds, and dried fruit.

"Look upon mine affliction and my pain; and forgive all my sins"
(Psalm 25:18).

This unusually shaped root is excellent at soothing and aiding digestive disorders and the intestinal tract. It also increases gastric juice secretion, which in turn facilitates proper digestion, helps to relieve gastrointestinal irritation, and stimulates the appetite along with saliva flow and bile production. With these improvements, the food is digested quicker and thereby creates an unfriendly environment for unhealthy bacteria. By stimulating pancreatic and gastric enzyme secretions, ginger improves the assimilation and absorption of essential nutrients. Ginger is also instrumental in boosting the immune system and healthy gut bacteria. The volatile oils in ginger have a powerful bacteria-killing capacity, and these volatile oils can kill bacteria along the digestive tract and also help with food poisoning. Ginger is known to promote gastrointestinal peristalsis and kidney function and also helps to flush out the system. It also relieves stomach ache, promotes digestion, and is known to be efficacious in many digestive disorders. Studies have confirmed that ginger has shown dramatic results for non-alcoholic fatty liver disease, which can be caused by over-eating.

"The LORD is righteous in all His ways, and holy in all His
works" (Psalm 145:17).

Ginger root kills ovarian cancer cells with zero toxicity. It is an outstanding herb for annihilating ovarian cancer cells, which die by apoptosis. This ability effectively and significantly inhibits the proliferation of ovarian cancer cell growth, which is the most lethal gynaecological malignancy. Most primary ovarian cancers arise from malignant transformation of the surface epithelium. Inflammation, which is a precursor to ovarian cancer, is controlled by the action of ginger root. Studies show that ginger inhibits the growth and modulates the secretion of angiogenic factors in ovarian cancer cells.

"He only is my rock and my salvation; He is my defence; I shall not be greatly moved" (Psalm 62:2).

The phenolic compounds in ginger root are stimulating and promote healthy circulation, which is beneficial for the whole body. Ginger's naturally warming effect and perspiration-inducing properties may also be useful with fevers, as warming the body encourages the release of toxins. It is a protective agent and viable antidote against fatal poisoning from toxic substances such as heavy metals, medications, fungal toxins, environmental pollutants, and pesticides. It also has protective effects against chemical and radiation-induced toxicities.

"But as it is written, Eye hath not seen, nor ear heard, neither have entered into the heart of man, the things which God hath prepared for them that love Him" (1 Corinthians 2:9).

Ginger is known to be significantly more powerful than toxic drugs at defeating inflammation and cancer and has also been used medicinally for decades for its anti-inflammatory properties in treating a variety of cardiovascular conditions. Toxins that enter the bloodstream are also associated with the onset of heart disease, strokes, and multiple sclerosis. However, ginger improves blood circulation, which in turn helps to rid the body of deadly toxins. As an anti-clotting agent, ginger helps the blood platelets to become less sticky, which inhibits the platelets from clumping together in the bloodstream, thereby thinning the blood and reducing the risk of blood clots. Blood clots that can trigger heart attacks and strokes dissolve when exposed to ginger because it interferes with the long sequence of events necessary for blood clots to form. This helps to avert clots that can lodge in narrowed coronary arteries and trigger a heart attack. Thromboxane synthesis (any of several compounds that stimulate platelet aggregation and vasoconstriction) initiates clot formation, and ginger is a potent inhibitor of this process. Ginger inhibits blood clots more effectively than garlic or onion, and as a cardiotonic agent, it also increases the production of energy and the strength of the heart.

"The LORD is nigh unto them that are of a broken heart; and saveth such as be of a contrite spirit" (Psalm 34:18).

One of many healing compounds found in ginger root is the sleep-regulating hormone melatonin, which conducts several important functions in the body. Melatonin is known to act as a powerful antioxidant, and even small amounts of it are able to aid in raising glutathione levels. Ginger root contains about 500 picograms of melatonin per gram (1,000,000 picograms = 1 milligram). Melatonin is produced by the pineal gland, which is responsible for regulating sleep and wake cycles and is often considered to be the natural pacemaker of the body. The pineal gland is so called because it resembles the shape of a pinecone. It is a tiny endocrine gland that is located deep in the centre of the brain and is influenced by light. It plays an instrumental role in signalling the time of the day and year, thereby helping to regulate the internal body clock. Other melatonin-producing food sources that significantly assist with boosting the circulating melatonin are tart cherries, raspberries, tomatoes, almonds, sunflower seeds, rice, corn, and fennel.

"Upon this I awaked, and beheld; and my sleep was sweet unto me" (Jeremiah 31:26).

Research reveals that in every case where ginger powder was used to treat cancer cells, the cells all died as a result of being exposed to this herb. Studies have shown that ginger kills cancer cells in two ways: through apoptosis and autophagy. In apoptosis, the cancer cells are programmed to commit suicide while leaving the surrounding healthy cells untouched. In autophagy, cancerous cells are tricked into digesting themselves because when ginger is present the cancer cells attack each other. Whole ginger extract has powerful death-inducing and growth-inhibiting effects on a range of cancer cells as a result of interrupting cancer cell-cycle advancement, impairing cancer reproduction, and modulating apoptosis.

"Seek the LORD, and His strength: seek His face evermore" (Psalm 105:4).

The health benefits of this super-herb extend beyond cancer. A clinical trial showed that ginger improved insulin sensitivity and lowered insulin levels in adults with diabetes. It helps to regulate blood sugar by stimulating pancreatic cells and may assist in the prevention of the progression of type 2 diabetes through its hypoglycemic effects. Ginger also has a protective effect on diabetes complications, including protecting the diabetic's central nervous system, liver, kidneys, and eyes. It is not known to contain any measurable amounts of oxalates or purines.

"And all these blessings shall come on thee, and overtake thee, if thou shalt hearken unto the voice of the LORD thy God" (Deuteronomy 28:2).

Ginger also works well for repetitive strain injury, of which carpal tunnel syndrome is one example. Repetitive strain injury occurs when movements of the body are frequently repeated, thereby causing a strain in an area. Ginger can be taken internally in therapeutic doses and also applied externally as a poultice to a problem area. Consuming high levels of antioxidants, such as berries, has proven to be an effective therapy for this painful affliction, as it also reduces the inflammatory response.

"But the LORD is my defence; and my God is the rock of my refuge" (Psalm 94:22).

This knobbly root has been proven to be an effective miracle healer when treating prostate cancer as it is known for its ability to shrink tumours and has been proven to target and destroy cancer cells and cancer stem cells. Studies on a spectrum of prostate cancer cells show that whole ginger extract brings to bear powerful death-inducing and growth-inhibiting effects with zero toxicity. Studies have shown that ginger extract blocks lipoxygenase-5 (LOX-5) enzymes and cyclooxygenase-2 (COX-2) enzymes. LOX-5 enzymes are the only food for prostate cancer cells, which die in one to two hours without these enzymes. It also inhibits the COX-2 enzymes, which produce prostaglandins that promote inflammation and pain. Stem cells, being the root cells, can form various types of cancers. These stem cells further form offspring cells which invade the body. A tumour comprises mostly of offspring cells. Prostate cancer can be due to a mineral deficiency and is one of the most over-treated cancers. By the age of fifty, nearly half of all men already have prostate cancer and will likely never even know about it. If they are treated with conventional interventions, their prognosis can worsen, as the slow-growing and often benign cancer can change into the deadly type. An authoritative, recently-published study showed that the PSA (prostate-specific antigen) blood test is very unreliable and gives false positives 80% of the time, and any benefits that are claimed for it are outweighed by its potential harm.[21] Other researchers agree with these findings, recognizing that the test can lead to a high rate of biopsy complications, known

---

[21] "Prostate-Specific Antigen (PSA) Test," National Cancer Institute, https://1ref.us/1p6 (accessed June 6, 2021).

side-effects from over-treatment and a high risk of over-diagnosis. Many will succumb to various health issues and even death from the conventional treatments of their tiny tumours, that would never have killed them in the first place if the cancer had been left alone without any intervention.

"What man is he that desireth life, and loveth many days, that he may see good?" (Psalm 34:12).

Components in ginger root are full of antioxidant power and have been proven to stimulate the vasomotor and respiratory nerve centres. Two of these antioxidant compounds protect the lungs against damage and inflammation. Gingerols help to clear the lungs by reducing the amount of mucous that they produce. Regular consumption of ginger encourages the release of mucus, making it beneficial for pulmonary-related issues such as protection against respiratory viruses. Shagaol, the compound that gives ginger its flavour, prevents bronchial tubes from restricting and keeps the airways open, thereby allowing for better airflow. Because ginger enhances bronchodilation, it has benefits for asthma, which are attributed to the potent antioxidant activity of gingerols, shogaols, and zingerones. These compounds have shown particular anti-inflammatory and analgesic properties. Ginger is not a commonly allergenic food, but it can help to treat allergies as an antihistamine.

"The Spirit of God hath made me, and the breath of the Almighty hath given me life" (Job 33:4).

Gingerols and curcumin, two of ginger's most important antioxidants, have been shown to inhibit and even reverse the deposition of amyloid plaques in the brain that are associated with Alzheimer's disease. Furthermore, zingerone, another of gingers' antioxidants, neutralizes the powerful oxidant peroxynitrite, which has been implicated as an aggravating factor in Alzheimer's disease and other neurodegenerative diseases. These antioxidants protect against the premature degeneration of brain neurons. The neuron is the basic working unit of the brain. It is a specialized cell that is designed to transmit information, and these powerful antioxidants have many neuro-protective effects. Current research shows that ginger protects the brain against oxidative stress, neurological afflictions, and improves cognitive ability by enhancing memory and mental clarity.

"Thou wilt keep him in perfect peace, whose mind is stayed on thee: because he trusteth in thee" (Isaiah 26:3).

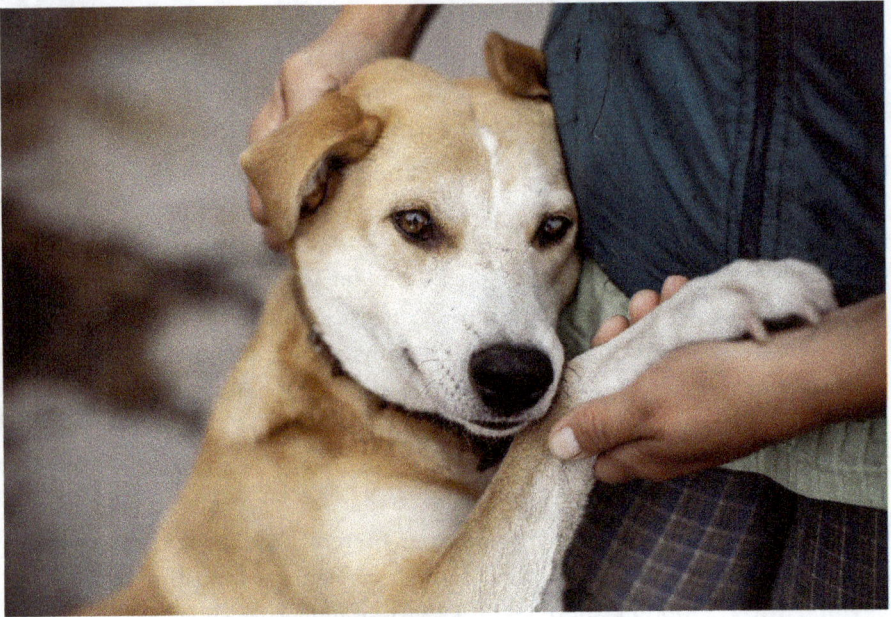

Ginger is a compound that boosts the metabolism and may temporarily increase thermogenesis in the body. The body burns stored fat to create heat, which has beneficial effects on fat storage and metabolism. Research suggests that by consuming thermogenic ingredients such as ginger, turmeric, and cayenne pepper, fat burning may increase by up to 16% and boost the metabolism by up to 6%. During weight loss, it may also help to counteract the decrease in the metabolic rate. Ginger also promotes satiety, which helps to control hunger.

"Beloved, think it not strange concerning the fiery trial which is to try you, as though some strange thing happened unto you"
(1 Peter 4:12).

Not only is ginger beneficial for the human population, but it is also effective for canines in a number of respects, including pain, cancer, and heartworm, as its properties are anti-carcinogenic, analgesic, anti-parasitic, and vermifugal. Ginger has excellent anti-cancer effects with major benefits for reducing canine tumours. It has been shown to decrease tumour necrosis factor-alpha, which is a chemical signal in a dog's body that stimulates cancer cell growth. It also has immune-stimulating ability and is able to remove toxins. Ginger has been shown to be effective against heartworms, and injections of ginger extract have been tried with good success, but it does take time. Ginger, turmeric, and garlic, all have the potential to reduce inflammation and damage caused by parasite infestations. Raw, organic pumpkin seeds have also been used successfully to eliminate hookworms and tapeworms. The recommended dose is one teaspoon of the ground seed daily per 4½ kilos (approximately 10 pounds) of the animal's body weight, as the ground seeds perform as ground glass to worms. Raw organic pumpkin seeds are also a super source of vitamin A and zinc and contain more protein than almost any other seeds. They are also valuable for eliminating tapeworms and their eggs in humans. For beneficial effects, half a cup of these ground seeds can be added to various foods in a variety of ways. The presence of a natural fat and cucurbitin in the seeds is toxic to tapeworms and their eggs.

"Thou art my God, and I will praise thee: thou art my God, I will exalt thee" (Psalm 118:28).

This wonderful warming herb has so many beneficial qualities that its regular use is potent for all-round protection against many maladies that inflict humans and animals alike. It also enhances many sweet and savoury dishes with its delicious flavour. Enjoy it as one of the powerful God-given superfoods that support abundant health.

"And then shall appear the sign of the Son of man in heaven: and then shall all the tribes of the earth mourn, and they shall see the Son of man coming in the clouds of heaven with power and great glory" (Matthew 24:30).

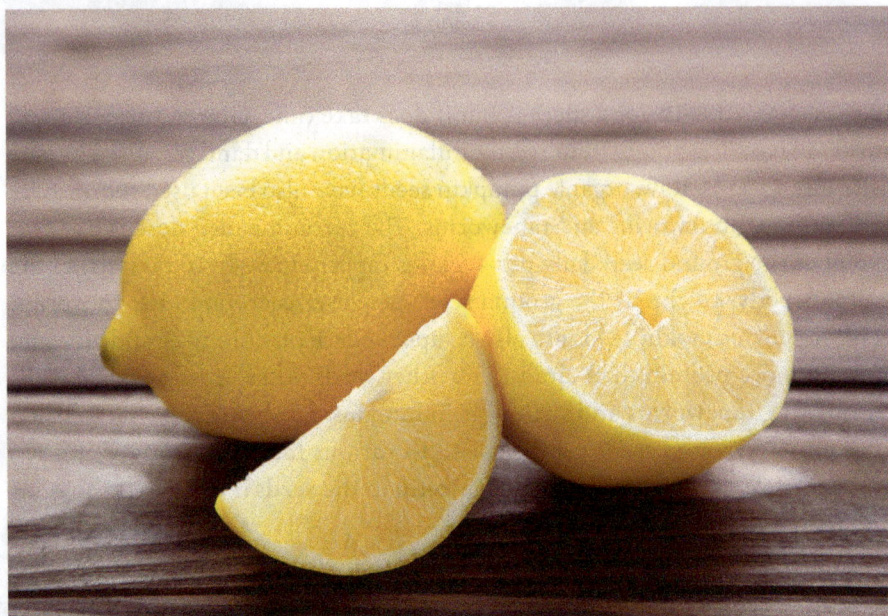

Chapter 6

Lemons

"THE FOOD THAT YOU EAT CAN EITHER BE THE MOST POWERFUL AND SAFE FORM OF MEDICINE OR THE MOST INSIDIOUS FORM OF POISON."

Lemons are an important medicinal plant of the genus Rutaceae, to which all citrus fruits belong. They were originally developed as a cross between the sour orange and the citron and have a documented history of cultivation spanning more than 4,000 years.

Powerful lemons have long been appreciated for their health qualities. Ancient populations from Mesopotamia and regions of India and China cultivated and regularly used them to treat a wide variety of health conditions. Ancient Egyptians used antiseptic lemon juice to embalm their mummies and often put lemons in their tombs with dates and figs. Lemons are depicted on a wall painting in the tomb of Nakht, who was the priest and scribe of Pharaoh Thutmoses IV, an eighteenth dynasty king of ancient Egypt who reigned around the fourteenth century BC. In Media and Persia, there was a tree called the Persian apple, or Median-apple (the citron), whose fruit was not edible but had an exquisite aroma. These same fruits were known early to the Greeks and Romans, as lemons were transported to ancient Greece, followed by Rome, Persia, and the majority of the Mediterranean civilizations. In Rome, Emperor Nero regularly consumed them, as he was obsessed with the possible danger of poisoning. A mosaic-tiled floor, likely from the second century AD, has been found in a Roman villa at Carthage. It depicts recognizable fruit-bearing lemon trees and branches of citron. A vaulted ceiling in a mausoleum built by the emperor Constantine the Great (AD 274–337) conspicuously portrays a mosaic with oranges, citrons, and lemons, all of them attached to branches covered with green leaves. Lemon leaves were also utilized as a protection against moths in clothing.

"Keep my commandments, and live; and my law as the apple of thine eye" (Proverbs 7:2).

There are references to the citron in early European literature, and lemons were first introduced to Europe by Arabs who brought them to Spain in the eleventh century. They were also introduced into Northern Africa at about the same time. During the Middle Ages, they were used for the prevention of various epidemics. In the fifteenth century, sailors who were at sea for long periods of time and were living on foods that were lacking in vitamin C, discovered that lemon and lime juice treated and prevented the dreaded scurvy (a nutrient deficiency disease), which had horrendous symptoms that sailors were dying from at a rate of 50% prior to this discovery. A scurvy cure was first published in *The Surgeons Mate* in 1617 by John Woodall, who was an English military surgeon, but it was completely ignored by the medical community. In 1734, Johannes Bachstrom, a Dutch physician, invented the term *antiscorbutic* (without scurvy), which he used to describe fresh vegetables. Then, in 1753, James Lind (1716–1794), a naval surgeon and pioneer of naval hygiene in the British Royal Navy, published his discovery in *A Treatise of the Scurvy*, which unfortunately was also ignored. The medical establishment of the day insisted that the discovery of eating citrus fruits to reverse scurvy was not based on scientific evidence. After Lind had persevered with his conclusion for nearly fifty years, citrus fruits were finally accepted and used for the prevention and treatment of scurvy on sailing vessels and changed the course of world history. Tragically, after its first discovery, this citrus fruit scurvy cure was ignored by the medical establishment for over 300 years, which resulted in horrendous suffering and many unnecessary deaths. Lemons were also used for food preservation and for protection from the contamination of rats, which are repelled by them.

"And God said, Behold, I have given you every herb bearing seed, which is upon the face of all the earth, and every tree, in the which is the fruit of a tree yielding seed; to you it shall be for meat (food)" (Genesis 1:29).

Lemons are rich in nutrients such as potent flavonoids, which are a group of phytochemicals. Abundant antioxidant flavonoids not only help to boost the potency of vitamin C but they also improve blood flow, help to maintain a normal pulse pressure, and powerfully reduce inflammation. Lemons are also a good source of B-complex vitamins such as pantothenic acid and pyridoxine. They also contain beta-carotene, calcium, copper, folate, iron, magnesium, manganese, phosphorus, potassium, pectin (an appetite suppressant), and selenium. The acids contained in lemons are ascorbic acid, citric acid, malic acid, and glucaric acid, which aids digestion. Citrus fruits are principally composed of citric acid, which is one-third oxygen. Lemon bioflavonoids include chrysoeriol, diosmetin, diosmin, eriocitrin, eriodictyol, hesperidin, isolimocitrol, isorhamnetin, limocitrin, limocitrol, neohesperidoside, naringin, naringenin, narirutin, neodiosmin, neohesperidin, nobiletin, rutin, rutinoside, and tangeretin. Lemon essential oils contain carotenoids and coumarins.

"Build ye houses, and dwell in them; and plant gardens, and eat the fruit of them" (Jeremiah 29:5).

Lemons contain powerful properties and are alkalizers, anaesthetic, analgesic, anti-ageing, anti-allergenic, anti-asthmatic, anti-arthritic, anti-atherogenic, antibacterial, antibiotic, anti-carcinogenic, anticatarrhal, anti-depressant, anti-diabetic, antifungal, antigripal, antihemorrhagic, antihistamine, anti-infective, anti-inflammatory, anti-ischaemic, antimalarial, antimicrobial, antioxidant, anti-parasitic, antiphlogistic (prevents or relieves inflammation), antipyretic, antiseptic, antispasmodic, anti-toxin, antivenom, anti-ulcer, antiviral, anxiolytic, apoptotic, astringent, carminative, a cholagogue, cicatrizant, cleansing, a coagulant, cytotoxic (to cancer stem cells), a decongestant, detoxifying, a disinfectant, a diuretic, epigenetic, hemostatic, immune-protective, neuroprotective, neurorestorative, remineralizing, and a vermifuge.

"Oh that men would praise the LORD for His goodness, and for His wonderful works to the children of men!" (Psalm 107:31).

The powerful health benefits of lemons also include their use as a treatment for cancers, viruses, rheumatism, asthenia, diarrhoea, dyspepsia, indigestion, haemorrhages, stress, hyperuricemia, constipation, depression, edema, epilepsy, stomatitis, pharyngitis, fever, coughs, arthritis, colds, obesity, gout, tetanus, typhoid, nausea, rabies, cardiovascular disease, flu, tonsillitis, headache, heart disease, cholera, infections, including urinary tract infections, leprosy, diphtheria, meningitis, chronic fatigue, allergies, eczema, pain, urolithiasis, Parkinson's disease, diabetes, inflammation, insomnia, malaria, otitis, scurvy, asthma, epithelial and endothelial dysfunction, hemorrhoids, blepharoconjunctivitis, macular degeneration, cataracts, digestion, snake bites, joint pains, liver problems, capillary fragility, bleeding gums, receding gums, sensitive teeth, nosebleeds, burns, dry skin, respiratory disorders, eye diseases, skin, wrinkles, immune system deficiencies, stroke and aneurysm protection, eliminating organ stones, capillary protection, blood circulation, Alzheimer's disease protection, cognitive decline, and for burn patients when taken internally.

"And He came down with them, and stood in the plain, and the company of His disciples, and a great multitude of people out of all Judaea and Jerusalem, and from the sea coast of Tyre and Sidon, which came to hear Him, and to be healed of their diseases" (Luke 6:17).

The humble yet powerful God-given lemon is accessible, time-tested, affordable, and potent. It is also many times more powerful than nefarious drugs that are used to treat cancer. Ineffective and injurious treatments cannot reach to the root cause of the problem, which is the cancer stem cells. These chemical carcinogens are themselves dangerous toxic poisons which weaken the whole system, and the blood cell count declines during this damaging treatment. The use of these poisons causes fewer red blood cells, which means that less oxygen is transported around the body. This also causes less white cells, which weakens the immune system, which is the body's natural defence system against invading elements. The body cannot be poisoned into health but needs to have the cause of the problem removed, the noxious substances flushed out, and the whole system built up with sound nutrition, such as a whole plant-food diet, together with healthy lifestyle practices. After receiving pernicious radiation and chemical cancer drug protocols, the pectin from lemons and other fruits and plants can remove remnant traces of radiation from the bloodstream and tissues of the body by binding radioactive residues, purifying the blood, and helping to strengthen the immune system. Pectin works as a natural chelating agent and is a structural polysaccharide, which is found in the cell walls of plant cells.

"Behold, God will not cast away a perfect man, neither will He help the evil doers" (Job 8:20).

Unfortunately, all humans are born with the inability to manufacture vitamin C. The ascorbic acid molecule of vitamin C is an organic acid, and when it was discovered in 1937 by Albert Szent-Györgyi von Nagyrápolt, ascorbic acid was the only identified component of the complex, and therefore ascorbic acid was named vitamin C, but ascorbic acid is not a vitamin. His discovery was one of the foundations of modern nutrition. The molecular formula for ascorbic acid is $C_6H_8O_6$. Other components of this complex have been found since that time, but the definition of vitamin C has remained the same. Vitamins are biological complexes and not individual molecular components. They are biochemical interactions that can only be activated when the whole vitamin complex is functioning together. Albert Szent-Györgyi von Nagyrápolt was also responsible for coining the term vitamin P, which is not a vitamin at all but a term given to a group of remarkable healing plant substances that are better known as bioflavonoids, which are important elements found in thousands of plant species. Vitamin C is an exceptionally powerful antioxidant which enables the body to efficiently utilize protein, carbohydrates, and fats. The complete vitamin C molecule also contains J, P, and K factors. The J factor assists the oxygen-carrying capacity of the blood; the P factor assists with strengthening the blood vessels, thereby preventing strokes, aneurysms, bleeding gums, and bruising; and the K factor assists with blood coagulation. In addition, the whole vitamin C molecule contains at least fourteen known bioflavonoids, various ascorbagens, the tyrosinase (organic copper) enzyme, rutin, magnesium, iron, phosphorus, five copper ions, selenium, zinc, manganese, and ascorbic acid. Ascorbic acid is the antioxidant portion of the vitamin C complex, which protects the other important components from oxidation. For vitamin C to be complete, all of the components are required and not just ascorbic acid, which has two electrons to donate instead of one, making it twice as powerful. The amount of natural ascorbic acid in lemons is around 50 milligrams per 100 grams, which is the same amount as in oranges and double the amount contained in limes. Natural ascorbic acid is much more synergistically bioavailable and active when it is still in the whole food and not as effective when detached from the whole food. The body absorbs almost 100% of the vitamin C as part of a whole food, whereas barely 10% of isolated ascorbic acid is absorbed. Isolated ascorbic acid is also ten times more acidic than the naturally buffered vitamin C that is found in natural raw foods. When isolated ascorbic acid is removed out of its nutritional context of whole vitamin C, it behaves more like a drug, as mineral co-factors need to be available in the correct amounts, otherwise, the body must supply the difference by drawing from its own reserves.

Vitamins and minerals function together as a complex team, and if any components are absent, the whole sequence of metabolic processes will malfunction. The abundant ascorbic acid in citrus fruits promotes wound healing and is also an essential nutrient for the maintenance of healthy bones, connective tissue, and cartilage. The majority of artificial ascorbic acid is produced using fermented corn syrup, which is often genetically modified. To extract the ascorbic acid it is treated with solvents such as sulphuric acid, acetone, or sodium hydroxide. This results in an artificial ascorbic acid which has a much shorter life within the body than whole vitamin C, which is absorbed more slowly and is available to the cells for significantly longer. Just one gram of ascorbic acid can immediately and invisibly chemically neutralize 100 gallons of water containing one part per million of chlorine. Albert Szent-Györgyi von Nagyrápolt was a brilliant physiologist and researcher who not only identified ascorbic acid but isolated it as well. He was born in Budapest, Hungary, in 1893 and died in 1986. His discovery of the metabolic mechanism that enables ascorbic acid to be used within the cells was recognized with a Nobel Prize in physiology in 1937, and he is accredited with saying: "Life is a wondrous phenomenon. I can only hope that some day man will achieve a deeper insight into its nature and its guiding principles and will be able to express them in more exact terms. To express the marvels of nature in the language of science is one of man's noblest endeavours."

"Behold, I will bring it health and cure, and I will cure them, and will reveal unto them the abundance of peace and truth" (Jeremiah 33:6).

In the early 1940s, Dr. F. R. Klenner was the first physician to aggressively utilize ascorbic acid to successfully reverse many diseases including measles, chickenpox, tetanus, mumps, polio, and cancer, to name a few. He discovered that by frequently injecting massive amounts of ascorbic acid into patients who tested positive for polio, over a seventy-two hour period, the infection was healed with zero paralyses. He also saw the same consistent results with a great variety of bacterial and viral diseases. Dr. Klenner prescribed his patients at least 350 milligrams of IV ascorbic acid per kilogram of body weight per day, or approximately 25–30 grams in divided doses per day for the average-sized adult, or the same amount every two hours if required. He also prescribed a variety of other nutrients with varying delivery methods for various diseases.

"And He sent them to preach the kingdom of God, and to heal the sick" (Luke 9:2).

Modern research has concluded that an unhealthy gut environment impacts the immune system and leads to a myriad of diseases. Because lemons are such a powerful anti-inflammatory, they are effective at purifying and cleansing the skin, liver, pancreas, intestines, and the lymph and also squelch inflammatory conditions wherever they occur in the body. The lymph system, which is the largest circulatory system in the body, is twice as large as the arterial system and is responsible for flushing out waste and toxins from the body. The regenerative potential of lemons also have an anti-microbial effect against bacterial infections and fungi and are also effective against internal parasites. Parasites thrive in an acidic environment and drinking lemon water helps to flush them out. Lemons are rich in potassium, a mineral that can help to nourish brain function and nerve cells. Potassium is vital for the function of the heart and helps to prevent heart-related illnesses, such as an irregular heartbeat. Because lemons are high in potassium, citrate levels in the urine are also higher, which discourages stone formations in the kidneys and gallbladder. Skeletal tissue contains 90% of the citrate that is found in the body. There is also a citrate transporter in the membranes of stem cells. Additionally, lemons act as an anti-depressant and combat stress and nervous disorders. Their unique flavonoid compounds are rich in antioxidants and anti-cancer properties, which are known to neutralize free radicals that oxidize cells in the body. Lemons also help to reduce the pain and inflammation of joints. They prevent the growth and multiplication of pathogenic bacteria that cause infections and diseases. Having powerful antibacterial properties against pathogens, experiments have demonstrated that fresh lemon juice destroys the bacteria of cholera (Vibrio cholerae), typhoid, diphtheria, and other deadly diseases. Drinking a lemon juice mixture can help to treat a fever by bringing it down faster, as it helps to break fevers by increasing perspiration. Lemon water (a diluted solution of fresh lemon juice) helps to alkalize the system, thereby balancing acidity levels and keeping the body hydrated, which is very important for overall health. Lemon and lime juice stimulate the peristaltic action of the colon, thereby increasing the efficiency of the digestive system. Lemon juice has an atomic structure that is similar to gastric juices, which tricks the liver into producing bile. It is always more beneficial to use the juice as soon as possible after extracting it as it loses its nutritional value after a while. As an aromatic and antiseptic agent, fresh lemon juice is also useful for soaking and relaxing the feet when it is added to warm water. This should bring instant relief and muscle relaxation.

"Blessed be the name of the LORD from this time forth and for evermore" (Psalm 113:2).

Powerful vitamin C is the primary water-soluble antioxidant in the body and is one of the most essential antioxidants in nature. As the human body cannot make or store it, adequate amounts need to be ingested during the day for optimal results. The abundance of vitamin C in lemons helps to strengthen the immune system as it possesses anti-fibrotic effects, helps to eliminate radioactive contaminants from the body, cleanses the stomach, and is considered a powerful blood purifier of the whole body. Vitamin C is needed by the phagocytes and T cells of the immune system to perform their tasks. The adrenal glands and the eyes also need plenty of vitamin C. Macular degeneration can be prevented and corrected by sufficient antioxidants, including powerful vitamin C and healthy fats such as Omega-3 and unrefined coconut oil. Vitamin C travels through the body neutralizing any free radicals that it comes into contact within the aqueous environments of the body, both inside and outside of the cells. Free radicals are missing a critical molecule and can interact with the healthy cells of the body by stealing an electron from them and damaging their membranes to quench that need. Good health occurs when there is an ample flow and interchange of electrons in the cells. Poor electron flow and interchange equates with a diseased state, and when the flow and interchange ceases the cells die, as free radical oxidation involves the loss of electrons and all toxicity is caused by oxidation. A nutrient is only nutritious after it has been broken down and metabolized to its basic molecular level of antioxidant power.

"So Jesus had compassion on them, and touched their eyes: and immediately their eyes received sight, and they followed Him" (Matthew 20:34).

Free radicals can also cause much inflammation and painful swelling in the body. The birth and death of cells in the body is a continuous process twenty-four hours a day. This process is necessary to keep the body healthy. Oxidation is a process that happens during normal cellular functions. The body metabolizes oxygen very efficiently, but 1 or 2% of cells become damaged in the process and convert to free radicals. When free radicals are on the attack, they do not just kill cells to acquire their missing molecule but often injure the cell and damage proteins in the cytoplasm and the DNA, which creates the seeds for disease. Some of these cytoplasm proteins are enzymes, which are responsible for triggering thousands of chemical reactions in the body. When enzymes are destroyed, the reactions that they would normally catalyze do not occur. When the internal and external cell membranes are impaired they no longer efficiently receive nutrients or expel waste. For necessary appropriate physiological function, a balance is needed between antioxidants and free radicals. When free radicals overwhelm the ability of the body to regulate them, then oxidative stress occurs, which causes cells to weaken and malfunction and adversely alters the DNA, the proteins and lipids, and provokes diseases. There are two major reactive oxygen species, the hydroxyl radical and the superoxide radical, which are continuously being formed in a process of reduction of oxygen to water. Free radical reactive oxygen species and also reactive nitrogen species are generated by the various endogenous systems of the body because of exposure to pathological states or physiochemical conditions created by herbicides, stress, tobacco smoke, inflammation, X-ray radiation, low magnesium levels, and environmental toxins.

> *A nutrient is only nutritious after it has been broken down and metabolized to its basic molecular level of antioxidant power.*

Collagen is a ubiquitous structural protein that comprises about one-third of the total protein in the body. Optimal vitamin C is needed to support collagen production as it interacts with amino acids within collagen cells to provide oxygen and hydrogen to make collagen. Vitamin C is a very powerful antioxidant which assists with oxidative stress, and insufficient intake can cause very serious health issues, but sufficient quantities have been demonstrated to reverse osteoarthritis, rheumatoid arthritis, cancer, and many other diseases. It is not only vital to the function of a strong immune system, which protects the body from illness, but it immobilizes free radicals, which are the cause of many ailments. Vitamin C enhances the level of the powerful glutathione master antioxidant, which is a tri-peptide found in every cell of the body. Its unique intracellular ability maximizes the performance of all other antioxidants, eliminates toxins from the cells, and protects from the damaging effects of environmental pollutants, toxic metals, oxidative stress, radiation, and chemicals. Elevated levels of glutathione within the cells constitute a healthier body, whereas low levels are conducive to disease. Vitamin C and glutathione work together as a team. Glutathione recycles vitamins C and E and helps to detoxify potentially dangerous substances. Vitamin C is an essential nutrient in the maintenance of good health and recovery from stress and injuries, and there are no known toxins that it cannot neutralize. Researchers have found that this powerful antioxidant can also be utilized to improve hormone issues, due to its high antioxidant properties, as hormones can degrade, become toxic and cause cancer, due to lifestyle factors. Vitamin C is able to regenerate these hormones by donating electrons to steroid hormones thereby neutralizing cancer-causing free radicals. It can also be recycled in the body, as there are various cells that will utilize the used form of vitamin C, which is known as DHA, and recycle it so that it can be used elsewhere. There are various cells that can only uptake this DHA, which include red blood cells, nerve cells, and some bone cells. If there has been any damage caused by toxins (including vaccines), vitamin C will begin to repair that damage. Adding vitamin C-rich fresh lemon juice to green vegetables also improves the absorption of iron by a factor of four. Iron plays an important role in the proper functioning of the immune system and protects the body from disease. It is crucial to absorb this essential iron trace element, as it performs an extremely important role in the cytokine-mediated immune response, and an insufficiency can either cause inflammation or significantly weaken the immune system. Lemons are rich in super-antioxidant bioflavonoids, which are found in many natural foods. They give lemons their yellow colour and are sometimes referred to as vitamin P. They complement vitamin C and are found in many of the same foods that contain vitamin C, thereby enhancing its effect on the body.

"And in that day shall ye say, Praise the LORD, call upon His name, declare His doings among the people, make mention that His name is exalted" (Isaiah 12:4).

Inflammation has been recognized as a disease and injury indicator for thousands of years. References to physical symptoms of inflammation date back to a medical treatise written by the scholar Aulus Cornelius Celsus in the first century AD. Because lemons are anti-inflammatory, they also naturally help to protect the cardiovascular system from the dire consequences of leaks. Inflammation in the body is measured by levels of cytokines (also called C-reactive proteins). Adequate vitamin C strengthens blood vessel walls and squelches inflammation before it becomes a major life-threatening issue. Inflammation is the body's response to a perceived threat, is part of the natural healing process, and is a component of every major degenerative disease. However, when the body becomes imbalanced, such as being in a state of acidosis, it loses its ability to produce counteracting anti-inflammatory chemicals, which is why it is vitally important to maintain a healthful pH and lifestyle. Those with a vitamin C deficiency are at an increased risk for lethal strokes, aneurysms, cancer, heart attacks, and peripheral artery disease, to name a few.

"Wherefore by their fruits ye shall know them" (Matthew 7:20).

Sepsis (blood poisoning), also known as septicemia, is a very deadly form of bacterial infection that kills millions of people worldwide every year. This very serious life-threatening condition is initiated by a bacterial infection and characterized by an excessive immune system response which causes a systemic inflammatory response, damaging healthy tissues and organs. Vitamin C combats infections by terminating this oxidation process. Certain bacteria produce toxins which cause cells to release substances that initiate inflammation. Sepsis can be caused by the following bacteria: Escherichia coli (E. coli gut bacteria); Klebsiella pneumoniae (gut bacteria); Pseudomonas (common soil and water bacteria); Staphylococcus Aureus (nostrils and skin bacteria); and Streptococcus (a bacterial infection that enters the bloodstream). Rarely, sepsis can be caused by fungi, such as Candida. Vitamin C prevents the formation of blood clots by thinning the blood and raising the level of nitric oxide in the body. Low levels of vitamin C and vitamin B1 (thiamine) are aggravating factors in this condition. Foods containing vitamin B1 include asparagus (a good source), nuts, whole grains, oranges, seeds, legumes, yeast, cauliflower, and kale. The frequency and amount of vitamin C that should therefore be taken needs to be appropriate to the seriousness of the condition because the severity of the inflammation dictates the amount and frequency, as the inflammation, similar to a fire in the system, needs to be quenched. Whole vitamin C can be taken orally in high amounts as the body will either utilize it or dispose of it. Ascorbic acid does not stay in the body for as long as whole vitamin C, and large amounts of ascorbic acid may cause diarrhoea as the gut cannot tolerate large amounts of this isolated substance. Liposomal encapsulated vitamin C can be taken orally in high doses or in an IV if required, as this bypasses the digestive system. Intravenous vitamins C and B1 have successfully been used in the following amounts to combat sepsis: 1,500 milligrams of vitamin C every six hours for four days (higher and more frequent doses may be required if necessary), plus 200 milligrams of vitamin B1 every twelve hours for four days. Vitamin C is very safe at high doses.

"In my distress I cried unto the LORD, and He heard me"
(Psalm 120:1).

Vitamin C, which is found abundantly in lemons, is a much safer and effective way to withdraw from drug addictions without the withdrawal symptoms. It quickly causes the symptoms to be reversed and shows enormous promise for overcoming addictions to hard drugs such as heroin. Heroin addictions are often related to addictions to prescription opioid painkillers. Opioids greatly increase the risk of obesity by adversely impacting the metabolism. It is well known that heroin addictions are difficult to overcome because of the considerable withdrawal symptoms that are associated with attempting to reject this toxic addictive narcotic drug. The symptoms of withdrawal can continue for quite some time and include sweating, cravings, mood swings, abdominal pain, nausea, trembling, muscle spasms, agitation, depression, anxiety, and more. A deficiency of vitamin C and malnutrition are also sizable components of drug addictions. Vitamin C administered at high doses rapidly reduces the desire for opioid use and produces profound healing effects without the negative side effects associated with dangerous conventional protocols, which commonly have relapses and cravings.

Charcoal can also help to decrease the detoxification workload of the liver. Vital nutrients and an oral intake of 30–90 grams of sodium ascorbate (a milder buffered mineral salt of ascorbic acid), taken in segmented doses every day, with tapering off at about 20–35 grams per day, have completely reversed heroin addictions. Symptoms of recovery begin to improve within twelve hours of ingesting the first dose, and just a week of this treatment can expedite a profound reversal of symptoms. Taking ascorbic acid orally in high doses can result in diarrhoea, but utilizing liposomal encapsulated vitamin C negates this problem as it by-passes the digestive system. Ingesting large doses of ascorbic acid on a regular basis lowers copper levels, which can compromise the immune system. Whole vitamin C not only stays in the body much longer, but it is also more nutritious and beneficial as it includes other synergistic components of this most important nutrient. Vitamin C not only works for drug addictions but with the addition of vitamin B3 (niacin) it also works for cigarettes, food, and alcohol addictions. These two vitamins are very safe. Studies show that vitamin C therapy restores

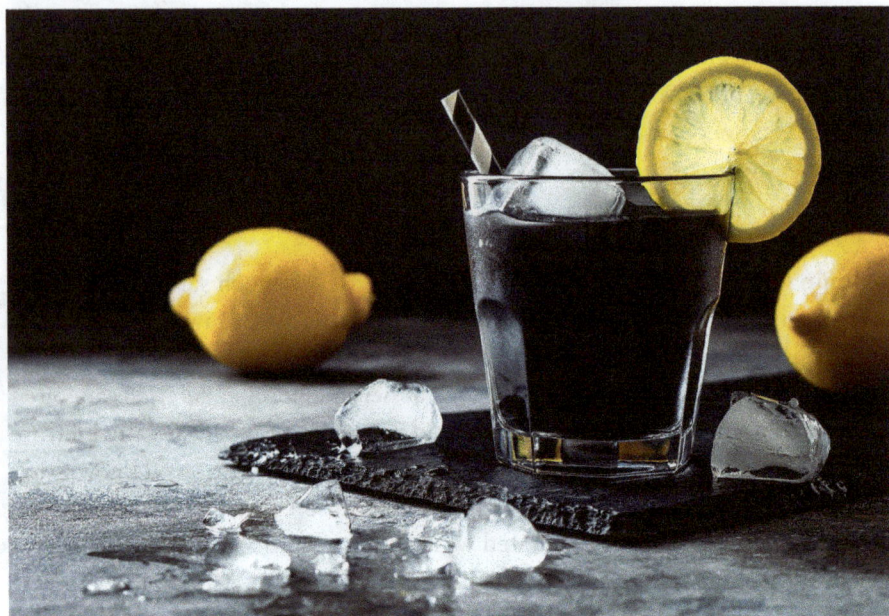

restful sleep patterns because of its anti-inflammatory action in the brain. It also assists with the return of appetite. Vitamin C is a potent analgesic and vitamin C therapy of around ten grams a day, administered intravenously, has proven effective at halting pain for terminally-ill cancer patients who discover that they no longer need morphine or have withdrawal symptoms and they recover from their cancer because vitamin C halts the rapid progression of cancer as it is selectively cytotoxic to cancer cells when administered intravenously at high doses. By bypassing the digestive tract, IV administration results in blood levels exponentially higher than what can be achieved via the oral route. Vitamin C has powerful detoxifying properties and is very effective at reversing opioid addictions as it can emulate morphine and fits into the opiate receptor sites of the cells, which deceives the body into no longer desiring drugs. It is very effective and can be lifesaving, not only for reversing many cancers but also for a whole host of other deadly diseases. This vital lifesaving information has been well documented for many decades. Vitamin C actually targets and kills cancer stem cells by starving them and blocking the process of glycolysis, which is responsible for glucose metabolism and fuels energy production in the mitochondria. Its inhibition prevents the mitochondria of the cancer stem cells from obtaining essential energy needed for their survival.

Morphine suppresses natural killer cell activity, and many cancers have morphine receptor sites on their surfaces. When morphine and its derivatives are used in the treatment of pain, these receptor sites are activated and cancer grows and spreads more quickly. When morphine is discontinued vitamin C can assist in overcoming the malignancy. Vitamin C has the ability to selectively target cancer cells because of its delivery mechanism, which involves the generation of hydrogen peroxide, and this is what ultimately destroys cancer cells. A study has shown that tumour cells are much less capable of removing the damaging hydrogen peroxide than normal cells, thereby exhibiting that cancer cells are much more prone to damage and death from a high amount of hydrogen peroxide. This explains why extremely high vitamin C levels are selectively cytotoxic to cancer cells whilst leaving normal cells unharmed. Normal tissues are unharmed by the high levels of generated hydrogen peroxide because healthy cells have several ways of removing it effectively, thereby preventing a toxic level of build-up. A study demonstrated that a very high intake of vitamin C not only lowers the damaging effects of refined sugar but also reduces blood sugar levels. Because humans cannot make their own vitamin C as animals do, for preventative maintenance a healthy, whole plant-food diet containing adequate vitamin C is essential. As well as citrus, beneficial amounts of vitamin C can also be found in the following healthy whole plant-foods: peppers, kale, broccoli, cauliflower, Brussels sprouts, papayas, mangos, strawberries, blueberries, raspberries, blackberries, cherries, grapes, blackcurrants, pineapple, and kiwi fruit. As an anti-toxin, vitamin C is also effective against the bites of poisonous snakes, scorpions, and spiders.

"Gracious is the LORD, and righteous; yea, our God is merciful" (Psalm 116:5).

Vitamin C has been determined to have protective effects against the damaging effects of unnatural fluoride (fluorosilicic acid), which is a by-product of fertilizer manufacturing. Vitamin C can also be synergistically enhanced with magnesium and calcium-rich foods for extra protection against fluoride. Experiments have demonstrated that adequate vitamin C increases fluoride excretion from the body, including the bones, and can also reverse dental fluorosis when absorbed with sufficient vitamin D3 and dietary calcium. Poisonous fluoride causes dental fluorosis. Vitamin C also eradicates other poisons from the body.

"But the Lord is faithful, who shall stablish you, and keep you from evil" (2 Thessalonians 3:3).

Super-antioxidants support strong cell formations and also fight cell oxidation as well as free radical damage, which are the primary causes of cancer. Bioflavonoids, which are naturally abundant in lemons, also naturally stimulate the production of insulin in the body, which in turn balances blood glucose levels. Most people with cancer and diabetes have a very acidic body pH. The high soluble fibre and vitamin C content in lemons have been found to have beneficial properties for those with diabetes, as the acid slows digestion and prevents sudden spikes in blood glucose levels. Research has shown that symptoms of eye disorders, including diabetic retinopathy, improve due to the rutin found in lemons. Most diabetics have low stomach acidity and impaired digestive enzymes, meaning that they absorb fewer nutrients from nutritious food. However, lemons increase stomach acidity, thereby aiding digestion. Vitamin C foods also contain bioflavonoids, which are required for vitamin C absorption and both work together. Bioflavonoids also interact with cell membranes and make them less insulin resistant, which is partly due to the vitamin C content. Vitamin C also has other significant benefits for the diabetic as it increases collagen production, which strengthens blood vessels, an important issue for diabetics as many diabetics have problems with arterial damage and circulation.

"But we have this treasure in earthen vessels, that the excellency of the power may be of God, and not of us" (2 Corinthians 4:7).

Hydrochloric acid is a critical ingredient needed by the stomach for proper digestion, the assimilation of nutrients, and the expulsion of waste. Drinking warm vitamin C rich lemon water, especially first thing in the morning, assists the gut and promotes good digestion by stimulating the stomach to increase the production of hydrochloric acid. It also improves peristalsis throughout the entire digestive tract. Improved digestion means better nutrient absorption and less bloating. Lemon water is alkaline water and is also a good remedy for constipation as water helps to lubricate the digestive system. The citric acid in lemons helps to stimulate the system and flush out toxins and undigested waste from the colon. Not only does lemon water help to hydrate the body but it also replenishes lost vitamins and minerals caused by stress. However, drinking lemon water on an empty stomach shortly before retiring for the night may produce unnecessary hydrochloric acid in the stomach which can lead to uncomfortable heartburn symptoms as lemon increases stomach acid.

"But whosoever drinketh of the water that I shall give him shall never thirst; but the water that I shall give him shall be in him a well of water springing up into everlasting life" (John 4:14).

Lemon peel consists of two layers: the outermost zest layer and the inner layer. The outer layer contains 6% essential oils, 90% of which is d-limonene and 5% citral, plus glycosides, carotenoids, coumarins, sitosterol, alpha-Terpineol, a small amount of citronellal, linalyl, and geranyl acetate. The inner layer contains no essential oils but instead has a variety of bitter flavone glycosides and coumarin derivatives. Not only is the peel of citrus fruits a rich source of flavones but also many polymethoxylated flavones, which are very rare in other plants. Polymethoxylated flavones help to maintain overall cardiovascular function and contain biologically active molecules that have metabolic properties. Two of these flavones are tangeretin and nobiletin, which are the most researched. The potent phytonutrient tangeretin has been proven to be effective for neurological disorders such as Parkinson's disease. Tangeretin is an anti-inflammatory, anti-cancer flavone that is mainly concentrated in the peel of tangerines and other mandarin oranges and in smaller amounts in some other citrus fruits. Nobiletin is an anti-inflammatory, anti-cancer, and a neuroprotective brain-boosting flavonoid. Flavonoids contained in the citrus peels help to counter cancerous cell divisions. Lemon peel contains five to ten times more vitamins than the lemon juice itself,

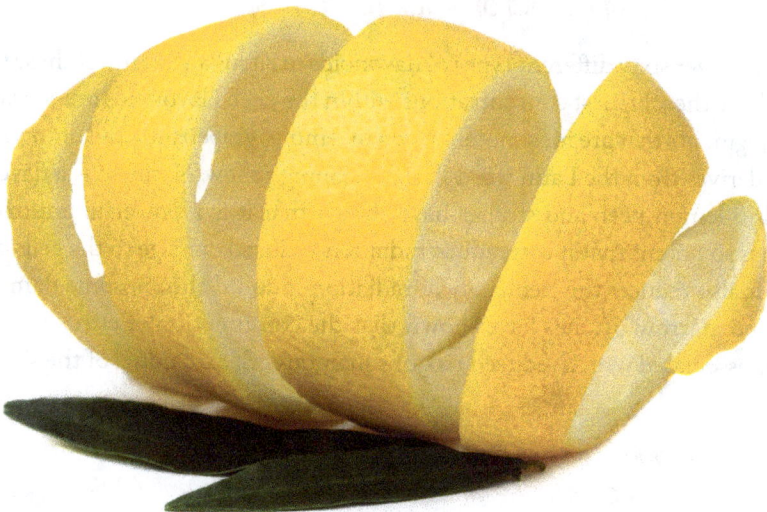

and most of the pectin and dietary fibre are found in the white pith just under the skin. All citrus fruits contain high levels of pectin in their rinds and are anti-parasitic. Pectins are prebiotic fibres which help to promote the growth of beneficial microbiota in the colon, and studies suggest that pectins may also help to prevent colon cancer. When ingested, pectin becomes an effective detoxification compound which is capable of excreting heavy metals that have been deposited in the body.

"And the land shall yield her fruit, and ye shall eat your fill, and dwell therein in safety" (Leviticus 25:19).

All citrus peels contain considerable amounts of the phytochemical d-limonene, a monoterpene which is a known anti-cancer agent that flushes away carcinogens from the body. D-limonene is found in the essential oils extracted from the peels of citrus fruits and is currently being used in clinical trials to dissolve gallstones. It also increases the levels of liver enzymes involved in detoxifying carcinogens, thereby decreasing the damaging effects of carcinogens. Citrus essential oils are mechanically cold pressed using the rind of the fruit, and the expressed oil is extremely potent and condensed. It takes approximately seventy-five lemons to make one 15 millilitre bottle of lemon essential oil, which can be 60–72% d-limonene. The amount depends somewhat on many other factors including the growing conditions of the fruit trees.

"I made me gardens and orchards, and I planted trees in them of all kind of fruits" (Ecclesiastes 2:5).

There are over sixty different types of flavonoids in citrus and many of these flavonoids have their highest concentrations within the peel. Flavonoids are the yellow plant pigments that are most notably seen in lemons, grapefruits, and oranges. The name derives from the Latin word *flavus*, meaning yellow. Naringin is a flavonoid found in lemon peel, and studies have shown that it is a powerful antioxidant which is so potent that it can reduce radiation-induced damage to the cells of the body. It also reduces the frequency of radiation-induced chromosome damage in the bone marrow. Studies have shown that the consumption of citrus peels and juice is associated with a reduced risk of squamous cell carcinoma of the skin.

"Now when the sun was setting, all they that had any sick with divers (various) diseases brought them unto Him; and He laid his hands on every one of them, and healed them" (Luke 4:40).

Limonoids are phytochemicals which are natural gallstone dissolving compounds present in lemons and other citrus fruit peels. They are responsible for the bitter taste of the peel and are unique to citrus as they are not present in any other fruits or vegetables. Limonoids impede breast cancer growth, which points to the importance of citrus fruit for breast cancer prevention. They are capable of slowing cancer cell growth and inducing apoptosis. They also induce increased activity of the detoxifying enzyme glutathione-S-transferase. Citrus limonin, which is a limonoid, is an intensely bitter limonoid that widely occurs in citrus juices and has been shown to help fight a variety of cancers. Limonin is from a parent compound—limonin glucoside—which is present in citrus juices in quantities approximately equal to the amount of vitamin C. Research shows that limonin is easily accessed by the body when citrus juice is consumed, as it enters the body as part of a sugar molecule. When oranges are consumed the digestive system separates the sugar from the limonin, which is then absorbed into the bloodstream and operates as an active antioxidant, thus preventing the breakdown of cell DNA.

"Then I will give you rain in due season, and the land shall yield her increase, and the trees of the field shall yield their fruit"
(Leviticus 26:4).

These powerful little yellow fruits pack a lot of nutritional punch and are one of the most alkalizing foods for the body, and both the ascorbic and citric acids, which are weak acids that are easily metabolized by the body, allow the mineral content of lemons to help alkalize the blood. Lemons have a very powerful and positive alkalizing effect on the body because the minerals from them disassociate to make the body alkaline as the body absorbs them. Even though lemon is acidic in itself, when it enters the bloodstream the alkalizing salts override the presence of acids during the metabolic processes. Other healthy foods including pineapple, grapefruit, and blueberries also have an acid pH but are alkaline in the body. Citric and ascorbic acids occur naturally in citrus fruits but there is no vitamin C in citric acid. Citric acid enhances the body's ability to naturally flush out unwanted toxins and lemon peel is rich in citric acid. Citric acid also helps to maximize the enzyme function which stimulates the liver, aids in detoxification, and helps not only to flush toxins from the liver but also from the gallbladder and colon that otherwise would be absorbed by the body. Chemically, the only difference between citric and ascorbic acids is that citric acid has one extra oxygen atom. Citric acid is also responsible for the sour taste of lemons and can help to eliminate calcium deposits from the arteries as well as dissolving gallstones, pancreatic, and kidney stones. Citrus rind is high in oxalates, which can crystallize and become stones. But lemon juice can eliminate the occurrence of swelling, gout, and stones by forming urinary citrate, which prevents the formation of crystals and the build-up of uric acid inside the body. Oxalates are present in cooked citrus such as marmalades because oxalates are resistant to cooking. Other fruits high in oxalates include grapes, blackberries, rhubarb, raspberries, blueberries, figs, and kiwifruit. Epsom salt baths displace oxalates. To lower oxalate levels while enjoying oxalate containing foods, consuming calcium-rich foods together with high-oxalate foods will prevent the oxalate from being problematic by binding to the calcium in the digestive tract. Calcium and oxalates bind together and leave the body together. But reduced calcium intake will cause oxalates to be absorbed back into the system, which leads to higher oxalate levels in the body. Citrus fruits are powerful and are most protective against stomach, mouth, larynx, and pharynx cancers.

"Hope deferred maketh the heart sick: but when the desire cometh, it is a tree of life" (Proverbs 13:12).

The organs of the body, and especially the kidneys, help to balance the body's pH levels. Restoring the pH to normal alkaline levels of at least 7.0 is of tremendous importance for those with cancer, as levels of pH below 7.0 are acidic. When the body becomes acidic it is more prone to disease, as cancer thrives in an acidic body. In its natural state, lemon juice, although acidic by nature, is anionic (negatively charged) and therefore produces an alkalizing effect on the body. It has a pH of about 2.0, but once lemon juice is fully digested and metabolized in the body it has an alkalizing effect with a pH well above 7, as its antioxidant vitamin C content does not create acidity in the body. Lemons are one of the most alkaline-forming foods in the world, and consuming them on a regular daily basis, especially with the rind, will help to increase the pH levels in the body. If the body is alkaline to a level of 7.4 pH and above, this higher pH level makes it more difficult for cancer cells to survive due to the amount of oxygen present. The majority of those with cancer have acidic pH levels of below 6.5, which makes it more difficult for normal cells to breathe properly. This causes the mutation of cells which can later become cancerous. A beneficial way to help balance the pH level is to drink warm water with fresh lemon juice to alkalize the body and lower acidity levels. Studies have shown that people who maintain a more alkaline diet do lose weight faster.

Lemons

Lemons

"The Spirit of God hath made me, and the breath of the Almighty hath given me life" (Job 33:4).

For a healthy start to the day, freshly squeezed lemon juice in warm water should be the first thing that goes into the stomach in the morning before having breakfast or any other liquid. Consuming lemon water at least half an hour before a meal gently detoxifies the liver and thereby the entire body. It will also help to break down waste and flush out toxins from the gut. For a higher dose of vitamin C, simply add fresh orange juice and fresh red grapefruit juice to lemon water, which will also impart a sweeter flavour with added nutrition. The high amounts of vitamin C in lemons aids the body with synthesizing toxic materials into substances that can be absorbed by water.

"Then they cry unto the LORD in their trouble, and he bringeth them out of their distresses" (Psalm 107:28).

Lemons can energize and enhance the mood. The energy that is received from food comes from the atoms and molecules that are in that food. A reaction occurs when the positively-charged ions from food enter the digestive tract and interact with the negatively-charged enzymes. Lemons are one of the few foods that contain more negatively charged ions, thereby providing the body with more energy when it enters the digestive tract. Negative ions increase the flow of oxygen to the brain, resulting in more mental energy, higher alertness, and decreased drowsiness. Other health benefits of lemon juice include relief from mental stress and depression. Nutrients have a powerful impact on brain function and mood. The nervous system, together with the rest of the body, requires the full spectrum of minerals, vitamins, fatty acids, and amino acids to function properly. Trillions of gut bacteria directly communicate with the nervous system. Not only does lemon juice often help to improve the mood, but it can also improve the functions of the mind such as memory, judgment, and perception. In cases of insomnia, fresh lemon juice also helps to improve sleep because of its anti-inflammatory properties, as insomnia is caused by inflammation of the brain.

"For if we believe that Jesus died and rose again, even so them also which sleep in Jesus will God bring with Him" (1 Thessalonians 4:14).

According to The Reams' Biological Ionization Theory, the lemon is the ONLY food in the world that is anionic, which is an ion with a negative charge. All other

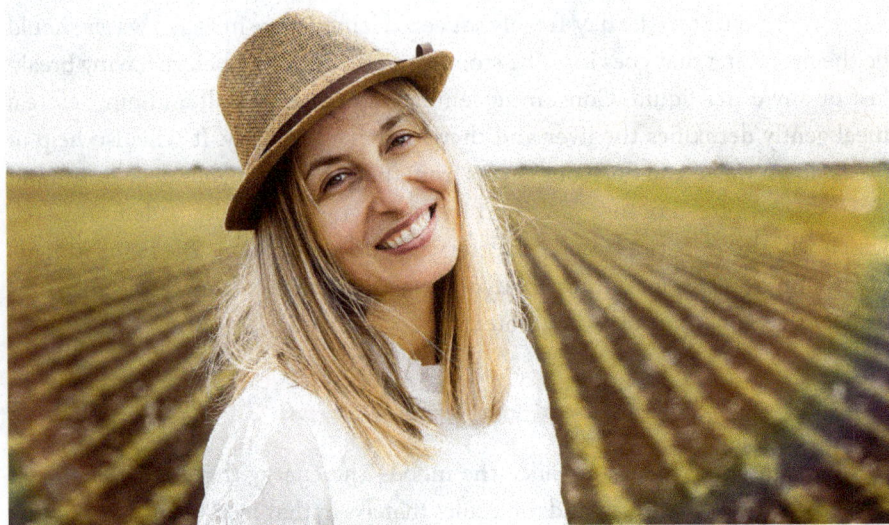

foods are cationic, which is an ion with a positive charge. This makes it extremely useful for good health, as it is the interaction between anions and cations that ultimately provides all cell energy for life.

"Jesus saith unto him, I am the way, the truth, and the life: no man cometh unto the Father, but by me" (John 14:6).

Salvestrols are essential for wellbeing and are found across the diversity of the plant kingdom. They are naturally occurring phytonutrients that have a significantly powerful disease-fighting impact. There are 100 salvestrols which have been found to be 30% higher in organic produce. They are classified as alpha, beta, delta, gamma, and omega and it is the omega salvestrols that ultimately destroy tumours. Salvestrol Q40 is a most potent cancer cell fighter and is found in high concentrations in lemons, in other citrus fruits, and also cruciferous vegetables. Once inside cancer cells, it is activated into anti-cancer metabolites and destroys cancer from inside the cell. All cancer cells have the enzyme beta salvestrol activase, and when salvestrols are absorbed by cancer cells, deadly chemicals are released which kill tumour cells. Salvestrols are extremely important in the body, and after reaching the liver, they return to the system and are re-delivered to a tumour. Salvestrols only eliminate damaged cells and not healthy ones and they are more active than antioxidants, which protect the cells from DNA damage but are ineffective once the damage has occurred.

"Many, O LORD my God, are thy wonderful works which thou hast done, and thy thoughts which are to us-ward: they cannot be reckoned up in order unto thee: if I would declare and speak of them, they are more than can be numbered" (Psalm 40:5).

For a post-workout recovery, there are excellent health benefits to drinking lemon water. Lemons are rich in electrolytes and can be included in a post-work-out recovery drink. A useful recipe includes pure water, lemon juice, Himalayan crystal salt, and raw honey. This provides a safer alternative beverage to unhealthy, commercial *energy* drinks which can contain some very questionable substances. During workouts, the body can become very acidic—especially if the workout is intense. Lemons are a very good neutralizer of high acidity within the body and are also natural energy boosters, especially if a little natural raw honey is added. Greek athletes were known for consuming honey to boost their performance. Drinking lemon water instead of plain water improves muscle endurance during workouts, as it alkalizes the body and helps to maintain a healthy pH. Adding natural raw honey or maple syrup can raise the body's acidity levels, so it is beneficial to use these sweeteners sparingly in an energy drink during and after exercise. Also ingesting natural sweeteners while the stomach is still digesting food may cause fermentation and interfere with digestion, so it is wise to ingest these on an empty stomach. When exercising, there is a rise in adrenaline, dopamine, and serotonin, which improve the blood flow and mood. These internal movements move the immune cells throughout the body, which more effectively targets cancer cells. Carbohydrates such as fruits, vegetables, legumes, and whole grains, have been used for thousands of years to enhance exercise and athletic performance, as they are the most efficient fuel for creating energy.

"How sweet are thy words unto my taste! yea, sweeter than honey to my mouth!" (Psalm 119:103).

The super-healthy coconut fruit belongs to the Arecaceae family and the Cocoideae sub-family. Its unadulterated and unheated enzyme-rich, pure coconut water is also a healthy alternative refuelling drink which is harvested from fresh young green coconuts that are about six months old. An average green coconut contains about a half to one cup of coconut water. It is a natural mineral-rich drink that packs quite a nutritional punch while it rehydrates the body, and is more nutritious when consumed in its freshest form. The coconut is a drupe (a stone fruit) and not a nut, and takes about a year to fully mature. As a coconut matures, some of the coconut water remains liquid, which helps to nourish it while the rest ripens into the firm white coconut flesh. Coconut water has a beneficially high electrolyte content and contains electrically charged ions, which assist cells in maintaining and transmitting electrical impulses (voltages) across and between their membranes and across to other cells. Electrolytes have the capability to conduct electricity and are inorganic compounds which become ions in solution. This essential cellular communication maintains the electrical signalling to the bioelectrical systems of the nervous system, heart, muscles, and brain. Fresh coconut water has the highest concentration of electrolytes of any natural food, and in an emergency can be transferred directly into an IV catheter, providing that it is in its natural state, as it has the same electrolytes that are completely compatible with the human body—phosphorus, calcium, potassium, magnesium, and sodium. Many bodily processes rely on electrolytes to function, and an imbalance can have dire consequences. Documented studies show that fresh coconut water has been successfully used by physicians as an IV fluid for over sixty years for the treatment of dehydration and malnutrition, showing that it is more effective than standard IV saline solutions. Coconut water is also rich in antioxidants, organic acids, amino acids, phytonutrients, and enzymes. It is also rich in natural vitamins, especially the B vitamins, minerals, and trace elements including manganese, copper, sulphur, selenium, iodine, and zinc. It also contains some vitamin C. Vitamins are necessary for the enzymatic reactions that cells need to function properly. Coconut water is also a nutritional source of quick energy. It helps to combat cancer, is an aid in kidney function, and helps to prevent and dissolve kidney stones. It is also a UTI remedy, an anti-inflammatory, and an anti-microbial—killing bacteria, fungus, yeasts, and viruses while feeding friendly gut flora. It kills tapeworms, assists with muscle cramps, increases exercise performance, helps to balance blood glucose and insulin levels, aids weight loss, promotes cardiovascular health, and helps to prevent heart attacks. It is also an enzyme-rich digestive tonic which improves the digestion and absorption of other nutrients, including vitamins, minerals, and amino acids. It has an alkalizing effect on the body, strengthens the bones, boosts endurance and energy, is a remedy for diarrhoea and constipation, supports immune function, and contains numerous anti-ageing benefits. It also contains the plant hormone trans-Zeatin, which is a member of the cytokinins plant growth hormone family and the primary active ingredient in coconut milk. Trans-Zeatin can be used to treat

Alzheimer's disease and dementia. Cytokinins are phytohormones, or plant hormones, that support cell division, and coconut water is the richest natural dietary source of cytokinins. Nature contains the greatest medicine.

"I went down into the garden of nuts to see the fruits of the valley, and to see whether the vine flourished, and the pomegranates budded" (Song of Solomon 6:11).

Shingles is an infection which results from the varicella-zoster virus. It is commonly known as herpes zoster and generally manifests in areas supplied by the spinal nerves. The infection is usually characterized by a blistering skin rash with debilitating and phenomenal pain. The activated shingles virus originates from an underlying weakened immune system. The primary virus infection is usually isolated from the shingles outbreak and commonly occurs during a childhood contraction of chickenpox, as the virus can remain dormant in the body for a number of years. Taking 3,000milligrams of IV vitamin C every twelve hours for at least three days, supplemented by 1,000milligrams of whole oral vitamin C with warm lemon water every couple of hours, should result in complete pain relief within the first few hours. More can be taken if necessary. The same treatment can also be applied to chickenpox. Vitamin C has a general acute virus-inactivating effect if taken in large enough doses for a long enough time period.

"For we know that the whole creation groaneth and travaileth in pain together until now" (Romans 8:22).

One of the best natural treatments for asthma are lemons because they are rich in the primary antioxidant vitamin C. They also help to clear out mucus from the air vessels. Dehydration produces much more lung mucus than a well-hydrated body. Lemons also help to deal with long-term respiratory disorders as they can improve the oxygenation of the body. Because lemon juice assists in relieving respiratory problems, it has the ability to bring soothing relief to those suffering from an asthma attack. This condition may not cause pain, as some internal organs do not relay pain. Asthma is caused by inflammation of the airways and is reversible. When immune cells generate an inflammatory process, it is usually associated with free radical damage and oxidative stress. These issues cause asthma symptoms such as the swelling of airway walls, smooth muscle contraction, and airway constriction. Allergies can cause asthma, and chronic systemic inflammation is not confined to any particular tissues but involves many internal organs and systems and the lining of blood vessels. When inflammation occurs, chemicals from white blood cells are released into the blood or affected tissues to protect the body from foreign substances. This release of chemicals increases the blood flow to the area of infection or injury, which can result in warmth and redness. The polyphenol hesperidin (vitamin P), primarily found in citrus fruits, fights allergic reactions by blocking the release of histamine. It can also decrease histamine release from mast cells by strengthening cell membranes. A lack of this bioflavonoid in the diet has also been linked to abnormal capillary leakiness. While a lemon, natural raw honey and warm water drink can be soothing for coughs, colds, and sore throats, asthmatics can also benefit by adding ginger, which can assist with opening the airways, while the vitamin C helps with the healing process. The citric acid that is present in lemons and natural raw honey also helps to dissolve phlegm.

"In whose hand is the soul of every living thing, and the breath of all mankind" (Job 12:10).

When there is insufficient oxygen and difficulty in breathing, such as when mountain climbing or being at an elevated altitude, lemons are very helpful as they improve the oxygen levels in the body. Lemons contain a small amount of iron and also increase the absorption of iron from other foods. Iron combines with specific proteins to become haemoglobin in the red blood cells, which carries oxygen around the body. Oxygen helps to convert food into energy. Vitamin C-rich foods increase the absorption of non-haem iron (from plant sources). The first man to reach the summit of Mt. Everest, Sir Edmund Hillary, said that his success on Mt. Everest was greatly due to the use of lemons.

"Every valley shall be exalted, and every mountain and hill shall be made low: and the crooked shall be made straight, and the rough places plain" (Isaiah 40:4).

As lemon is a diuretic it helps to flush out excess fluid from the body and thereby reduces inflammation, which is associated with all diseases. Inflammation is a crucial component of the immune system and is the body's natural response to an infectious agent or a traumatic or chemical injury. Inflammatory cells generate free radicals that destroy genetic material. Inflammation is a direct cause of cancer and creates an environment for its formation by creating toxins in the body which can damage the DNA and create cells that can grow into cancer. The anti-inflammatory power of lemons enables the body to prevent and fight cancer by inhibiting the spread of cancer cells.

"The LORD shall fight for you, and ye shall hold your peace"
(Exodus 14:14).

The liver has more than five hundred functions and its most important role is to filter the blood of waste products. At a molecular level, lemons are similar to saliva, and they encourage the liver to produce bile, which is the fluid needed to carry neutralized toxins to the intestines for safe disposal of these wastes. Lemon is a liver stimulant and a powerful cholagogue, which is a substance that stimulates gallbladder contraction to promote bile production into the duodenum. The liver is an important fat-burning organ. It regulates fat metabolism, breaks down fats, and removes them via the large intestine. Lemons play an enormous role in helping to detoxify the body. Not only do they aid digestion, but

> *The first man to reach the summit of Mt. Everest, Sir Edmund Hillary, said that his success on Mt. Everest was greatly due to the use of lemons.*

they also help to cleanse the colon, which is essential for the detoxification process. They protect the liver so that it can function properly, and they also encourage it to produce Phase I and Phase II enzymes, which supports it in removing toxins from the body. This promotes good health and helps to keep the skin clear. Lemon water not only stimulates liver function but also fat loss, and strengthens the liver by providing energy to the liver enzymes. The antiseptic properties of vitamin C stimulate the liver to flush out not only uric acid but also other impurities. The citrus bioflavonoid hesperidin in lemons also has the ability to protect the liver from toxic damage.

"And Jesus went forth, and saw a great multitude, and was moved with compassion toward them, and He healed their sick"
(Matthew 14:14).

Scientists have long known that the abundance of vitamin C in lemons plays a key role as a co-factor in building and protecting collagen, which is a protein family that glues cells together. Collagen is an important part of the cartilage and cushions moving joints. It is also required to help wounds heal and to produce glutathione, the master antioxidant, which is needed to detoxify the liver. Collagen is also involved in bone matrix formation and maintenance, and a lack of vitamin C can cause unstable bone structure, or bone scurvy, as vitamin C is essential for the biosynthesis of collagen, which is also beneficial for arterial walls. The antioxidant properties of lemons help to achieve more radiant skin from the inside out by repairing damaged cells, flushing out toxins, and killing free radicals that can ruin the skin. Vitamin C is a normal constituent of the skin and is normally transported through the bloodstream. It is found at high levels in both the epidermis (outer skin layer) and the dermis (second skin layer) and its role in collagen synthesis make it a vital molecule for healthy skin. Transport proteins specific for vitamin C are found on cells in every layer of the skin. By consuming as little as 10 milligrams of vitamin C daily, symptoms of scurvy, such as skin lesions, can be prevented. Because the body is unable to make or store vitamin C, signs of a deficiency can appear within one month of little to no intake of vitamin C (below 10 milligrams per day). These manifestations of scurvy result from a decline in collagen synthesis, which leads to the fragility of the blood vessels and a disruption of connective tissue. Skin lesions can be remediated by a sufficient intake of vital vitamin C and Omega-3 fatty acids, which can be obtained by an adequate and varied whole plant-food diet.

"And I will lay sinews upon you, and will bring up flesh upon you, and cover you with skin, and put breath in you, and ye shall live; and ye shall know that I am the LORD" (Ezekiel 37:6).

To help protect tooth enamel, the mouth should be thoroughly rinsed out directly after consuming lemon because the acid can literally eat away at the protective enamel coating of the teeth. It is beneficial not to brush the teeth until at least half an hour after consuming lemon as citric acid softens the enamel, and brushing immediately, even after rinsing with water, can remove some of the enamel. This also applies if consuming sugar. A deficiency in vitamin C can lead to problems with the gums and teeth such as sensitive teeth, gingivitis (inflammation of the gums, which is an initial stage of gum disease and a dangerous precursor to other serious issues), bleeding, and aching gums. Vitamin C can help to prevent these problems if adequate quantities are consumed. According to a *British Medical Journal* study, tooth decay and cavities can potentially be reversed with a healthy diet.

"How sweet are thy words unto my taste! yea, sweeter than honey to my mouth!" (Psalm 119:103).

The vitamin C in lemons also helps to thin the blood and a lack of water results in the thickening of the blood. It is essential to keep well hydrated throughout the day as a lack of water in the body causes the system to go into preservation mode, which means that the body will retain every last drop of water. It is also important to consume sufficient vitamin C on a regular basis. Blood vessels are strengthened by the vitamin P bioflavonoids in lemons, thereby preventing internal haemorrhage.

"But whosoever drinketh of the water that I shall give him shall never thirst; but the water that I shall give him shall be in him a well of water springing up into everlasting life" (John 4:14).

Urinary tract infections can be caused by E. coli bacteria that exist in the bowel but find their way into the urethra. A UTI may also occur when kidney stones are present, or the urine flow is blocked, which causes the urine to pool in the bladder, creating an ideal environment for bacteria growth. Lemons help to prevent and reverse urinary tract infections, providing the lemons are not consumed in excess, otherwise, the pH can be altered to an overly alkaline state. When a UTI is present, drinking sufficient pure water with added lemon juice will flush out toxins and help to facilitate a healing process. Lemon juice is a natural probiotic that kills the bacteria inside the bladder and urethra, which will naturally help to relieve any pain. Pain is caused by inflammation and adequate vitamin C extinguishes inflammation. Lemon cleanses the system, helps to flush out unwanted materials, and increases the rate of urination in the body. Therefore, toxins are released at a faster rate, which helps to keep the urinary tract healthy. There are those who drink fermented apple cider vinegar for their urinary tract infection because they perceive that they will reap benefits from it, but the resulting appearance of its influence is due to the fact that this acid is alkaline in the system, as are healthy lemons.

"And the LORD shall guide thee continually, and satisfy thy soul in drought, and make fat thy bones: and thou shalt be like a watered garden, and like a spring of water, whose waters fail not" (Isaiah 58:11).

When dealing with bee stings, the stinger can be gently scraped from the skin with the edge of a bank card or something similar, then a piece of fresh lemon can be applied to the afflicted area of the skin and secured in place until the venom becomes neutralized. The natural acid in lemons acts as a blood purifier and helps the body to naturally eliminate venom. Applying lemon juice to poison ivy or insect bites can soothe the skin, as it not only has anti-inflammatory properties but also anaesthetic effects. Lemon juice can also be applied to reduce the pain of sunburns, and because it is antifungal, it can clear up a mild case of athlete's foot when applied topically.

"O death, where is thy sting? O grave, where is thy victory?" (1 Corinthians 15:55).

Astringent lemons have antiseptic and coagulant properties, which can stop internal bleeding. Lemon juice can put a rapid stop to internal and external hae-morrhages, as does cayenne pepper, and a combination of the two proves to be very effective in cases of bleeding. To stop nosebleeds, fresh lemon juice can be applied to a small cotton ball and placed inside the nostril, or very firm pressure can be applied for a few minutes to the side of the bridge of the nose where the nostril is bleeding. Unless they have occurred as a result of an accident, nose-bleeds can be caused by bodily inflammation.

"But if we walk in the light, as He is in the light, we have fellow-ship one with another, and the blood of Jesus Christ His Son cleanseth us from all sin" (1 John 1:7).

Citrus peels that remain after consuming the fruit can easily be dried and added to many recipes and dishes for added vitamin C and other vital nutrients. Organic citrus is best. A dehydrator or a low-temperature oven can be used to dry the citrus peels with the pith (white inner lining) attached. The peels need to be dehydrated for about twenty-four hours or until crisp and thoroughly dried out. These can then be stored in a covered container in a cool dry place for about a year. To use the peels as a nutritious flavouring, they can be ground to a powder and sprinkled onto any number of dishes. Two level teaspoons or more of the dried, powdered rind per day will supply the body with a good quality vitamin C complex including healthy hesperidin, rutin, and bioflavonoids.

"And God said, Let the earth bring forth grass, the herb yielding seed, and the fruit tree yielding fruit after his kind, whose seed is in itself, upon the earth: and it was so" (Genesis 1:11).

Vitamin C can also be found in sprouted produce. For sprouting dehydrated produce, such as dried corn, or for dehydrating damp sprouted produce, such as grains, which can then be ground into flour, it is vital to know that heat can denature vital enzymes in plants if they are heated to more than 48°C (118° F). This temperature can be proven by soaking grains, nuts and seeds for several hours and then dehydrating them at 48°C for four hours, after which they can be sprouted, which proves that the enzymes are still alive. Enzymes are essential for sprouts to grow. Some vitamin C is still available after this ground flour is baked into bread.

"For the earth bringeth forth fruit of herself; first the blade, then the ear, after that the full corn in the ear" (Mark 4:28).

Frozen whole organic lemons can be finely grated or shredded without being peeled, bearing in mind that the seeds can be bitter and absorb the most pollutants. This can then be sprinkled on healthy fruit salads, vegetable salads, soups, ice creams, curries, cereals, vegetables, noodles, spaghetti sauce, and more, resulting in a fantastic flavour as fresh lemon is an excellent flavour enhancer.

"And he shall be like a tree planted by the rivers of water, that bringeth forth his fruit in his season; his leaf also shall not wither; and whatsoever he doeth shall prosper" (Psalm 1:3).

The amazing God-given lemon, from its rind to its juice, is a rich source of nutrients and antioxidants that help to flush out toxins, prevent diseases, and promote healing in the body. Adding lemons to the diet will greatly help to balance the body's pH levels and prevent it from being too acidic. In an acidic environment, bacteria, parasites and cancer cells tend to thrive.

"But the day of the Lord will come as a thief in the night; in the which the heavens shall pass away with a great noise, and the elements shall melt with fervent heat, the earth also and the works that are therein shall be burned up" (2 Peter 3:10).

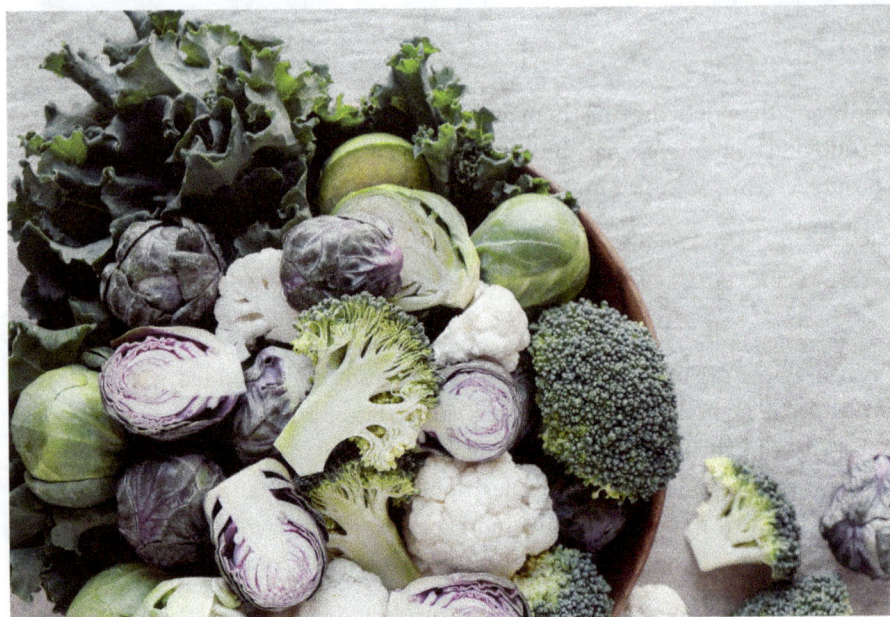

Chapter 7

Cruciferous Vegetables

"TO EAT IS A NECESSITY, BUT TO EAT INTELLIGENTLY IS AN ART."

Cruciferous vegetables belong to the genus Cruciferae. Although appearing to be very different, broccoli, Brussels sprouts, cabbage, cauliflower, kale, and kohlrabi are botanically the same species of plant and have the same common wild cabbage ancestor. These crucifers were selectively bred thousands of years ago to emphasize different characteristic traits. The only differences between them are the traits that were introduced over many centuries of selective plant propagation and cultivation. This group of vegetables was named for the four equal-sized petals in its flowers that could be seen as forming a cross-like shape. The word cruciferous means *one who bears a cross*. The human body contains untold numbers of the cross-shaped protein adhesion molecule called laminin, which is the glue of the body and holds it together. Cells organize themselves into specific molecular structures which determine which proteins they will be. Laminin is organized into this special cross-shaped structure, which instructs it as to what role it will play in the body. Laminin keeps cells in position by gluing the cells to a foundation of connective tissue and helping them to function properly. The arms of laminin associate with one another to form sheets which bind to cells. Defects in the laminin structure result in health disorders as it can become unstable if its shape is lost.

"And Pilate wrote a title, and put it on the cross. And the writing was, JESUS OF NAZARETH THE KING OF THE JEWS" (John 19:19).

Preserved crucifer seeds have been unearthed in Pakistani villages dating back to 2000 BC, and also in some ancient Chinese villages dating back thousands of years. Chinese and Sanskrit writings mention the use of crucifers in the first and second millennium BC, while other reliable references to crucifers are shown in Arab writings from AD 1200–1300. Cruciferous vegetables were disseminated across Europe and around the Mediterranean region as a result of the Crusades. Crucifers such as cabbage, mustard, horseradish, radish, and turnip were thriving throughout Europe by the sixteenth century. They continued to spread throughout the world, and the first American settlers took European crucifers to Jamestown.

"Thou wilt shew me the path of life: in thy presence is fulness of joy; at thy right hand there are pleasures for evermore" (Psalm 16:11).

The crucifers considered in this book are broccoli, Brussels sprouts, cabbage, cauliflower, kale, and kohlrabi. They are accessible, affordable, time-tested and potent. The cruciferous vegetable family is quite large and includes arugula, bok choy, broccoli, broccoli sprouts, Brussels sprouts, cabbage, cauliflower, Chinese cabbage, collard greens, horseradish, kale, kohlrabi, land cress, maca root, mustard greens, napa cabbage, radishes, red cabbage, rutabaga, shepherd's purse, swedes, turnips, wasabi, and watercress. This crucifer group have amazingly high nutrient profiles that are hard to equal and include vitamin A, vitamin B1, vitamin B2, vitamin B3, vitamin B5, vitamin B6, vitamin C, vitamin E, vitamin K, calcium, carotenoids, chlorophyll, chromium, copper, fibre, folate, iron, kaempferol, magnesium, manganese, Omega-3 fatty acids, phosphorous, potassium, protein, selenium, and zinc. The high concentration of vitamin A, carotenoids and vitamin E in crucifers, with their unusually high content of vitamin C and manganese, are important components of this antioxidant vegetable class. The vitamin K and chlorophyll content of cruciferous vegetables, especially collards and kale, help to regulate the inflammatory response that can increase the risk of cancers and many other diseases. Chlorophyll can also maintain levels of active CoQ10, which is also known as ubiquinol. These vegetables contain a vast array of nutrients that are necessary for optimal health. Although spinach is not a crucifer it does kill cancer stem cells, along with other leafy greens and crucifers.

*Then shall thy light break forth as the morning, and thine health shall spring forth speedily: and thy righteousness shall go before thee; the glory of the LORD shall be thy rereward"
(Isaiah 58:8).*

Powerful crucifers have many health-promoting properties, including analgesic, anti-ageing, anti-allergenic, anti-angiogenic, anti-arthritic, anti-asthmatic, anti-atherogenic, anti-bacterial, antibiotic, anticarcinogenic, anti-depressant, antidiabetic, antifungal, anti-inflammatory, anti-ischaemic, anti-malarial, anti-metastasis, antimicrobial, antimutagenic, antioxidant, anti-parasitic, anti-phlogistic (prevents or relieves inflammation), anti-rheumatic, anti-tumourigenic, anti-ulcer, anti-viral, anxiolytic, apoptotic, cytotoxic (to cancer stem cells), detoxifying, diuretic, epigenetic, immune-protective, immune-stimulating, neuritogenic, neuroprotective, neurorestorative, and radioprotective.

"O LORD, thou art my God; I will exalt thee, I will praise thy name; for thou hast done wonderful things; thy counsels of old are faithfulness and truth" (Isaiah 25:1).

Various health issues that cruciferous vegetables benefit include cancers (including leukaemia), inflammation, cardiovascular disease, arthritis, endothelial and epithelial dysfunction, Alzheimer's disease, eczema, jaundice, scurvy, rheumatism, multiple sclerosis, autism, diabetes, lupus, asthma, haemorrhoids, anaemia, colds, flu, allergies, gastric ulcers, infections, macular degeneration, cataracts, constipation, heart disease, Candida, obesity, rabies, tetanus, headaches, epilepsy, gout, chronic fatigue, cystic fibrosis, urinary tract infections, kidney disease, liver disease, fevers, detoxification, eye disorders, brain health, skin disorders, respiratory disorders, and bile production.

"And Jesus went forth, and saw a great multitude, and was moved with compassion toward them, and He healed their sick" (Matthew 14:14).

Potent cruciferous vegetables are immensely superior to dangerous pharmaceutical drugs at defeating cancer. Such drastic chemical measures weaken and debilitate the whole system, from which it very often never recovers. Pernicious drugs kill normal healthy cells, and may only kill some less harmful cancer cells, and the cells that remain are the more lethal cancer stem cells that are resistant to these nefarious drug treatments. Toxic man-made drugs can never replace the efficacy of the superior, natural healing virtues of God-given nutrients in healing plants. Pharmaceuticals deplete the body of many nutrients and are thereby a threat to health. Crucifers are known to have high anti-cancer properties, which influence the environment of the cell which then modifies its genes in order to accommodate these changed environments (epigenetics). Fruits and vegetables are the highest nutrient-dense foods, with dark green leafy vegetables being the most nutritious. They are also cost-effective and tasty without the horrendous side effects. Health-giving plants were designed for the well-being of the human race since time immemorial, and it is the right of every human being to seek out the life forces of these amazing plants for the restoration of good health.

"And to you who are troubled rest with us, when the Lord Jesus shall be revealed from heaven with His mighty angels, In flaming fire taking vengeance on them that know not God, and that obey not the gospel of our Lord Jesus Christ: Who shall be punished with everlasting destruction from the presence of the Lord, and from the glory of His power" (2 Thessalonians 1:7–9).

Radiation transforms healthy cells into induced cancer stem cells, but broccoli and other crucifers have been shown to kill cancer stem cells. The diindolylmethane (DIM) in crucifers can protect against the effects of radiation, before and after exposure, whatever the source. DIM is produced in the stomach after cruciferous vegetables are consumed. Radiation hardly affects the platelets and red and white blood cells when DIM is present. DIM can boost cellular responses that repair damaged DNA, and radiation damages DNA.

"And the Lord shall deliver me from every evil work, and will preserve me unto his heavenly kingdom: to whom be glory for ever and ever. Amen" (2 Timothy 4:18).

It is unusual to find another plant-food group, other than crucifers, of which as many different parts of the plant are consumed. Among the cruciferous vegetable class, the flowers of the plant, such as the broccoli and cauliflower florets, the leaves, stems, and stalks are all consumed. The unique benefits of consuming this cruciferous vegetable food group may be partly related to the inclusion of so many different plant parts, as plants distribute nutrients differently in their particular anatomical sections. Commonly included in diets are so many different parts of the cruciferous plants that they may help to broaden the diversity of phytonutrients received from this special food class. Because different parts of the cruciferous plants are consumed, it is important to recognize that these different parts may require different cooking times and methods.

"The LORD is good, a strong hold in the day of trouble; and he knoweth them that trust in Him" (Nahum 1:7).

Scientific research on cruciferous vegetables has identified over 100 different glucosinolates with unique hydrolysis (breakdown) products. Hydrolysis is the chemical breakdown of a compound due to its reaction with water. With a lack of these vegetables in the diet, the body will be deficient in these essential compounds, which are powerful cancer preventatives. Crucifers contain isothiocyanates, thiocyanates, nitrile, and epithionitrile, which are a defence system of compounds that protect the plant against insects, pathogens, and herbivores. Active compounds that prevent cancer cell growth are indoles (also called benzopyrrole), a class of phytochemicals that are associated with cancer prevention; thiocyanates (a complex anion, or negatively charged ion); and isothiocyanates (sulphur-containing phytochemicals). Isothiocyanates are anti-cancer nutrients that activate cancer-fighting genes and are biologically active hydrolysis products of glucosinolates. They have also been found to induce apoptosis and inhibit proliferation in a number of cancer cell lines. Anti-cancer compounds operate in several ways: by triggering the body's own detoxification systems, by slowing the growth of cancer cells, and by supporting DNA repair. In epidemiological studies, a high consumption of cruciferous vegetables is associated with a decreased risk of various cancers.

"And to every beast of the earth, and to every fowl of the air, and to every thing that creepeth upon the earth, wherein there is life, I have given every green herb for meat (food): and it was so" (Genesis 1:30).

Members of the cruciferous family of vegetables pack a powerful punch when it comes to cancer prevention. Crucifers contain a diversity of anti-cancer nutrients, which have been shown to both systemically overcome cancer cells and prevent them from forming potent mechanisms, thereby inhibiting developing cancer cells. Research acknowledges that various elements of cruciferous vegetables stop cancer cell growth in breast tumours, lung cancer, colon cancer, liver cancer, and cancers of the uterine lining and cervix. They also shield the intestines from disease-causing micro-organisms. These vegetables are a rich source of phytochemicals, glucosinolates, and their hydrolysis products, including isothiocyanates and indoles, and have powerful anti-cancer properties. Crucifers contain the protective aryl hydrocarbon receptor protein (a protein-coding gene), which mediates toxicity. They also contain an impressive plethora of nutrients and a significant amount of fibre. These are elements that many scientists believe aid in the prevention of cancers. Not only are they impressive in terms of their nutrient content but are even more renowned for their phytonutrients. Many studies have shown that the nutrients present in cruciferous vegetables can arrest all cancer cell lines by inhibiting the fuel that is necessary for the cancer cells to multiply. The antioxidant abundance in cruciferous vegetables has also been explicitly mentioned in several studies as one of the strong contributors to the risk-lowering impact of these vegetables on numerous forms of cancer. These amazing vegetables have been found to improve the survival rates of those with cancer and have been demonstrated to reduce the risk of many other degenerative diseases and health conditions. The benefits of a diet rich in these vegetables have been well documented in medical literature.

"Fear thou not; for I am with thee: be not dismayed; for I am thy God: I will strengthen thee; yea, I will help thee; yea, I will uphold thee with the right hand of my righteousness" (Isaiah 41:10).

A characteristic and striking chemical property of all cruciferous vegetables is their high concentration of the powerful natural and unique organo-sulphur compounds glucosinolates, which are the precursors of isothiocyanates and which have the power to make changes on a genetic level and exert protective anti-cancer characteristics. They can activate genes that fight cancer, deactivate other genes that fuel tumours, and are water-soluble sulphur-containing compounds that are responsible for imparting the pungent aromas and slightly bitter taste of crucifers. The sulphur in glucosinolates induces enzyme expression, activates detoxification, and works as a detoxifier and antioxidant in the body. Glucosinolates, whose healing virtues have been extolled, have amazing health benefits and are made from several plant amino acids and glucose. When cruciferous vegetables are prepared, the enzyme myrosinase (or thioglucosidase), which accompanies the glucosinolates, is released. This myrosinase enzyme, which is distributed in myrosin cells, is responsible for hydrolyzing glucosinolates into isothiocyanates. Glucosinolates and their isothiocyanate hydrolysis products are well-known defenders against cancer development, and consuming plenty of these vegetables has the ability to lower the risk of different types of cancer. In the absence of myrosinase, when the vegetables are cooked and the myrosinase enzyme is inactivated by heat, the body can efficiently convert glucosinolates to isothiocyanates through the action of microflora in the gastrointestinal tract. When converted into the isothiocyanate molecules, the glucosinolates have an amazing record of lowering the risk of specific cancers as they contain high amounts of nitrogen and sulphur. In crucifer plants, the glucosinolate compounds accumulate inside their cells and are used by the plants as a form of natural defence. When these cells are damaged the glucosinolates mix with special enzymes kept separately within the cells (which is a similar feature of garlic), breaking them down into isothiocyanates. This phenomenon not only deters insects but provides crucifers with their distinctive taste and nutrition.

"But we see Jesus, who was made a little lower than the angels for the suffering of death, crowned with glory and honour; that He by the grace of God should taste death for every man" (Hebrews 2:9).

Research indicates that glucosinolates are able to stimulate the body's own natural antioxidant systems, or Phase II enzymes, which in principle are part of the cellular biotransformation machinery. Glucosinolates perform as indirect antioxidants by provoking the liver to produce detoxifying enzymes, which prevent free-radical attacks on the DNA. Once this process has occurred, a cascade of antioxidant activity repeatedly cycles within the body and continues to protect the body's system for up to four days after the glucosinolate-containing food was initially consumed. Excellent glucosinolate sources include broccoli, broccoli sprouts, Brussels sprouts, cabbage, red cabbage, cauliflower, kale, and kohlrabi. Consuming these crucifers increases the amount of glucosinolate in the system, adding to the enzyme production in the liver. These natural enzymes help to flush out carcinogens and other toxins from the body,

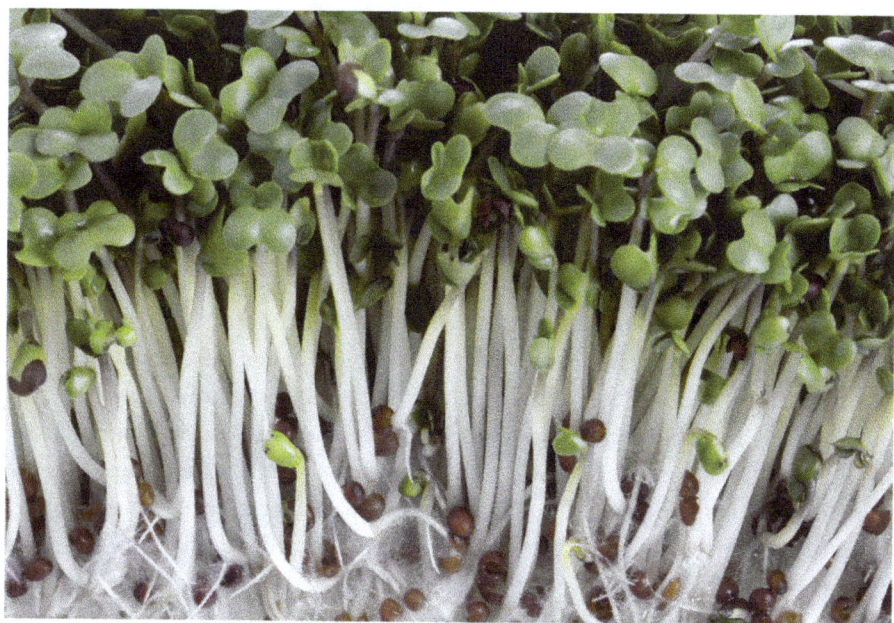

which can significantly lower the risks associated with cancer. Glucosinolates are utilized for DNA repair and help to prevent cancer by slowing cancer cell growth. All crucifers contain glucosinolates and thereby have amazing health benefits. They are important phytonutrients for health because they are the chemical starting points for a variety of cancer-protective substances.

"And a great multitude followed Him, because they saw His miracles which He did on them that were diseased" (John 6:2).

The indole diindolylmethane (DIM) is a natural substance that is produced when the body breaks down indole-3-carbinol (I3C), a compound present in crucifers and well known for its anti-cancer effects. I3C is a benzopyrrole and is only formed when the isothiocyanates derived from glucobrassicin are further broken down into non-sulphur containing compounds. I3C is a member of the glucosinolate family, which is a group of compounds that also contains other indoles and isothiocyanates such as sulphoraphane (an anti-inflammatory phytochemical). These are known antioxidants and natural detoxifying enzymes. The active cancer-protective properties of crucifers are attributed to the fact that these foods contain substantial quantities of the phytonutrients isothiocyanates, specifically I3C and sulphoraphane. These compounds help the body to fight disease by reducing inflammation and helping to prevent DNA damage. Inflammation promotes cellular proliferation and inhibits apoptosis, thereby increasing the risk of developing cancer. Research on I3C shows that it helps to deactivate a potent oestrogen metabolite that promotes tumour growth, especially in oestrogen-sensitive breast cells. Oestrogen is a family of hormones, and I3C partially blocks oestrogen receptor sites on cell membranes. Research also indicates that I3C may protect the liver by converting highly active oestrogen by-products to much safer compounds. It has also been shown to reduce and reverse breast tumour cell growth and cancerous cell metastasis. I3C can alter the activity of a number of enzymes involved in the cancer process as well as change the chemical metabolism of carcinogens, such as aflatoxin. Research has also shown that I3C not only inhibits the action of some carcinogenic aflatoxins but also prevents aflatoxin-induced liver cancer, leukaemia, and colon cancer. Cell cultures demonstrate that I3C inhibits human papilloma virus (HPV) proliferation and the development of pre-cancerous lesions and cysts. There is also evidence that I3C increases apoptosis and may help to prevent the recurrences of respiratory papillomatosis. This derived form of glucobrassicin blocks receptor sites that would otherwise be prone to chemical attacks, subsequently causing serious problems inside the cells. It also returns alpha and beta-receptor site expression to normal levels, directly kills cancer cells, and blocks other cancer-enhancing receptor sites.

"And Jesus went forth, and saw a great multitude, and was moved with compassion toward them, and He healed their sick" (Matthew 14:14).

Research demonstrates that there is a definite place in the diet for cruciferous vegetables in their raw sprouted, cultured, and cooked form. When consumed in their raw, uncooked, sprouted form the greater potential health benefits involving specific proteins that are very efficient catalysts for specific biochemical reactions. The myrosinase enzyme (which fights cancer and stomach ulcers), provides a better opportunity for having phytonutrients, such as glucosinolates, converted into uniquely health-supportive molecules such as isothiocyanates. Nutrients from these uncooked cruciferous vegetable sprouts are also more likely to be absorbed in the upper digestive tract and then transported to the liver where they are made available to other tissues in the body that may benefit from their availability. All cruciferous vegetables contain significant amounts of powerful sulphoraphane. However, gram for gram, broccoli sprouts have several orders of magnitude higher concentrations of sulphoraphane than the mature broccoli plant. Culturing is another healthy option and one of the oldest ways of preserving foods. Properly prepared cultured raw vegetables are beneficial for the gut and create desirable gut probiotics, which are extremely important. These micro-organisms create lactic acid, which acts as a preservative. The same bacteria predigest specific food components, which makes the digestion and absorption of nutrients easier. For example, culturing cabbage increases cancer-fighting glucosinolate compounds.

"Therefore my heart is glad, and my glory rejoiceth: my flesh also shall rest in hope" (Psalm 16:9).

Crucifers that can be cooked and contain high amounts of sulphoraphane are broccoli, Brussels sprouts, cabbage, cauliflower, mustard greens, and collards. After cutting sulphoraphane containing crucifers into pieces for cooking, it is advisable to thoroughly pierce them with a sharp knife before leaving them to rest for about thirty minutes prior to cooking, as this allows the powerful sulphoraphane compound to be released. This is a similar reaction to garlic and is designed as a defence mechanism against microbial pathogens, which attack the vegetables. When cruciferous vegetables are consumed in a cooked form and have not been pierced and allowed to rest prior to cooking, there is unlikely to be very much enzyme activity and the digestive products of these vegetables are more likely to pass unabsorbed through the upper digestive tract and on into the lower digestive tract. In the colon, the cruciferous vegetable nutrients are likely to be further metabolized by bacteria. If the vegetables have been

Having a healthy digestive system with a well-functioning gut microbiota is vital for obtaining and maintaining the most health benefits.

overcooked the microbiota in the digestive tract can salvage some important cancer-preventive agents. Having a healthy digestive system with a well-functioning gut microbiota is vital for obtaining and maintaining the most health benefits. Cooking crucifers not only supplies more beta-carotene, which the body converts to vitamin A but also produces indole, which helps to prevent malignancies. To boost the bacteria in the colon and enhance the anti-cancer effects of sulphoraphane, it is beneficial to feed the desirable bacteria in the gut with plenty of prebiotics such as fibre, to encourage their proliferation. Research has proven that this natural chemical compound sulphoraphane in cruciferous vegetables is transferred directly from the digestive system into the body through beneficial gut bacteria. Intestinal microbiota consume and break down glucoraphanin, the parent compound of sulphoraphane, and deliver it into the bloodstream where it provides a direct anti-cancer effect. When the body is operating at optimal capacity it is able to absorb the most organo-sulphur and reap its considerable anti-cancer benefits. Boiling green vegetables with added bicarbonate of soda in the water to keep them bright green kills their vitamin C content.

"Comfort ye, comfort ye my people, saith your God"
(Isaiah 40:1).

There is overwhelming evidence that cruciferous vegetables have an enormous, valuable, unique, and powerful role in the widely recognized protective effects of natural plant foods against cancer. The biologically active compounds from sprouted, cultured, and cooked green vegetables enhance the natural defences of the human body and shield against DNA damage. They also fuel the body's ability to block the replication and growth of cells that are already damaged.

"Every word of God is pure: He is a shield unto them that put their trust in Him" (Proverbs 30:5).

The sulphur-rich sulphoraphane compound in crucifers has the potential to prevent and treat at least 200 different health conditions. Cruciferous vegetables use the extracted carbon dioxide from the air to build life-saving sulphoraphane molecules which have a molecular structure of $C_6H_{11}NOS_2$. Research indicates that crucifers, and sulphoraphane specifically, kills cancer stem cells, as it has been shown to have potent anti-cancer properties. As a powerful anti-cancer nutrient it also performs a number of beneficial functions in the body as it possesses many health benefits, such as high bioavailability. It is also known to have anti-diabetic and anti-microbial properties. The organo-sulphur in crucifers blocks parasites by competing for receptor sites on mucous membranes, as parasites that are unable to attach themselves are flushed out of the system. It has been determined that sulphoraphane also helps to protect the health of the stomach lining by preventing a bacterial overgrowth of Helicobacter pylori in the stomach. Having healthy gut flora can also help to release sulphoraphane. Researchers have ascertained that this active phytochemical effectively eradicates cancer cells, while not harming healthy cells, by entering cancer cells and reacting with specific internal proteins to induce apoptosis. Sulphoraphane supports the body's process of detoxification and assists in the protection from, and the elimination of, pesticides and arsenic, as sulphoraphane activates Nrf2, which performs a crucial task in the metabolism and excretion of poisonous substances. Sulphoraphane also supports healthy joint cartilage, the bladder, the prostate, the gut, and cell health, together with the production of enzymes that protect the blood vessels. It participates in activating over 200 different genes and helps to support DNA methylation, normal cell division, and growth. Sulphoraphane has also been demonstrated to reduce incidences of autistic behaviour by reducing brain inflammation. It protects muscles from exercise-induced damage and also DNA, tissues, and cells from free radical damage. A study has demonstrated the capability of sulphoraphane to search out and selectively strike at potential threats to the body. It targets prostate cancer and other hormone-dependant cancers while also leaving healthy cells unaffected. Sulphoraphane triggers anti-inflammatory activity in the cardiovascular system, which helps to prevent and reverse blood vessel damage. Researchers have discovered preliminary evidence of the ability of crucifers to lower the risk of cardiovascular damage, including ischaemic heart disease and heart attack. They were also able to reverse multiple sclerosis without toxic pharmaceutical drugs by having subjects consume a diet high in organic sulphur-rich foods such as crucifers. Because cruciferous vegetables are rich in the potent anti-cancer nutrient sulphoraphane, even minimal amounts are capable of thwarting disease.

"Sing unto the LORD; for He hath done excellent things: this is known in all the earth" (Isaiah 12:5).

It was believed for decades that it was not possible for the brain to regenerate. However, sulphoraphane, which is a neuritogenic substance, has been documented to stimulate new nerve growth in the brain. The brain is now considered to be resilient and pliable. Evidence indicates that the brain is in a continual dynamic state of self-repair and self-regeneration, in which damaged and aged tissue is replaced and repaired by neural stem cells. A new study reveals that sulphoraphane contains significant therapeutic elements that are remedial for the underlying pathological disturbances found in neurodegenerative diseases. Researchers have discovered that exposing neural stem cells to sulphoraphane resulted in their differentiation to neurons, which provides compelling evidence and gives powerful support to the hypothesis that sulphoraphane is able to stimulate brain repair in degenerative disorders. It is also neuroprotective and improves cognitive function after traumatic brain injury.

"That ye may with one mind and one mouth glorify God, even the Father of our Lord Jesus Christ" (Romans 15:6).

According to research, potent sulphoraphane has the capability of boosting the capacity of the liver to detoxify harmful cancer-causing compounds. Specifically, sulphoraphane raises the activity of the liver's Phase II detoxification enzymes. These enzymes are noted for their ability to dispose of a wide range of toxic elements from the body, including many carcinogens and reactive oxygen species, which are a particularly destructive type of free radicals. By boosting these important detoxification enzymes, the compounds in crucifers contribute to protection against cancer cell mutations and many other detrimental effects that would otherwise be caused by these toxins. Scientists have clearly demonstrated that sulphoraphane targets prostate and breast cancer cells and has an amazing ability to induce specific enzymes to act, which is performed by signalling genes in the cell nucleus. These particular enzymes activate the antioxidant and detoxification process as sulphoraphane stimulates enzymes in the body that detoxify carcinogens before they can damage cells. This powerful element improves the liver's ability to detoxify carcinogens and other toxins. The synergistic combination of two other cruciferous constituents, crambene and I3C, also appears to vigorously activate detoxification enzymes.

"The LORD is their strength, and He is the saving strength of his anointed" (Psalm 28:8).

All leukaemias begin in the bone marrow, which is substituted by unnaturally proliferating neoplastic (malignancy) cells. Leukaemias are malignant neoplasms (tumours) that involve cells primarily originating from haematopoietic (related to the formation of blood cells) precursor cells. Neoplastic cells can leak out of the bone marrow into the blood, resulting in leukaemia. Researchers are still uncovering the amazing medicinal power of sulphoraphane, which was recently discovered to prevent and treat leukaemia. Specific aspects of sulphoraphane's haematologic cancer-fighting properties reinforce its viability as a natural and safe compound for cleansing the blood. Sulphoraphane has been shown to induce cytotoxic effects on acute leukaemia cells and also in a variety of tumour cells.

"In whom we have redemption through His blood, the forgiveness of sins, according to the riches of His grace" (Ephesians 1:7).

The molecules in sulphoraphane work via a process known in biochemistry as a redox reaction, that is, a reaction of reduction and oxidation. A redox reaction happens when two chemical compounds exchange electrons. One molecule donates electrons and the other molecule receives electrons. This chemical reaction occurs when an alkaline molecule provides negatively charged electrons to acidic molecules to neutralize an acid. Cruciferous vegetables can manipulate genes as sulphur is the key. Many antioxidants do this but sulphoraphane also alters the epigenetic endpoints. Epigenetics involves influencing the cellular environment surrounding the genes. Healing sulphur works through redox reactions and alters the cellular environment. The sulphur-containing part of the plant cells in broccoli has been demonstrated to be an indirect antioxidant.

"Such knowledge is too wonderful for me; it is high, I cannot attain unto it" (Psalm 139:6).

Researchers have discovered that a remarkable compound in cruciferous vegetables targets cancer stem cells and helps to prevent the recurrence and spread of cancers. The anti-inflammatory compound phenethyl isothiocyanate (PEITC) is a naturally occurring phytochemical found abundantly in cruciferous vegetables. PEITC is produced from its precursor gluconasturtiin by the action of the myrosinase enzyme. For more protection against cancers, and to increase the availability of enzyme breakdown in the upper digestive tract, preparing cruciferous vegetables as aforementioned allows time for the production of PEITC, which forms when cruciferous vegetables are cut. PEITC has been demonstrated to have preventative activity against a range of cancers, including prostate cancer, breast cancer, ovarian cancer, colon cancer, pancreatic cancer, and cervical cancers. PEITC is known to prevent the initiation phase of the carcinogenic process and also inhibits the progression of tumourigenesis. Researchers discovered that it significantly reduced the proliferation of both cervical cancer cells and cervical cancer stem cells and is significantly superior at abrogating cervical cancer stem cell proliferation than extremely harmful toxic cancer drugs. They also found that the concentrations of PEITC used in their study can be achieved through a diet rich in cruciferous vegetables and especially land and watercress. Watercress is known to be a rich dietary source of nasturtin, which is a precursor of PEITC, and is one of many compounds found in these vegetables that has been reported as a potential anti-cancer agent. It has been shown to inhibit cancer cell growth and the induction of apoptosis in many cancer cell lines. Research indicates that the PEITC from nasturtin may suppress breast cancer cell development. It also slows or stops Phase I enzymes found in the liver, which are known to activate many carcinogens that trigger cancer cell growth. Nasturtin induces the liver's Phase II enzymes, which enhance the excretion of carcinogens, thereby preventing DNA damage and inhibiting cancer cell growth. When PEITC and turmeric are combined, these two nutrients significantly reduce tumour growth and the ability of cancerous cells to metastasize.

"And Jesus went about all the cities and villages, teaching in their synagogues, and preaching the gospel of the kingdom, and healing every sickness and every disease among the people" (Matthew 9:35).

The average adult body contains more than five litres of blood, which carries oxygen and nutrients (such as fatty acids, amino acids, and glucose), to all living cells, removes their waste products (such as carbon dioxide, lactic acid and urea), protects the body from foreign bodies, produces proteins, and delivers immune cells to fight infections. Its platelets can prevent blood loss by plugging damaged blood vessels. Blood adapts to the needs of the body through the circulatory system. The green chlorophyll in crucifers is almost identical to the haemoglobin protein inside the red blood cells, which has, as its primary function, the transport of oxygen from the lungs to other parts of the body. The only difference between chlorophyll and haemoglobin is that chlorophyll has a magnesium nucleus while haemoglobin has an iron nucleus. The chlorophyll in plants contains magnesium, oxygen, carbon, nitrogen, and hydrogen; while the haemoglobin in blood contains iron, oxygen, carbon, nitrogen, and hydrogen. Interestingly, chlorophyll has been used in times of war instead of blood plasma.

"For the life of the flesh is in the blood" (Leviticus 17:11).

Green leafy vegetables are one of the most potent allies for cleansing the liver. These cleansing foods are powerfully protective of the liver, and incorporating green vegetables into the diet helps to increase the creation and flow of bile, which removes waste from the blood and organs. Dark green leafy vegetables are the primary source of lutein and zeaxanthin, which can reduce the risk of macular degeneration and cataracts. Greens are incredibly high in plant chlorophylls; they absorb environmental toxins from the bloodstream and have the distinct ability to neutralize heavy metals, pesticides, and chemicals. Greens contain thylakoids, which trigger satiety signals to help regulate food intake, promote weight loss, and prevent weight gain. Inside the leaves of a plant are numerous organelles which function together to create and collect energy, and the thylakoid is one of the most important places that this occurs. Thylakoids are tiny compartments found inside chloroplasts which help to absorb sunlight for photosynthesis to occur. All of a plant's chlorophyll is contained in the thylakoid membranes of chloroplasts, which in turn allows for sunlight absorption. On the surface of plant leaves, there are a large number of tiny pores known as stomata, in which the thylakoid membrane vesicles are located. Chlorophyll, the photosynthetic pigment of green leaves, harnesses the energy from sunlight for photosynthesis to occur.

Photosynthesis occurs when carbon dioxide is drawn in from the air and enters the plant leaves through the stomata. This is chemically combined with water and minerals that the plant draws from the ground to create oxygen and carbohydrates (which are stored in the plant as food). Two categories of carotenoids found in plants are xanthophyll and carotene, which operate as additional pigments in photosynthesis by absorbing light energy at wavelengths inefficiently absorbed by chlorophyll. They further safeguard plants

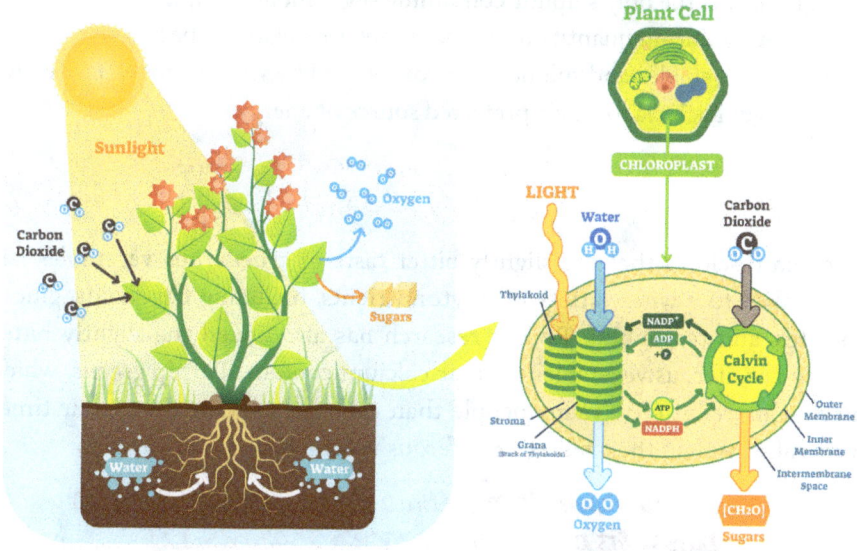

PHOTOSYNTHESIS

from being overexposed to sunlight by absorbing excess light energy as heat. It is a well-established fact that as CO2 in the atmosphere increases, the rate of photosynthesis also increases, as confirmed by NASA. Higher CO2 levels are a major contributor to the vast global regreening that has been observed for a few decades. NASA acknowledges that CO2 is responsible for a world-wide increase in vegetation by 50%. CO2 is a most vital molecule for sustaining global plant life, and without plants, there would be no oxygen and therefore no humans. To balance nature, God designed humans and other living creatures to breathe in oxygen and breathe out carbon dioxide to produce energy, and plants to take in carbon dioxide and give out oxygen to produce energy. The entire process of photosynthesis can be explained by this chemical formula: $6CO_2 + 12H_2O + Light \rightarrow C_6H_{12}O_6 + 6O_2 + 6H_2O$.

"Truly the light is sweet, and a pleasant thing it is for the eyes to behold the sun" (Ecclesiastes 11:7).

A study suggests that leafy greens are an essential food source for beneficial gut bacteria. Researchers have discovered a unique sugar, known as sulphoquinovose, that is produced through photosynthesis. A special enzyme named YihQ is used by gut bacteria to change the sulphoquinovose in leafy greens into an available supply of carbon and sulphur. Sulphur is recycled by gut organisms that utilize YihQ to feed on the considerable quantity of sulphoquinovose. Sulphoquinovose is unique as it is the only sulphur containing sugar molecule, and sulphur builds proteins. A significant quantity of sulphoquinovose sugars can be consumed from leafy green vegetables and sulphoquinovose is used by vital strains of protective beneficial gut bacteria for their preferred source of energy.

"Who giveth food to all flesh: for His mercy endureth for ever" (Psalm 136:25).

Research discloses that the slightly bitter taste of cruciferous vegetables has been linked to a wide variety of phytonutrients, including flavonoids, gluco-sinolates, and terpenoids. Recent research has also linked the slightly bitter taste of cruciferous vegetables to their calcium content. Turnip greens, which taste far more bitter to many people than cabbage, contain about four times more calcium than their fellow cruciferous vegetables.

"The LORD will give strength unto His people; the LORD will bless His people with peace" (Psalm 29:11).

As with other vegetables, crucifers are good sources of a variety of nutrients and phytochemicals, which may work synergistically to help prevent cancer. Spinach and leafy cruciferous vegetables, such as broccoli and kale, contain high amounts of the natural antioxidant alpha-lipoic acid (ALA). ALA captures free radicals and also binds with heavy metals such as arsenic and mercury, effectively eliminating them from the circulation. These phytochemicals have unique abilities to modify hormones, detoxify compounds, and prevent toxic substances from binding to DNA, thereby preventing toxins from causing DNA damage that could lead to cancer.

"If ye be willing and obedient, ye shall eat the good of the land"
(Isaiah 1:19).

Medical science (University of California) now confirms that crucifers should preferably be consumed cooked, as when these coarse vegetables are eaten raw they can remove iodine from the body and impact thyroid function as they contain goitrogens. But when they are cooked most of their goitrogenic chemicals are lost. It is difficult to properly break down any raw, coarse vegetables just by chewing, and cooking them makes their plant cell walls less rigid and easier to digest. They need to be cooked until just tender for their nutrients to be released and absorbed, as the nutrients are in the coarse fibres. All coarse vegetables are abounding in healthful nutrients when properly cooked. Ellen G. White is the most prolific translated woman writer in the entire world history of literature and the most translated American author. Her Godly inspired writings cover many topics. In her book entitled *Education*, she states the following: "...coarse vegetables...fail of supplying proper nutriment" (ch. 22, p. 100.3).

"And whosoever doth not bear his cross, and come after me, cannot be my disciple" (Luke 14:27).

BROCCOLI

Broccoli (Brassica oleracea var. italica) was derived from a wild cabbage-like relative by selective breeding in pre-Roman times around 600 BC. It comes from the Mediterranean region, was eaten by the Romans and its name derives from *little sprouts* in Italian. The Italians regarded this quintessential green vegetable as a good source of nutrition. Interestingly enough, the Romans, who nailed Jesus Christ to a cross, consumed crucifers. Broccoli is known for its resemblance to a tree, and Jesus died on a tree; broccoli gives life, and Jesus gives life. Broccoli could be called a tree of life because of its life-giving qualities. Sprouting broccoli was cultivated in Italy in ancient Roman times and was introduced into England around 1720. Its heritage name comes from the Italian *broccolo*, which relates to the flowering top of a cabbage. Broccoli has been selected for its edible, immature flower heads which comprise of a proliferation of clusters of tiny green or purple flower buds that group onto the undeveloped stalks. Broccoli is picked before these flower bud heads are open.

"The righteous shall flourish like the palm tree: he shall grow like a cedar in Lebanon" (Psalm 92:12).

Scientists have long demonstrated the antioxidant properties of broccoli, which is rich in vitamins A, C, and E, the primary free radical scavenger vitamins. Broccoli contains twice the amount of vitamin C that is found in citrus fruits, which helps with the absorption of iron and calcium. It also contains large amounts of vitamin B and calcium as well as chromium, chlorophyll, fibre, folate, iron, Omega-3 fatty acids, and potassium.

According to research, the sulphoraphane in broccoli is the most potent natural Phase II enzyme-inducer known. This is one of the detoxification systems of the liver. It is a most essential vegetable for health and nutrition because of its nutrient density. Broccoli has an especially powerful type of sulphoraphane, which researchers believe gives it its unique superfood cancer-fighting properties. Interestingly, a close-up look at the tiny green tips on a broccoli head looks like a myriad of cancer cells. Broccoli is an exceptional source of sulphoraphane and produces more than any other known plant in the world. However, none of the sulphoraphane is available until the plant is cut. In one part of the broccoli cells there is an enzyme called myrosinase, and in another part there is glucoraphanin, which is an important phytonutrient in broccoli, and broccoli is the only crucifer to have any significant quantity of it. Glucoraphanin belongs to the category of compounds called glucosinolates, which are enzymatically converted into isothiocyanates that are active anti-cancer nutrients in the body. This enzymatic conversion is performed by myrosinase, which is found naturally in crucifers. Myrosinase-like activity occurs in the intestinal microflora, and if glucoraphanin is consumed by itself the gut microflora will convert a portion of it into the potent cellular protector and antioxidant, sulphoraphane. Glucoraphanin, the glucosinolate precursor of sulphoraphane, also influences the process of mutagenesis and carcinogenesis. Glucoraphanin has also been proven to eliminate carcinogens and environmental pollutants through the urine. The naturally occurring presence of glucoraphanin in broccoli corresponds to a healthier regulation of fats in the liver. Broccoli inhibits the input of too much fat into the liver by decreasing the liver's input of lipids and increasing its output of lipids, demonstrating its ability to protect against fatty liver disease, which is usually associated with obesity and over-eating in general, thus providing benefits that may be crucial to the protection of the liver. When the cells of broccoli are cut, the enzyme myrosinase converts glucoraphanin and produces sulphoraphane. Sulphoraphane is unobtainable without myrosinase, which all crucifers contain. After cutting broccoli into florets as aforementioned, this allows the sulphoraphane to be released. Once the sulphoraphane has been produced by the myrosinase enzyme, this enzyme is no longer required, as it has already performed its needed task and the broccoli can be cooked until tender, thus destroying the myrosinase enzyme while still retaining its powerful sulphoraphane content. Steaming broccoli florets optimizes its sulphoraphane content by eliminating the epithiospecifier protein, which is a heat-sensitive sulphur-capturing protein that inhibits the formation of anti-cancer sulphoraphane. This attests that cooked broccoli is more nutritious than raw. Broccoli also contains more folate when cooked.

In addition to sulphoraphane, broccoli also contains high amounts of carotenoids and other antioxidants and has been shown to protect against breast cancer, cervical cancer, colon cancer, laryngeal cancer, lung cancer, oesophageal cancer, oral cancer, ovarian cancer, pharyngeal cancer, prostate cancer, and stomach cancer. Broccoli is a diuretic and is also efficacious for eye infections, fevers, and toxin removal, including inhaled air pollutants. It also contains the necessary ingredients to switch on genes that prevent cancer development and switch off other genes that help it to proliferate. Accumulating research discloses that everyday foods such as broccoli contain substances that stimulate the repair and renewal of nerve tissue. Frozen crucifers have the decreased ability to manufacture sulphoraphane due to the rapid destruction of the myrosinase enzyme during the blanching process prior to freezing for the purpose of deactivating enzymes. However, adding other crucifers such as horseradish, radishes, wasabi, or daikon radish to the same meal will add myrosinase due to their abundant myrosinase content. Mustard greens are also members of the crucifer family, and their myrosinase-rich seeds, which are high in selenium and magnesium, can also significantly boost sulphoraphane levels when adding them to crucifers as a ground powder.

"And being found in fashion as a man, He humbled himself, and became obedient unto death, even the death of the cross" (Philippians 2:8).

It has been demonstrated that the phytonutrient sulphoraphane is present in much higher concentrations in broccoli seeds and three-day-old broccoli sprouts. Broccoli and broccoli sprouts have the highest amount of isothiocyanates, and adding broccoli sprouts to the diet is an excellent way to reap the incredible benefits of isothiocyanates. Small quantities of fresh broccoli sprouts contain as much cancer protection as more substantial amounts of raw, mature broccoli. If consuming broccoli raw, about 12% of the entire sulphoraphane content is obtainable based on its progenitor compound, but substantially more nutrients are available when it is cooked. Many studies have demonstrated the ability of broccoli to fight cancer, and when raw broccoli is combined with broccoli sprouts, such as a salad, the two together can be doubly powerful as the sprouts possess greater amounts of antioxidants and provide greater protection against cancer. Studies show that to maximize the benefits of the anti-cancer component sulphoraphane in raw broccoli, the enzyme myrosinase is required from sprouts, radishes, or other myrosinase containing vegetables, which increases the absorption

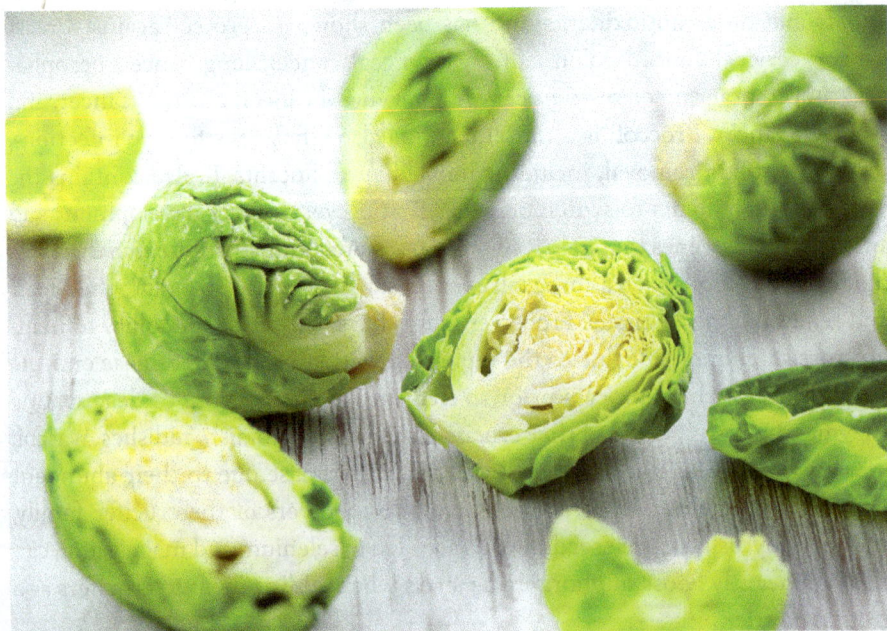

of sulphoraphane in the body. Thus, consuming these crucifers at the same time can double the cancer-preventive effects.

"And the earth brought forth grass, and herb yielding seed after his kind, and the tree yielding fruit, whose seed was in itself, after his kind: and God saw that it was good" (Genesis 1:1).

BRUSSELS SPROUTS

Although Brussels sprouts (Brassica oleracea var. gemmifera) have the wild cabbage as their ancient ancestor, they are thought to be native to a specific region near Brussels, the capital of Belgium, after which they are thought to be named. There are records of their being in the vicinity of Brussels as far back as the thirteenth century; although the French coined the name in the eighteenth century, as it was common to put a landmark on a food. The modern Brussels sprouts were first cultivated in large quantities in Belgium as early as 1587. They remained a local crop in this area until they spread across Europe during World War I. Although the sprouts resemble the structure of a small head of cabbage, they are produced in the leaf axils, starting at the base of the stem and working upwards.

The nutrients in Brussels sprouts include vitamin A, vitamin B, vitamin C, vitamin E, calcium, carotenoids, chlorophyll, choline, fibre, folate, iron, kaempferol, magnesium, manganese, molybdenum, Omega-3 fatty acids, phosphorus, potassium, and tryptophan. They are an extremely nutrient-dense food. Another important anti-inflammatory nutrient contained in Brussels sprouts is vitamin K, which is a direct regulator of inflammatory responses. It also promotes strong bones and has protective benefits against Alzheimer's disease.

Researchers have found that Brussels sprouts offer improved stability and unique protection to the DNA inside the white blood cells after daily consumption of these crucifers. This stability and protection are due to their antioxidants, which have the ability to block the activity of sulphotransferase enzymes that are responsible for catalyzing the transfer of a sulpho-groups from a donor molecule. Brussels sprouts are known to have the highest total glucosinolate content of cruciferous vegetables. Their total glucosinolate content has been shown to be greater than the amount in broccoli, turnip greens, cauliflower, mustard greens, kale, or cabbage. The glucosinolates in Brussels sprouts can also help to protect the lining of the stomach and digestive tract. Four

Specific glucosinolates are found in a unique combination in Brussels sprouts and these are glucobrassicin, glucoraphanin, gluconasturtiian, and sinigrin.

> *The Omega-3 fatty acids in Brussels sprouts are fundamental components for one of the body's most effective groups of anti-inflammatory messaging molecules.*

Equally important are sulphoraphane, isorhamnetin, kaempferol, ferulic, and caffeic acids, together with the relatively rare sulphur-containing compound 3H-1,2-dithiole-3-thione (D3T). Brussels sprouts contain a broad spectrum of antioxidant phytonutrients, including numerous antioxidant flavonoids. These crucifers also assist the digestive system by preventing the overgrowth of bacteria in the gut microflora. The sulphoraphane in Brussels sprouts triggers anti-inflammatory activity in the cardiovascular system and can help to prevent and reverse blood vessel damage. The Omega-3 fatty acids in Brussels sprouts are fundamental components for one of the body's most effective groups of anti-inflammatory messaging molecules. It has been demonstrated that the DNA is protected by naturally occurring elements in Brussels sprouts which can help to prevent adverse changes. The consumption of Brussels sprouts affords cancer protection and prevention for many types of cancers which include bladder cancer, breast cancer, colon cancer, lung cancer, prostate cancer, and ovarian cancer as Brussels sprouts help to activate cancer-fighting enzyme systems in the body. The sulphur compounds in Brussels sprouts also help to support both the Phase I and Phase II detoxification process, which removes toxins from the system, as they have a substantial amount of sulphur-containing nutrients and vitamin C. Their rich source of antioxidants is necessary for Phase I detoxification when toxins are disassembled into smaller particles and eliminated later during Phase II. Supporting both Phase I and Phase II detoxification with nutritious foods such as Brussels sprouts is important, as harmful substances can be broken down and regularly and safely be removed from the body. Conversely, disaggregated toxins can accumulate in the body if foods that support Phase I but not Phase II are consumed. Brussels sprouts provide special nutrient support for three body systems that are closely connected with cancer prevention and development. These are the body's antioxidant, detoxification, and anti-inflammatory systems, and any imbalances of any one or more of these systems can increase cancer risk. There are significantly more cancer risks when a greater number of these imbalances occur.

"But God forbid that I should glory, save in the cross of our Lord Jesus Christ, by whom the world is crucified unto me, and I unto the world" (Galatians 6:14).

CABBAGE

Cabbage (Brassica oleracea var. capitata) has a long history, both as a medicine and food. It was initially developed from the wild cabbage, which was closer in appearance to kale and collards and was composed of leaves that did not form a head. The cabbage was grown by ancient Greek and Roman civilizations which held it in high esteem as a general panacea that was capable of treating a multitude of health conditions. The first recorded use of the natural bioactive compounds found in crucifers was from the recommendation of Cato the Elder, who was a Roman statesman around 200 BC. He wrote that crushed cabbage leaves would heal breast cancer. Ancient Roman healers believed that they could heal breast cancer by rubbing cabbage poultices on the chest area. Studies show that when cabbage paste is rubbed on animals it can prevent tumour development. The cultivation of cabbage spread across northern Europe and into Poland, Germany, and Russia, where it became a very popular vegetable. It was the Italians who were known for developing the Savoy cabbage.

Cabbage is rich in nutrients including vitamin B1, vitamin B5, vitamin B6, vitamin C, vitamin K, vitamin U, calcium, carotenoids, chlorophyll, fibre, folate, iron, magnesium, manganese, Omega-3 fatty acids, phosphorus, and potassium.

Today's varieties of cabbage descended from cabbages that grew wild in Mediterranean regions thousands of years ago. Over 400 varieties of cabbage are now grown worldwide with varying shapes including round, oval, and cylindrical. There are interesting dissimilarities in the leaves of today's varieties and all have very short stems. The colours also vary, with some being nearly white; others are pale green, blue-green, and reddish-purple. Cabbage contains sulphoraphane, which has outstanding benefits for cancer prevention. It also reduces the likelihood of tumours, absorbs toxins, and squelches inflammatory conditions and fevers. Bruised cabbage leaves can also be used as a poultice and are very beneficial in cases of inflammation, pain, arthritis, and breast issues. Abundant evidence shows cabbage to be an amazing healer of stomach and external ulcers, due to its high phytonutrient content. Cabbage soup with a pinch of cayenne pepper is a wonderful healer of stomach ulcers. The vitamin U in cabbage has powerful healing properties which are not affected by heat if consumed cooked. Cabbage is a remarkable natural medicine and when it is well chewed it reduces the nitrates in the mouth to nitrites, which in turn converts to nitric oxide in the stomach and expands blood vessels. Ample proof shows that cabbage has more medicinal value than many other natural foods and also helps with constipation and liver disorders. The detoxification systems of the body necessitates generous supplies of sulphur to function effectively, and cabbage is abundant in sulphur-containing nutrients. Consuming cabbage helps to stimulate the activation of two crucial major liver detoxifying pathways inside the liver cells known as Phase I and Phase II enzymes, that help to flush out toxins. These pathways require specific nutrients to function efficiently. Folate, glutathione, vitamins A, B, C, and E are required for Phase I; and amino acids and sulphurated phytochemicals, such as those found in garlic and crucifers are required for Phase II, which eliminate the waste products of detoxification from the body via the bowel and urine. Cabbage has high amounts of some of the most powerful antioxidant phytonutrients found in crucifers which stimulate and is required by Phase I detoxifying enzymes. Sinigrin is one of the glucosinolates especially plentiful in cabbage, and Savoy cabbage, in particular, is an especially good source. Sinigrin can be converted into allyl-isothiocyanate (AITC). This isothiocyanate compound displays unique cancer preventive properties with regard to bladder cancer, colon cancer, and prostate cancer. Cabbage has also been shown to be protective against radiation. The sulphurous odour that is often associated with cooking cabbage only develops when cabbage is overcooked, as the strength of the odour is synonymous with the length of cooking time.

"Jesus said unto her, I am the resurrection, and the life: he that believeth in me, though he were dead, yet shall he live" (John 11:25).

The vitamin C antioxidant equivalent capacity of red cabbage is six to eight times higher than that of green cabbage and is one of the tastiest and most nutritious vegetables. Red cabbage sprouts contain six times more vitamin C and forty times more vitamin E than the fully mature plant. While green cabbage is the most commonly consumed variety of cabbage, red cabbage has added nutritional benefits that are not found in green cabbage, plus it has a hearty, robust flavour. The rich red colour of red cabbage reflects its concentration of anthocyanin polyphenols, which contribute to it containing significantly more protective phytonutrients than its green counterpart.

"Looking unto Jesus the author and finisher of our faith; who for the joy that was set before Him endured the cross, despising the shame, and is set down at the right hand of the throne of God" (Hebrews 12:2).

CAULIFLOWER

Cauliflower (Brassica oleracea var. botrytis) is another cultivated descendant of the wild cabbage which has undergone many transformations. The name cauliflower derives its name from the Latin word *caulis* which means *cabbage with a flower*. It has been an important vegetable in Italy and Turkey since at least 600 BC. Cauliflower gained popularity in France in the sixteenth century and was subsequently cultivated in the British Isles and northern Europe. There are in excess of eighty varieties of edible cauliflowers worldwide including light green, yellow, pale orange, and purple variants, which are said to be just as nutritious as the white type, with the purple cauliflower having been proven by several research studies to have exceptionally powerful antioxidant potential due to its abundant concentration of anthocyanins, which are mainly concentrated in the outer layers of the cauliflower head. As cauliflowers begin to grow, they resemble broccoli, and cauliflowers are believed to have been bred from broccoli. Yet, unlike broccoli, their flowers stop developing before any flower buds are produced, resulting in the immature flowering white heads. Cauliflowers form a compact head on a central stalk from the undeveloped flower buds, called a curd, which is shielded from the sunlight by the overshadowing heavy outside green leaves which are usually secured together over the emerging curds when growing. This also prevents over-maturity and protects its softness and flavour. It is because the leaves prevent chlorophyll from forming that the cauliflower heads are white. Even though they are of the same species these two crucifers look quite different. Their shape can resemble the brain and they also have neuro-protective properties. However, they do still share some characteristics such as a similar taste and aroma, similarly shaped flowers, and an arrangement of four petals in a cross-shape.

Cauliflower is a rich source of nutrients. Among these are vitamin B1, vitamin B2, vitamin B3, vitamin B5, vitamin B6, vitamin B7, calcium, carotenoids,

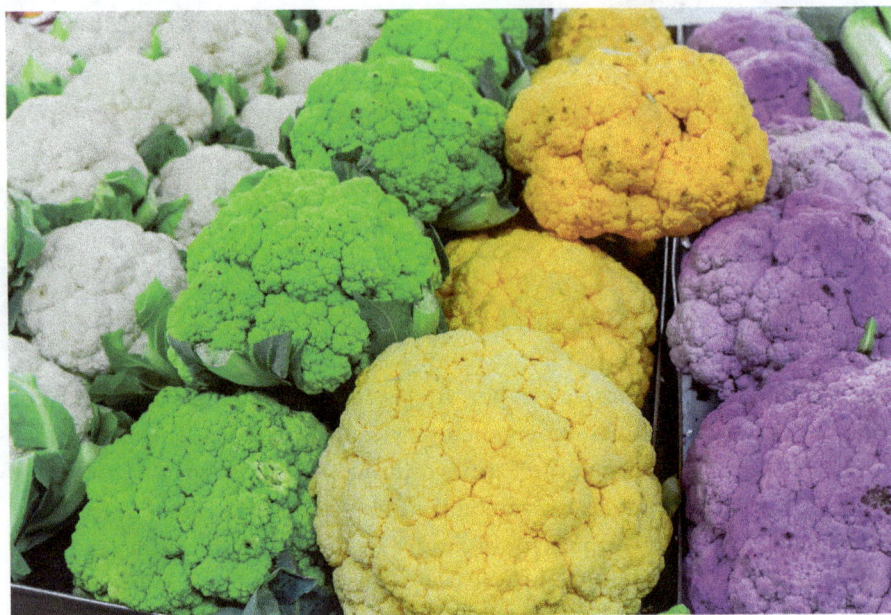

chlorophyll, choline, folate, iron, magnesium, manganese, Omega-3 fatty acid, phosphorus, and potassium. Cauliflower also has a very high vitamin C content and is an excellent source of vitamin K and fibre. As an excellent source of vitamin K, cauliflower provides anti-inflammatory nutrients which act as a direct regulator of an inflammatory response. Cauliflower heads contain numerous phytonutrients including allicin, indole-3-carbinol, and sulphoraphane. Amongst cauliflower's most important antioxidant phytonutrients are beta-carotene, beta-cryptoxanthin, caffeic acid, cinnamic acid, ferulic acid, kaempferol, lutein, quercetin, rutin, and zeaxanthin.

This broad-spectrum antioxidant support assists in lowering the risk of oxidative stress in the cells. By providing such a broad array of antioxidant nutrients cauliflower helps to lower the risk of cancer. Cauliflower has prostate cancer preventing capabilities, especially when consumed with turmeric. It also inhibits prostate cancer recurrence. There have been several dozen studies linking cancer prevention to diets containing cauliflower, particularly concerning bladder cancer, breast cancer, cervical cancers, colon cancer, lung cancer, and ovarian cancer. Cauliflower contains antioxidants that support Phase I detoxification together with sulphur-containing nutrients which are important for Phase II detoxification. Cauliflower's glucosinolates can help to activate detoxification enzymes and regulate their activity. Three glucosinolates have been clearly identified in cauliflower and these are glucoraphanin, glucobrassicin, and gluconasturtiin. Cauliflower is also an important source of dietary fibre for digestive health. The indoles in cauliflower possess anti-obesity effects. Cauliflower also helps to stimulate fat-burning thermogenesis and aids weight loss. The powerful sulphur compound sulphoraphane contained in cauliflower has been shown to kill cancer stem cells. Scientists believe that the benefits of sulphoraphane are related to improved DNA methylation which is essential for proper gene expression and normal cellular function. The potassium content in cauliflower aids with the regulation of glucose metabolism as it is utilized by the pancreas for secreting the insulin hormone that combats high blood sugar. The abundant vital B vitamin nutrient choline is found in cauliflower and is important for brain function. When choline is combined with phosphorus they help to repair cell membranes. This results in better sleep, a sharper memory and better cognitive performance. Other health benefits of cauliflower include boosting the immune system, improving digestion, lessening heart and circulatory system issues, and keeping hormones in check.

"For the preaching of the cross is to them that perish foolishness; but unto us which are saved it is the power of God" (1 Corinthians 1:18).

KALE

Kale (Brassica oleracea var. sabellica) has been cultivated for well over 2,000 years and is another descendant of the wild cabbage which is thought to have originated in Asia Minor. Wild cabbages may have been brought to Europe around 600 BC by groups of Celtic peoples. Curly kale was a significant crop during ancient Roman times and evidence for the cultivation of cruciferous vegetables is recorded in the writings of the early Roman Empire. This blue-green, leafy vegetable continued to be grown for many hundreds of years. In a large part of Europe, kale was the most widely eaten green vegetable until the Middle Ages when the cabbages of that era became more popular. During the Middle Ages, curly kale was a popular vegetable eaten by peasants. Historically, it has been of particular importance in the colder regions of the world due to its frost resistance. Over time, preference for larger leaved varieties prevailed, and this continued preference for a larger leaved vegetable led to the development of kale, as it is now known. As time passed, a preference was expressed for kale plants with a large number of tender leaves in a tight cluster at the centre of the plant at the top of the stem, and these plants were frequently selected and propagated. Continued favouritism for these plants for many hundreds of successive generations resulted in the gradual formation of denser clusters of leaves at the top of the plant which eventually became so large that it dominated the whole plant and the cabbage head of today was born.

Kale is an excellent source of vitamin A, vitamin C, vitamin K, carotenoids, copper and manganese. It is also a very good source of vitamin B1, vitamin B2, vitamin B5, vitamin B6, vitamin E, calcium, chlorophyll, choline, fibre, folate, iron, magnesium, Omega-3 fatty acids, phosphorus, potassium, and selenium.

Kale studies have shown impressive bioavailability of lutein, zeaxanthin, beta-carotene, and retinol from this crucifer. Research studies also show rapid and significant increases in the blood levels of these important antioxidant nutrients in those who consume plenty of cruciferous vegetables. Researchers have identified over forty-five different flavonoids in kale with quercetin and kaempferol showing premium importance. Kale's flavonoids combine both anti-inflammatory and antioxidant benefits in a way that makes kale one of the dietary leaders in avoiding oxidative stress and chronic inflammation. The isothiocyanates in kale play a primary role in achieving these risk-lowering benefits. Kale provides comprehensive support for the body's detoxification system, and new research indicates that the isothiocyanates that it contains can help to regulate detoxification at a genetic level. Kale has unsurpassed health benefits because of its exceptional nutrient richness and its achievement is difficult for most foods to match. It has been studied more extensively in relationship to cancer than any other health condition. Research studies show cancer-preventive benefits from kale intake including bladder cancer, breast cancer, colon cancer, ovarian cancer, and prostate cancer. Its cancer-preventive benefits are clearly linked to its unusual concentration of two types of antioxidants—the flavonoids and the carotenoids. Within the flavonoids, kaempferol is the primary antioxidant in kale, followed by the flavonoid quercetin. The broad range of flavonoid antioxidants is vital to kale's cancer-preventive benefits. Within the carotenoids, beta-carotene, and lutein are kale's prominent antioxidants and have the ability to raise the blood levels of these key carotenoid nutrients. They protect the body from oxidative stress and health issues related to oxidative stress. An increased risk of atherosclerosis, cataracts, and chronic obstructive pulmonary disease are just three of these health issues. Also among these chronic health problems is cancer, as the risk of cells becoming cancerous is partly related to oxidative stress.

Consuming plenty of cruciferous vegetables may provide a significant survival advantage for women diagnosed with ovarian cancer, which is one of the most aggressive cancers.

"And He bearing His cross went forth into a place called the place of a skull, which is called in the Hebrew Golgotha" (John 19:17).

KOHLRABI

Kohlrabi (Brassica oleracea Gongylodes Group) is another vegetable that was cultivated from the wild cabbage and was in existence in the 1st century AD. Pliny the Elder mentioned a *Corinthian turnip*, which was a vegetable that closely resembled the growing habits of kohlrabi. It is native to northern Europe and highly valued for its nutritional content. Kohlrabi grows above the ground and was bred specifically as a hardier version of cruciferous vegetables which can grow in harsher conditions. Kohlrabi was commented on by Apicius in his cookbook, which was the oldest known book on cooking and dining in imperial Rome. In AD 800, Charlemagne was crowned Emperor of

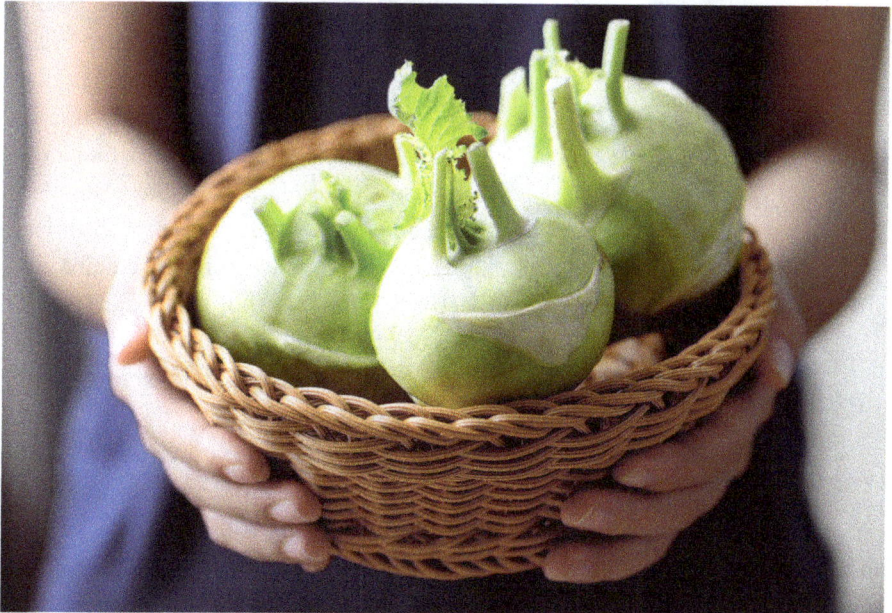

the Holy Roman Empire and he ordered kohlrabi to be grown in the lands over which he reigned. The home of Charlemagne was located in the western portion of Germany, which accounts for the German name of kohlrabi, which means *cabbage turnip*. From Charlemagne's era to the present day, kohlrabi has been commonly used throughout Germany, France, and Italy. It arrived in northern India during the Middle Ages where it was considered by the Hindus to be a predominant fundamental in their diet.

Kohlrabi is rich in vitamins and minerals which include vitamin A, vitamin B1, vitamin B2, vitamin B3, vitamin B5, vitamin B6, vitamin E, vitamin K, calcium, chlorophyll, choline, copper, folate, iron, Omega-3 fatty acids, phosphorus, potassium, manganese, and magnesium. It is also an exceptionally rich source of vitamin C—even more so than oranges.

The taste of the kohlrabi bulb is mild and mostly resembles that of the heart of a cabbage when cooked but much juicier and sweeter with a texture similar to broccoli stems. There are over twenty-two different varieties which vary in size, colour, shape, and flavour, with some having a longer shelf life—such as Gigante and Kossak kohlrabi. The most commonly seen are pale green, white, and purple, with the purple variety having a stronger flavour. They all have creamy coloured flesh underneath their surface. It is high in fibre and is a member of the cabbage family, although its appearance is more like a turnip. The whole plant is edible, except for its slender root. Its leaves are rich in iron and can be enjoyed as spinach, collard, and beetroot greens, with a taste that is reminiscent of collards and kale.

> *The different varieties of cruciferous vegetables have proven throughout the ages to be a powerful source of protection against life-threatening diseases. It is incredibly beneficial to consume them daily for optimal health and longevity as they are truly a gift from God.*

As with other crucifers, kohlrabi possesses sulphur-containing glucosinolates which are health-promoting phytochemicals that have anti-inflammatory, anti-cancer, anti-parasitic, anti-fungal, and antibacterial properties. Kohlrabi has the ability to help prevent cancer, anaemia, diabetes, stroke, obesity, heart disease, Alzheimer's, and other diseases. It promotes digestive health, boosts the immune and cardiovascular systems, increases circulation, maintains a healthy metabolism, supports optimal nerve and muscle functioning, promotes vision health, strengthens the bones, and assists with weight loss. It is also a diuretic and relieves the pain caused by urinary tract infections. It reduces C-reactive protein, which is produced in the liver and is among a group of proteins called *acute phase reactants* that rise in response to inflammation, which predisposes disease.

The different varieties of cruciferous vegetables have proven throughout the ages to be a powerful source of protection against life-threatening diseases. It is incredibly beneficial to consume them daily for optimal health and longevity as they are truly a gift from God.

"And God shall wipe away all tears from their eyes; and there shall be no more death, neither sorrow, nor crying, neither shall there be any more pain: for the former things are passed away" (Revelation 21:4).

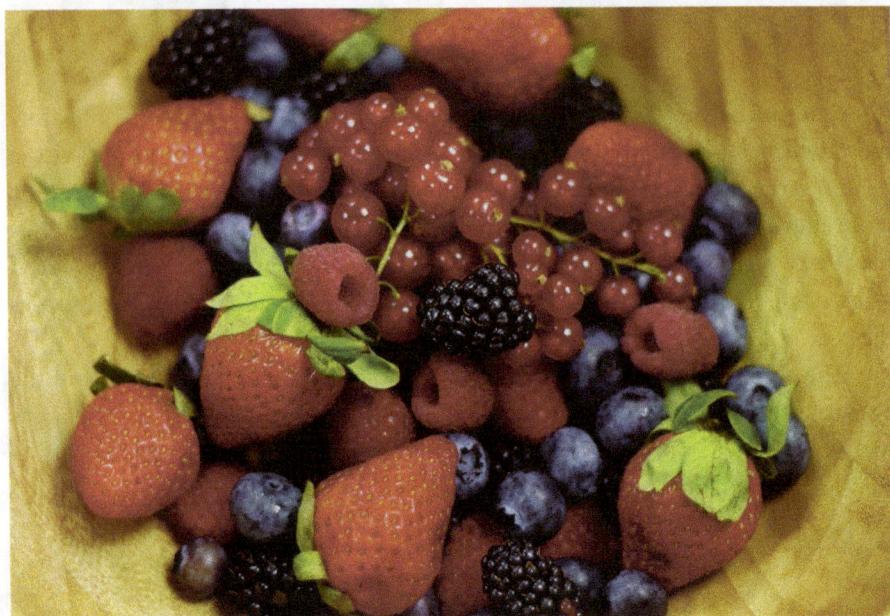

Chapter 8

Berries

"FOOD IS INFORMATION THAT CONTAINS MESSAGES THAT COMMUNICATE TO EVERY CELL OF THE BODY."

Berries are small fruits that originate from a single ovary that has multiple seeds. Cranberries, blueberries, gooseberries, blackcurrants, and redcurrants are berries; whereas, a likely lesser-known fact is that grapes, tomatoes, papaya, guava, bananas, and avocados are also botanically classified as berries. Many fruits commonly called berries, such as raspberries and blackberries, are not classified as berries but are classed as aggregate drupes, as they are made up of many tiny druplets clustered together. Cherries are also classified as drupes and strawberries are classified as fleshy receptacles. The berries that are considered in this book are blackberries, blackcurrants, blueberries, cherries, grapes, raspberries, and strawberries. Studies demonstrate that these are amongst the highest antioxidant fruits.

"Thus hath the Lord GOD shewed unto me: and behold a basket of summer fruit" (Amos 8:1).

These berries are time-tested, accessible, potent, and affordable. There is overwhelming evidence that all of these berries contain substances that are proven to have beneficial effects and protect cells against many types of cancers as they contain potent phytochemicals that directly inhibit the DNA binding of some carcinogens. Studies show that berry phytochemicals are also involved in the regulation of carcinogen-metabolizing enzymes, inflammatory cytokines, growth and transcription factors, tumour angiogenesis, apoptosis, subcellular signalling pathways of cancer cell proliferation, and xenobiotic-metabolizing enzymes (which primarily protect against environmental assaults). Many researchers recognize that regularly consuming richly-coloured berries can have a significant impact on health. Numerous studies have shown that they play a huge role in maintaining good health and warding off diseases. Berries are not only powerful anti-cancer foods but are also protective against viruses, bacteria, and many other pathogens while also boosting natural killer cell activity. The main component in berries is their rich and powerful anthocyanin content, which is responsible for their purple, red, and black colours. This deep-coloured pigmentation provides a broad indication of disease prevention activities. Anthocyanins have been shown to directly protect against the disease-causing effects of free radical damage, as each cell of the body receives approximately 10,000 oxidative assaults every day. Anthocyanins provide comprehensive antioxidant defence, regulate the control of inflammation, and influence gene and enzyme expression, as well as numerous other biochemical pathways.

"For they are life unto those that find them, and health to all their flesh" (Proverbs 4:22).

The risk of many degenerative diseases and cancers can be reduced with a diet that is rich in polyphenols, and the polyphenolics in berries have been demonstrated to retard and even reverse the deterioration of cognitive and motor performance. More than 8,000 different polyphenolic compounds have been identified and are extremely diverse and very abundant in nature. All polyphenols have similar chemical structures but there are some distinctive differences. Based on these differences, polyphenols are subdivided into several primary subclasses. These are flavonoids, phenolic acids, stilbenes, tannins, and diferuloylmethanes. The polyphenol group of nutrients is most essential in terms of its health benefiting biological properties, among which are anti-inflammatory, antioxidant, and anti-cancer, which can protect from oxidative stress and diseases. Cancer-fighting nitrilosides, a generic term for beta-cyanophoric glycosides (vitamin B17), are concentrated in fruit seeds, such as berries and cherries, as well as being contained in nuts, tubers, grasses, sprouts, grains, and beans. These are very stable substances which are reportedly not affected by cooking.

"Wherefore by their fruits ye shall know them" (Matthew 7:20).

These berries contain powerful anti-cancer potential that kills cancer stem cells. This can be linked to their myriad of bioactive antioxidant and anti-inflammatory phytonutrients. These include anthocyanins, beta-carotene, bioflavonoids, caffeic acids, carotenes, carotenoids, catechins, chlorogenic acid, cinnamic acid, coumaric acids, cyanidins, delphinidins, ellagic acid, ellagitannins, epicatechin, epigallocatechin, ferulic acids, fisetin, flavonoids, flavonols, gallic acids, gallocatechins, gallotannins, glycosides, hydroxy-benzoic acids, hydroxy-cinnamic acids, isoquercitrin, isorhamnetin, kaempferol, lambertianin, lignans, limonene, lutein, malvidins, myricetin, nitrilosides, pantothenic acid, pelargonidins, peonidins, peonidin-3-O-rutinoside, phenolic acids, piceatannol, proanthocyanidins, procyanidins, protocatechuic acids, pterostilbene, quercetin (natural anti-inflammatory), queritrin, resveratrol, rutin, salicylic acid, sanguiin, stilbenoids, tannins, terpenoids, tiliroside, triterpenoids, vanillic acid, and zeaxanthin.

"I will praise thee, O LORD, with my whole heart; I will shew forth all thy marvellous works" (Psalm 9:1).

Berries are good sources of vitamin A, vitamin B1, vitamin B2, vitamin B3, vitamin B5, vitamin B6, vitamin B7, vitamin C, vitamin E, vitamin K, ascorbic acid, calcium, choline, copper, folate, iodine, iron, magnesium, manganese, Omega-3 fatty acids, pectin, phosphorus, potassium, Omega-6 fatty acids, selenium, silicon, sodium, soluble fibre, and zinc.

"But seek ye first the kingdom of God, and His righteousness; and all these things shall be added unto you" (Matthew 6:33).

These powerful little fruits have been shown to be adaptogenic, analgesic, anti-ageing, anti-allergenic, anti-amyloid, anti-arthritic, anti-asthmatic, anti-atherogenic, anti-bacterial, anti-carcinogenic, anti-depressant, anti-diabetic, anti-flatulent, antifungal, anti-inflammatory, anti-ischaemic, anti-malarial, anti-microbial, anti-mutagenic, anti-parasitic, antiphlogistic (prevents or relieves inflammation), anti-psoriasis, antioxidative, anti-tumour, anti-ulcer, anti-viral, anxiolytic, apoptotic, cytotoxic (to cancer stem cells), epigenetic, immune-protective, immunomodulatory, neuroprotective, and neurorestorative.

"Thou wilt shew me the path of life: in thy presence is fulness of joy; at thy right hand there are pleasures for evermore" (Psalm 16:11).

Many diseases can be greatly alleviated through the consumption of berries. These include cancers, Alzheimer's disease, Parkinson's disease and other neurodegenerative diseases, cardiovascular disease, ulcerative colitis, epilepsy, Crohn's disease, rabies, macular degeneration, cataracts, diabetes, obesity, gout, stroke, thrombosis, meningitis, arthritis, glaucoma, varicose veins, hemorrhoids, peptic ulcers, insomnia, asthma, urinary tract infections, allergies, multiple sclerosis, obesity, bronchitis, coughs, colds, flu, tetanus, anaemia, immune diseases, heart disease, kidney infections, inflammatory bowel disease, parasites, diarrhoea, infections, fibromyalgia, whooping cough, tonsillitis, inflammation, including joint inflammation, eye strain, liver problems, menstrual issues, and gum disease. They may be used topically to treat insect bites and wounds. Berries also reduce the formation of unwanted blood clots which helps to prevent heart attacks and strokes.

"And His fame went throughout all Syria: and they brought unto Him all sick people that were taken with divers (various) diseases and torments, and those which were possessed with devils, and those which were lunatick, and those that had the palsy; and He healed them" (Matthew 4:24).

Powerful berries, as part of a healthy diet and lifestyle, are far superior as a disease preventative measure to the ineffective, horrendous poisons of contemporary medicine after a disease has made itself manifest. Genotoxic chemotherapy interactions cause DNA mutations and have many severe debilitating side effects on the body, which when already diseased is inundated with toxins from unhealthy lifestyle practices, environmental factors, and nutritional deficiencies. Chemotherapy devastates the immune system, after which the body is often incapable of recuperating enough to adequately protect itself from common health issues, as the use of chemotherapy often leads to death. As a serious carcinogen, it also causes hair loss, destruction of the erythrocytes (red blood cells), brain fog, constant nausea, vomiting, diarrhoea, pain, severe headaches, mouth ulcers, frequent dizziness, and the destruction of vital organs. These should be obvious signs that chemotherapy is highly dangerous and does not belong in the bodies of humans and animals as cancer cannot be cured by deadly poisons. A similar scenario would be to try and treat an alcoholic with the most potent alcoholic drink. Chemotherapy is an administered poison and an invasive treatment that kills all living matter. Its barbaric chemistry is unable to differentiate between cancerous cells and healthy cells and the surrounding healthy tissues. The lethal side effects of radiation, such as necrosis in the brain, kills the majority of its victims. High-powered radiation to the chest cavity increases the risk of heart disease and strokes. Radiation can have horrific long-term side effects that leave patients permanently mutilated and suffering in constant pain with the loss of bodily functions and they are often never the same again. When chemotherapy and radiation are repeatedly administered, the whole body gradually dies.

"The LORD preserveth all them that love Him: but all the wicked will He destroy" (Psalm 145:20).

Antioxidants are classified by their solubility and can be categorized as either water-soluble (hydrophilic) lipids or water-deterring (hydrophobic) lipids. The human body is composed of many different types of cells which are composed of many different types of molecules. The cell membranes are mostly comprised of lipids (fats) while the fluid interior of the cells are mostly comprised of water, as intracellular fluid contains lower density water with more potassium ions. Intracellular fluid bathes all of the biological molecules, including the nucleic acids and proteins. Bonds do not usually split in a way that leaves a molecule with an odd, unpaired electron. But when weak bonds do split free radicals are formed. Both types of antioxidants are needed for full protection from oxidative damage as free radicals can attack the fatty cellular membranes or the watery contents of the cells. Some free radicals are created during the course of normal metabolism and sometimes the cells of the immune system deliberately create them to neutralize bacteria and viruses. However, environmental factors can also create free radicals. Vitamin A, vitamin E, lipoic acid, and carotenoids are some examples of lipid-soluble antioxidants that protect the cell membranes from lipid peroxidation and these are mostly located in the cell membranes. Vitamin C acts primarily in cellular fluid and is the most abundant water-soluble antioxidant in the body. Glutathione and polyphenols are also examples of water-soluble antioxidants. These are found in aqueous fluids such as the fluids both around and within the cell's cytosol or cytoplasmic matrix (liquid matrix surrounding the organelles) and in the blood. Normally the body can cope with free radicals. However, if antioxidants are unavailable or if the free-radical production becomes excessive then free radical damage can occur. Antioxidant solubility can also be classed as non-enzymatic (produced in the body) and enzymatic (which break down and remove free radicals). Berries are abundant in the antioxidant phytochemical resveratrol, which has powerful antiviral effects and has also been shown to block the replication of respiratory viruses. In terms of detoxifying power, these antioxidants bind to heavy metals and aid in their removal from the body through the urine. They also fight inflammation caused by a toxic overload. The gallic acid contained in berries is an extremely effective antioxidant as well as a powerful antifungal and antiviral agent.

"Verily, verily, I say unto you, he that believeth on me hath everlasting life" (John 6:47).

Ellagic acid is a polyphenolic compound which is a known potent anti-carcinogen that has anti-bacterial, anti-inflammatory, and anti-viral properties, and berries are extremely rich in this naturally occurring constituent. Strawberries, blackberries, blueberries, red and black raspberries, cranberries, and grapes contain the highest quantities of ellagic acid, which is easily absorbed by the body and blocks and suppresses cancer cells and tumour growth. Wild strawberries may well contain the highest quantity of ellagic acid of all these fruits. The amount of ellagic acid found in raspberry seeds is 87.8%, while 12.2% is contained in the pulp. Blackberries contain approximately the same amount of ellagic acid as raspberries. The amount of ellagic acid found in strawberry seeds is 4.3%, while 95.7% is contained in the pulp. Ellagic acid is a protective phytochemical bioactive agent that is usually ingested in the

> *Berries are abundant in the antioxidant phytochemical resveratrol, which has powerful antiviral effects and has also been shown to block the replication of respiratory viruses.*

form of the biochemical ellagitannin. Plants produce ellagic acid and glucose which combine to form water-soluble ellagitannin compounds, whereby giving cancer cells a larger dose of anti-cancer ellagic acid than normal cells, as cancer cells consume approximately fifteen times more glucose than normal cells. Pecans also contain ellagic acid and belong to the same Juglandaceae family as walnuts, but they contain just slightly more than half of the ellagic acid that is found in walnuts.

"Let the heavens be glad, and let the earth rejoice: and let men say among the nations, The LORD reigneth" (1 Chronicles 16:31).

A number of parasites are killed by ellagic acid but it is better known for its ability to fight cancer than anything else. As a cancer inhibitor, it has the ability to cause the apoptosis process in cancer cells without damaging healthy cells. It prevents carcinogens from binding to DNA, strengthens connective tissue, which may prevent cancer cells from spreading, and can also inhibit mutations within the DNA of the cells. Viral infections can cause genetic mutations to the DNA but are unable to reproduce on their own. Viruses reproduce by hijacking the machinery of human cells, which subsequently turns them into virus manufacturing machines. However, ellagic acid inhibits viruses from entering cells. Ellagic acid also causes all types of bacterial DNA to unravel and inhibits a critical pathway in the lifecycle of fungi and yeast. It also impedes and stops mitosis (cancer cell division) in breast cancer, oesophageal cancer, skin cancer, prostate cancer, colon cancer, and pancreatic cancer cells. Studies have demonstrated that ellagic acid lowers the incidence of birth defects, reduces heart disease, promotes wound healing, reduces or reverses chemically induced liver fibrosis, protects the liver and liver function, reduces glucose levels, and binds with carcinogens and makes them inactive. This powerful phytonutrient contained in berries has been shown to help prevent the overactivity and overproduction of particular pro-inflammatory enzymes, including cyclo-oxygenase-2 (COX-2).

"He giveth power to the faint; and to them that have no might He increaseth strength" (Isaiah. 40:29).

Many scientific studies have determined that the natural pigments that give fruits and vegetables their vibrant colours also offer amazing health benefits. A leading class of compounds in this category are the powerful flavonoid antioxidants. Flavonoid antioxidants, such as those found abundantly in berries, are not only antioxidants but also have many beneficial effects by acting on signalling within the cells. They also activate natural detoxification enzymes of the body, block the growth of cancer cells, decrease inflammation, and engage in antiviral activity. Flavonoids also lower blood sugar levels, thus restricting angiogenesis, which is a process by which new lymphatic vessels and new blood vessels form as cancer cells depend on an adequate supply of nutrients and the removal of waste, but cancer cells can also adapt to low oxygen environments. Flavonoids can attach themselves to proteins, thus modulating the action of enzymes, including the kinase enzymes necessary for cell proliferation. When high amounts of flavonoids are ingested all cancer cell proliferation is inhibited without harming normal cells. Flavonoids utilize a multiplicity of neuroprotective actions within the brain, including the potential to protect neurons against damage induced by neurotoxins, the ability to suppress neuro-inflammation, and the potential to promote learning, cognitive function, and memory. The consumption of flavonoid-rich foods has the potential to limit neurodegeneration and to prevent and reverse loses in cognitive performance.

"Thou wilt keep him in perfect peace, whose mind is stayed on thee: because he trusteth in thee" (Isaiah 26:3).

The hormone melatonin, contained in cherries, grapes, and strawberries, is known to act as a powerful antioxidant, and even small amounts are able to assist with raising glutathione levels. Melatonin is a hormone produced in the pineal gland of the brain that is responsible for regulating sleep and wake cycles. It is often considered to be the natural pacemaker of the body and plays an instrumental role in signalling the time of the day and year, thereby helping to regulate the internal body clock.

"I will both lay me down in peace, and sleep: for thou, LORD, only makest me dwell in safety" (Psalm 4:8).

BLACKBERRIES

Blackberries are closely related to raspberries and belong to the flowering rose family (Rosaceae) of the diverse Rubus fruticosus genus. Although commonly called berries, the fruits of the Rubus species are technically aggregates of drupelets. Unlike the hollow fruits of raspberries, the distinguishing factor between the two is that the drupelets of blackberries remain attached to a juicy white core.

Beautiful blackberries were not cultivated in ancient times and were then considered wild. Today, they proliferate in almost all parts of the globe and there are more than forty known species of blackberries growing around the world. The Romans and Greeks used blackberries in their daily cooking and for medicine. Blackberries have been grown in Europe for over 2,000 years and are employed for medicinal purposes as well as a food. Native Americans also utilized them for medicine in addition to food. In medicinal applications, the leaf, the root, and the bark were used more than the beautiful berry.

Delightful blackberries are a superfood and notable for their strength as a powerful antioxidant. The humble blackberry contains considerably high levels of polyphenolic flavonoid phytochemicals such as anthocyanins, catechins, cyanidins, ellagic acid, ellagitannins, gallic acid, kaempferol, lutein, pelargonidins, quercetin, salicylic acid, tannins, and zeaxanthin.

Blackberries are much more than powerful antioxidants. They are also extremely high in some of the most potent forms of chronic disease and cancer-fighting compounds such as vitamin A, vitamin B1, vitamin B2, vitamin B3, vitamin B5, vitamin B6, vitamin C, vitamin E, vitamin K, copper, ellagic acid, folate, iron, magnesium, manganese, Omega-3 fatty acids, potassium, and selenium. They also have high levels of pectin and soluble fibre.

Appetizing blackberries have a wonderful flavour in addition to being rich in nutrients. They contain large quantities of anthocyanin plant pigments that are known to exert extremely powerful antioxidant properties. These antioxidant compounds in blackberries help to protect against unstable free radical molecules, which have been linked to the development of many degenerative diseases. The health benefits of blackberries include a strengthened immune system, memory loss improvement, better digestive health, assisting inflammatory conditions, a promising therapy for periodontal gum disease, healthy heart function, prevention of cancer and neurological diseases, strong bones, healthy skin, improved vision, and relief from endothelial and epithelial dysfunction. Blackberries are effective at treating the parasite Giardia duodenalis, which is a common cause of diarrhoea. They also dramatically reduce brain ageing by reducing immunoexcytotoxicity and microglial provoking and activation. The phytonutrient quercetin in blackberries not only has anti-inflammatory and antioxidant properties but also performs as a natural antihistamine.

"For I the LORD thy God will hold thy right hand, saying unto thee, Fear not; I will help thee" (Isaiah 41:13).

Powerful blackberries are rich in vital vitamins and minerals and are among the most potent cancer-fighting fruits. These nutrients provide a plethora of health effects. The vitamin A in blackberries is a large group of related nutrients and each nutrient provides health benefits, which may be quite different and may be provided in various ways. It is involved in immune function, reproduction, cell growth, vision, cellular communication, maintenance of organs, and much more. All of the B vitamins in blackberries are water-soluble, and vitamin B1, or thiamine, is an essential nutrient that is needed by all body tissues for proper functioning and also helps to turn food into energy in the form of ATP, which transports energy within the cells. Vitamin B2, or riboflavin, like other B vitamins, is involved in energy metabolism, and an abundance of B2 can turn urine yellow. Vitamin B3, or niacin, is also involved in energy production and is utilized to synthesize starch, which can be stored as an energy source in the muscles and liver. Vitamin B5, or pantothenic acid, is incorporated into coenzyme A, which is of the utmost importance for sustaining life and plays a key role in energy production. Vitamin B6, or pyridoxine, is used in the production of neurotransmitters, carbohydrate metabolism and red blood cell production. Vitamin B9, or folate, plays an instrumental role in making and repairing DNA and producing oxygen-carrying red blood cells. The vitamin C content of these powerful berries is essential for a healthy brain, a healthy gut, a healthy heart and blood vessels, healthy teeth, healthy gums, a strong immune system, and overall good health. Regular consumption of adequate vitamin C rich foods scavenges harmful, pro-inflammatory free radicals and assists the body in developing resistance against infections. It also helps to prevent respiratory problems such as lung cancer and asthma. The anti-viral nutrients in blackberries are effective for skin infections such as cold sores and the herpes virus. The vitamin E contained in blackberries improves the metabolic function of the body and its anti-inflammatory effects can combat rheumatism, asthma, arthritis, and other inflammatory disorders linked to chronic inflammation. Blackberries are also a very good source of vitamin K, which regulates blood calcium levels and builds strong bones. Vitamin K helps to regulate hormone function and potentially reduces the cramping pains of PMS, as does the calcium and manganese contained in blackberries. Vitamin K is important for the entire cardiovascular system as well as for preventing cancers. Blackberries and raspberries are rich in Omega-3 fatty acids, which should be taken on a regular basis. The manganese in blackberries also helps the body to make energy from food and when combined with vitamin C helps to protect cells from oxidative stress. The antioxidant polyphenols in blackberries are recognized for their cancer-fighting abilities and especially the high concentration of anthocyanins, which is a particularly potent polyphenol that opposes cell mutation and cancer development. The anthocyanin cyanidin-3-O-glucoside in blackberries is protective against endothelial dysfunction, which can cause many serious diseases and also death. Because of their high antioxidant content and antibacterial activity, blackberries also combat infections and boost immunity. Blackberries also contain alpha-cryptoxanthin, lutein, and zeaxanthin. In addition to their antioxidant properties, beta-carotene, lutein, and zeaxanthin all boost eye health. These nutrients can reduce the risk of macular degeneration and cataracts. Consuming unrefined coconut oil can also protect the eyes from macular degeneration.

"This is the LORD'S doing; it is marvellous in our eyes"
(Psalm 118:23).

Blackberries can prevent brain inflammation by protecting neurons from degenerating, which helps with short-term memory, increased brain performance, and memory loss. They change the way that brain neurons communicate, and it is these signalling changes that can prevent brain inflammation that contributes to neuronal damage. Manganese is vital to brain functioning and blackberries contain a substantial amount, with an elevated percentage found in the brain synapses where it is needed for proper synapse firing. A deficiency of manganese is connected to epilepsy, which also has brain inflammation as a major component.

"But the very hairs of your head are all numbered"
(Matthew 10:30).

Many of the health benefits of blackberries are not only attributed to their anthocyanins but also to their other powerful antioxidants which can help to keep skin looking young by neutralizing wrinkle-causing free radicals. They also help to prevent skin cancer by inhibiting the growth and spread of tumour cells. Elastin and collagen are two structural proteins that give the skin elasticity and support. Vitamin C boosts collagen production while the ellagic acid prevents the destruction of collagen in the skin. Wild and cultivated blackberries are one of the world's best dietary sources of ellagic acid. In studies, ellagic acid has been shown to enhance immune function, eliminate carcinogens, and induce apoptosis. The water-soluble flavonoid cyanidin-3-glucoside is the active compound that is responsible for the antioxidant benefits of blackberries and has a controlling effect over free radicals. Blackberries and blueberries also contain flavonoids that have anti-parasitic activity against Cryptosporidium parvum and Encephalitozoon intestinalis.

"Seek the LORD and His strength, seek His face continually"
(1 Chronicles 16:11).

A study by scientists has found that extracts from blackberry leaves have anti-cancer activity. These findings compare with the compelling results of other studies conducted on the health benefits of blackberry leaf tea.

"For every tree is known by his own fruit. For of thorns men
do not gather figs, nor of a bramble bush gather they grapes"
(Luke 6:44).

BLACKCURRANTS

Blackcurrants are the fruits of a small shrub belonging to the family of Grossulariaceae of the Ribes genus and its botanical name is Ribes nigrum.

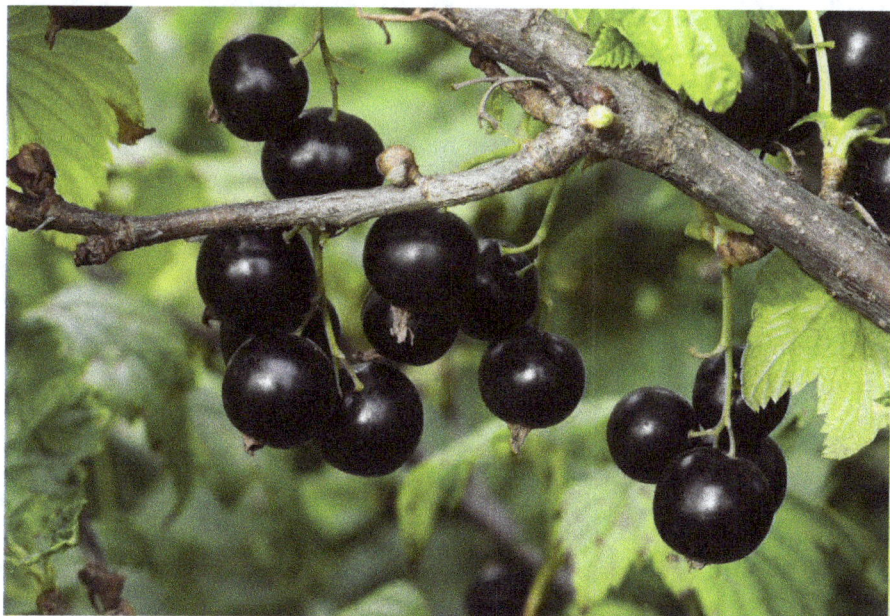

Powerful blackcurrants have been valued for centuries as a nutritious and ancient food in northern Europe. Blackcurrants emerged during the Middle Ages as a herbal medicine and were used by herbalists to treat liver disorders, bladder stones, lung ailments, coughs, and more. In the eighteenth century, the use of blackcurrants became widespread among physicians and herbalists. Blackcurrant preparations were used to treat gout, rheumatism, typhoid fever, urinary tract infections, skin infections, oral issues, and various intestinal conditions.

Life-enhancing blackcurrants contain significantly high amounts of the phenolic flavonoid phytochemicals, proanthocyanidins, and anthocyanins. They also contain other polyphenolic compounds and antioxidants such as catechin, cyanidin-3-O-glucoside, cyanidin-3-O-rutinoside, delphinidin-3-O-glucoside, delphinidin-3-O-rutinoside, epicatechin, epigallocatechin, lutein, peonidin-3-O-rutinoside, and zeaxanthin.

Health-giving blackcurrants can claim to be a superfruit and contain vitamin A, vitamin B1, vitamin B2, vitamin B3, vitamin B5, vitamin B6, and good quantities of iron for red blood cell production in the bone marrow. They protect cells and membranes from damage caused by free radicals and have very high levels of antioxidants with an especially high vitamin C free radical scavenger content. Blackcurrants, weight for weight, have a higher vitamin C content than an orange. The next highest levels are found in raspberries, blueberries, and strawberries. They are also a very good source of essential minerals such as calcium, copper, folate, magnesium, manganese, phosphorus, potassium, and zinc. Blackcurrant seeds are a rich source of both the Omega-3 fatty acid—alpha-linolenic acid and the Omega-6 fatty acid—gamma-linolenic acid.

"And when He sowed, some seeds fell by the way side, and the fowls came and devoured them up ... But other fell into good ground, and brought forth fruit, some an hundredfold, some sixtyfold, some thirtyfold" (Matthew 13:4 & 8).

Antioxidant-rich blackcurrants contain significant mental fatigue-busting compounds that can boost concentration and alertness. Scientific studies show that the consumption of blackcurrants have potential health benefits for cancers, Alzheimer's disease, asthma, diabetes, macular degeneration, cataracts, diarrhoea, arthritis, gout, tonsillitis, whooping cough, urinary tract infections, cardiovascular disease and associated illnesses, inflammation, kidney stones, gum disease, stiffness and muscle fatigue, ocular diseases, diabetic neuropathy, eye strain, neurodegenerative diseases, liver problems, and menstrual issues. They are also able to alleviate allergy-driven inflammation, which is a significant cause of asthma. Preliminary research has shown that the consumption of blackcurrants can increase insulin production by up to 50%. Studies on blackcurrant fruit extracts have confirmed that they have potent anti-viral activity, antioxidant effects, and the ability to inhibit the aggregation of blood platelets. They also have the ability to relax the aorta by enhancing the synthesis

Health-giving blackcurrants can claim to be a superfruit .

of nitric acid, which improves the functioning of blood vessels. These tasty little fruits can help to reduce the build-up of lactic acid in the blood, which causes painful muscles during vigorous exercise. Blackcurrants are also used topically to treat bites and wounds.

"But now in Christ Jesus ye who sometimes were far off are made nigh by the blood of Christ" (Ephesians 2:13).

The anthocyanins, contained primarily in the skin of blackcurrants, are effective at inhibiting tumour cells and increasing cancer cell death. They are water-soluble pigments that give blue, red, and purple fruits their colour, and their shade of pigment varies due to the pH level as anthocyanins can reversibly change colour with the pH. Researchers have discovered that anthocyanins are also extremely effective against influenza viruses. These tiny black fruits are amazingly powerful at boosting the immune system, and ground-breaking new research reveals that delicious blackcurrants can also help to promote healthy gut bacteria. This research has demonstrated that anthocyanins help to increase numbers of beneficial healthy bifidobacterium bacteria in the gut whilst stopping the growth of some species of harmful bacteria in the body, thereby helping to maintain a healthy, functioning digestive system, which reduces gut inflammation, and is important for disease prevention, weight management, and general health. The proanthocyanidins in blackcurrants stop bacteria from adhering to the walls of the urinary tract, thereby preventing them from causing urinary tract infections. Proanthocyanidins are compounds usually associated with pine bark and grape seed extracts.

"The meek shall eat and be satisfied: they shall praise the LORD that seek Him: your heart shall live for ever" (Psalm 22:26).

Blackcurrants are high in fibre and vitamin A, which is essential for maintaining healthy vision, reducing glaucoma, and maintaining the integrity of the skin and mucous membranes. These high potency berries also contain the flavonoids beta-carotene, zeaxanthin, and cryptoxanthin, which are compounds that are beneficial for eye health. Blackcurrants provide the building blocks of a substance called visual purple, which is a pigment that perceives light in the photoreceptor cells, thereby boosting night vision.

"To open their eyes, and to turn them from darkness to light, and from the power of Satan unto God, that they may receive forgiveness of sins, and inheritance among them which are sanctified by faith that is in me" (Acts 26:18).

Laboratory experiments have shown that extracts of blackcurrants inhibit enzymes such as elastase, which can cause the degradation of collagen. This can lead to a reduction in risk factors associated with inflammatory conditions.

"And the inhabitant shall not say, I am sick: the people that dwell therein shall be forgiven their iniquity" (Isaiah 33:24.)

BLUEBERRIES

Blueberries are one of the few fruits that are native to North America and were an important part of the Native American diet for many years. They are the fruits of a shrub that belong to the Ericaceae family of the Vaccinium genus.

Beautiful blueberries have a diverse range of phytonutrients including anthocyanins (derived from *cyan* in Greek, which means dark blue), caffeic acids, chlorogenic acid, coumaric acids, cyanidins, delphinidins, ferulic acids, flavonols, gallic acids, hydroxybenzoic acids, hydroxycinnamic acids, kaempferol, lutein, malvidins, myricetin, pelargonidins, peonidins, protocatechuic acids, pterostilbene, and high amounts of the powerful flavonoids quercetin, resveratrol, and zeaxanthin.

Appealing blueberries contain significant quantities of vitamin K, beta-carotene, and manganese. They also contain vitamin A, vitamin B6, vitamin C, vitamin E, calcium, choline, copper, fibre, folate, iron, magnesium, Omega-3 fatty acids, potassium, phosphorus, sodium and zinc. The vitamin K, calcium, iron, magnesium, manganese, phosphorous, and zinc contained in blueberries all contribute to building and maintaining the elasticity, structure, and strength of joints and bones.

"Behold, God is mighty, and despiseth not any: He is mighty in strength and wisdom" (Job 36:5).

Powerful blueberries contain a curative compound that is far more effective than anything that big pharma has available and which strikes at the very root of cancer malignancy. The pterostilbene component of blueberries operates as a potential anti-cancer stem cell agent that suppresses irradiation-mediated enrichment of hepatoma stem cells. Hepatoma is the most common type of liver cancer. Pterostilbene not only suppresses adverse changes associated with irradiation but is also a stilbenoid which is chemically related to resveratrol and is found in grapes as well as blueberries. Irradiation of hepatoma with the same type of radiation which is used to treat cancer patients results in the enrichment of highly malignant cancer stem cell sub-populations as well as cell properties and is associated with treatment resistance and increased invasiveness.

"And this is the condemnation, that light is come into the world, and men loved darkness rather than light, because their deeds were evil" (John 3:19).

Blueberries are also a superfruit, and vitamin A, vitamin C, and various phytonutrients function as powerful antioxidants that decrease inflammation, protect urinary-tract health, improve cognitive function, inhibit tumour growth, assist in protecting cells against free radical damage, and also help to impede and protect from several types of cancers. The folate contained in blueberries reduces DNA damage and contributes to DNA repair and synthesis, thereby preventing cancer cells from forming out of mutations to the DNA. In addition to exhibiting cancer-protective benefits, blueberries also boost the immune system, suppress harmful free radicals, and improve insulin resistance and glucose control, thereby helping to regulate blood sugar in those with type 2 diabetes. A study revealed that the daily consumption of blueberries increased natural killer cells, which are the white blood cells that perform a crucial role in the immune system's defence against foreign invaders such as tumours and viruses. These tiny hunters search the body for abnormal cells and destroy them before they can develop into cancers. Accumulating research reveals that the phytocompound resveratrol in blueberries has the ability to kill many lethal cancer types including targeting the cancer stem cells within them. Blueberries contain many substances with experimentally confirmed cancer stem cell-killing properties.

"How precious also are thy thoughts unto me, O God! how great is the sum of them!" (Psalm 139:17).

Of all the nutritional components of blueberries, gallic acid is outstanding. It has been thoroughly researched and the subject of almost 6,500 peer-reviewed scientific articles. It is a powerful antiviral and antifungal agent and an extremely effective antioxidant. As well as being an abundant source of vitamins, minerals and fibre, blueberries contain one of the highest amounts of antioxidant content than most other berries. Blueberries contain a large amount of bioactive compounds and virtually every body system benefits from the consumption of these amazing little fruits as these systems receive vital antioxidant support from them.

"If ye be willing and obedient, ye shall eat the good of the land" (Isaiah 1:19).

Studies have confirmed that delicious blueberries contribute to brain health by increasing specific neurotransmitters that expedite the transmission of impulses between neurons. Blueberries are well known for their enhancement of cognitive performance in Alzheimer's disease and also offer protection from other neurodegenerative diseases such as Parkinson's disease and the decline of memory and brain function by lowering the risk of oxidative stress on the nerve cells and maintaining healthy cognitive function. Blueberries have been shown to not only improve cognition in Alzheimer's disease but they also decrease the aggregation of platelets and enhance the immune system's breakdown removal of amyloid-beta plaques in the brain. Blueberries are also abundant in polyphenols, which are capable of crossing the blood-brain barrier to prevent and even reverse the deterioration of cognitive and motor performance. The Omega-3 antioxidants in blueberries are needed for brain health and help to protect against brain haemorrhage. Blueberries also improve circulation to the brain and extremities. In addition, the antioxidant capacity of blueberries can be attributed to anthocyanins, which blueberries possess in higher quantities than any other food and which can also slow and reverse brain ageing.

"For God hath not given us the spirit of fear; but of power, and of love, and of a sound mind" (2 Timothy 1:7).

Folate and vitamin B6 prevents the buildup of homocysteine, which can lead to heart problems and damage to the blood vessels when excessive amounts accumulate in the body. Heart health is supported by blueberries with vitamin B6, vitamin C, fibre, folate, potassium, and phytonutrients. Blueberries are extremely rich in a wide range of powerful heart-protective antioxidant flavonoids and carotenoids. Studies suggest that a diet high in these powerful little deep purple berries helps to protect the aorta, which is one of the body's most essential blood vessels. Blueberries also help to protect the myocardium and may prevent heart failure following myocardial infarction.

"Blessed are the pure in heart: for they shall see God"
(Matthew 5:8).

In keeping with the *doctrine of signatures*, which purports that foods resembling various body parts can be used to treat ailments of those same body parts, blueberries resemble the iris of the eyes, which are formed within 36 days of conception, and blueberries ingeniously increase the circulation to the eyes. Blueberries are recommended for a wide range of eye diseases and issues. The vitamin A contained in blueberries is particularly important for the eyes and a deficiency of this vital vitamin causes damage to the retina, which contributes to blindness. Macular degeneration and cataracts are a leading cause of visual impairment and acquired blindness but sufficient antioxidant nutrients lower the risk of these disorders. A link has been discovered between two processes in the retina, that when combined contribute to macular degeneration. Antioxidants disrupt this link and extend the lifetime of photoreceptors and other retinal cells. Antioxidant unrefined coconut oil also affords retinal protection. It has been demonstrated that even when cataracts have begun to cloud the vision, sufficient antioxidants can reverse this process and also other eye conditions. A lack of vitamin A causes the cornea (clear front surface of the iris and pupil) to become very dry, predisposing it to clouding, corneal ulcers and loss of vision. Omega-3 fatty acids can have a positive effect on the symptoms of dry eyes when taken in sufficient quantities. From a quarter to a half-million malnourished children worldwide become blind every year due to a vitamin A deficiency. This tragedy can be prevented with a healthful diet. There is abundant evidence to show that a healthy diet with sufficient antioxidants prevents the development of eye afflictions.

"The LORD openeth the eyes of the blind: the LORD raiseth them that are bowed down: the LORD loveth the righteous" (Psalm 146:8).

Lutein and zeaxanthin are fat-soluble antioxidants that belong to the group of carotenoids which are classified as xanthophylls. Lutein and zeaxanthin are two types of carotenoids with yellow, orange, and red pigments, which are extremely significant nutrients that can reduce the risk of macular degeneration and cataracts. These nutrients are revealed in elevated concentrations in the macula of the eye and research has identified that lutein and zeaxanthin can increase the optical density of the macula pigment. Studies demonstrate that increased quantities in the diet are associated with a lower occurrence of macular degeneration and cataracts. Lutein and zeaxanthin not only increase the opacity of the eye lens, but they also absorb slightly different light wavelengths in addition to neutralizing free radicals. Zeaxanthin is primarily located in the centre of the retina and lutein is more pronounced at the perimeter of the retina and in the rods of the eyes. Foods containing lutein and zeaxanthin include brightly coloured fruits

> *In keeping with the doctrine of signatures, which purports that foods resembling various body parts can be used to treat ailments of those same body parts, blueberries resemble the iris of the eyes.*

and vegetables such as oranges, sweet potatoes and leaves, lettuce, dandelion greens, butternut squash and leaves, beetroot greens, chard, basil, spring onions, coriander, asparagus, leeks, green and yellow beans, celery, rhubarb, tangerines, olives, sage, papayas, black pepper, carrots, red, yellow and green vegetables, goji berries, tomatoes, sweet corn, yellow-fleshed potatoes, red grapefruit, honeydew melon, peaches, kiwi fruit, parsley, peas, pistachio nuts, avocados, plums, pineapple, cucumber, apricots, blackberries, peppers, blackcurrants, blueberries, grapes, sweet and sour cherries, raspberries, strawberries, and bilberries, and are found in greater amounts in green leafy vegetables and crucifers. Corn and durum wheat also contain beneficial amounts. Interestingly, the chlorophyll in dark green vegetables conceals the lutein and zeaxanthin pigments, so that the vegetables appear green in colour. Consuming these foods with healthy fats improves the absorption of lutein and zeaxanthin.

"But as it is written, Eye hath not seen, nor ear heard, neither have entered into the heart of man, the things which God hath prepared for them that love Him" (1 Corinthians 2:9).

Studies clearly show that blueberries, as well as other berries, can be frozen and thawed without affecting the potency of their delicate cancer-fighting anthocyanin antioxidants. There are many antioxidant nutrients found in blueberries, and as anthocyanins are the source of their colourful pigments, the vibrant, deep colours of blueberries display that they are high in antioxidant compounds.

"O give thanks unto the LORD; for He is good: for His mercy endureth for ever" (Psalm 118:29).

Wild blueberries are one of the best foods for improving gut bacteria. They are particularly potent as they have less water and a higher skin-to-pulp ratio, which effectively doubles the antioxidant content and gives them a more intense flavour. They are approximately half the size of the cultivated varieties.

"The LORD is gracious, and full of compassion; slow to anger, and of great mercy" (Psalm 145:8).

CHERRIES

Cherries belong to the rose family (Rosaceae) of the Prunus genus. They are available in a variety of colours ranging from yellow to red to black. They also come in different shapes from round to heart-shaped. Cherries are classified as drupes and the sweet cherry variety belongs to the Prunus avium genus whilst the tart or sour variety belong to the Prunus cerasus genus.

Cheerful cherries are native to Asia and were eaten by the Chinese, Greeks and the Romans thousands of years ago. They only became popular in northern Europe in the late Middle Ages. In the seventeenth century, colonists took cherries to North America.

Beautiful and delicious cherries contain the following phytochemicals: anthocyanins, bioflavonoids, ellagic acid, flavonoids, lutein, quercitrin, isoquercitrin, limonene, proanthocyanidins, and zeaxanthin.

As an alkaline food, cherries help to maintain the body's ideal pH balance. They are a good source of vitamin A, vitamin B-complex, vitamin C, vitamin E, vitamin K, beta-carotene, calcium, choline, copper, fibre, folate, iron, magnesium, manganese, phosphorus, potassium, and silicon as well as a little Omega-3.

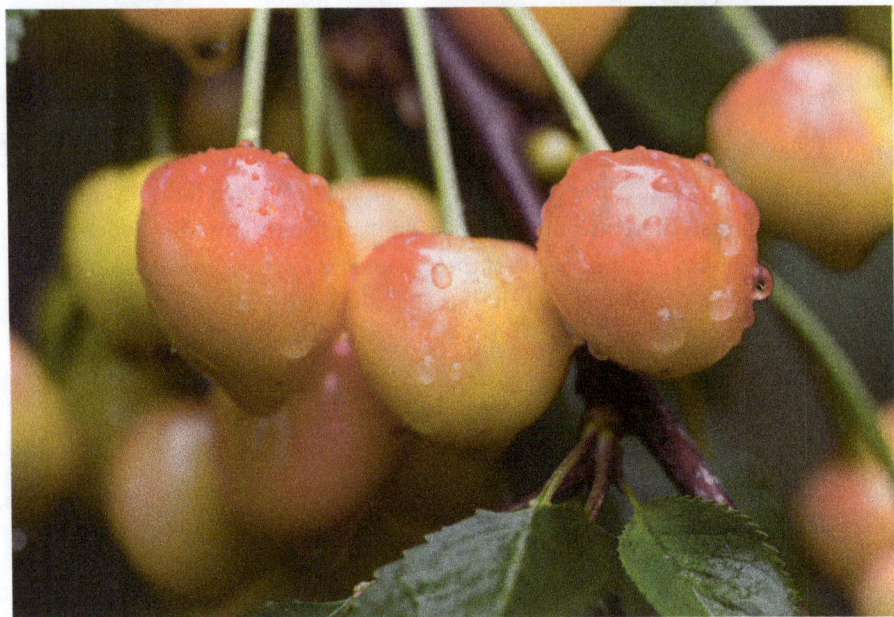

Powerful cherries are effective for adverse health conditions including cancer, urinary tract infections, gout, migraines, diabetes, insomnia, arthritis and associated pain, inflammation, neurological diseases, oxidative stress, and cardiovascular disease.

"For our heart shall rejoice in Him, because we have trusted in His holy name" (Psalm 33:21).

Cherries are not only among the most delicious and nutritious foods but they are also rich sources of flavonoids, specifically the ubiquitous molecules proanthocyanidins and anthocyanidins, which give cherries their deep red colour. Higher concentrations of flavonoids and nutrients are contained in the darker coloured varieties. The anthocyanins in cherries have proven anti-cancer properties which prevent the genetic mutations that cause cancer. They protect the body against the oxidative damage of free radicals by binding to DNA and also activate antioxidant and detoxification enzyme systems in the body. Cherry anthocyanins have been demonstrated to protect brain cells and blood vessels against oxidative stress, which is beneficial for neurodegenerative diseases. The compounds in cherries also help to combat migraine headaches. The high levels of bioflavonoids and anthocyanins in cherries are also related to reduced muscle and joint discomfort. Both cherries and grapes are amongst the most concentrated sources of polyphenols.

"Finally, be ye all of one mind, having compassion one of another, love as brethren, be pitiful, be courteous" (1 Peter 3:8).

Scrumptious cherries, as well as many other berries, are high in powerful anti-oxidants which help to prevent and repair the damage that is inflicted onto cells by free radicals. Due to their many anti-inflammatory compounds, cherries are traditionally associated with being remedies for gout and arthritis, as they bring relief to sufferers by lowering uric acid levels in the body that are associated with these conditions. These anti-inflammatory compounds contain the enzymes Cyclo-oxygenase 1 and 2, both of which slow down the progression of gout and arthritis, which are both acidic body conditions. Research has shown that they block the inflammatory pathways responsible for the pain associated with these conditions.

"The LORD will give strength unto His people; the LORD will bless His people with peace" (Psalm 29:11).

Two valuable cancer-fighting compounds contained in cherries are quercetin and ellagic acid. The powerful antioxidant quercetin is not only important for healthy veins but the high levels of it in cherries also destroy free radicals. Their rich ellagic acid content is an anti-carcinogenic compound that is very effective at combating cancerous conditions. This antioxidant flavonoid has been shown to promote tissue and cell health. It can inhibit the growth of cancer cells and can directly kill existing cancer cells without affecting healthy cells.

"To Him be glory and dominion for ever and ever. Amen" (1 Peter 5:11).

Sweet cherries have been shown to block the inflammatory processes involved in heart disease. This is especially beneficial for those with diabetes who face a higher risk of heart disease. Both tart and sweet cherry varieties have exhibited powerful anti-diabetic and cardiovascular effects through their ability to reduce blood levels of insulin and glucose.

"The light of the eyes rejoiceth the heart: and a good report maketh the bones fat" (Proverbs 15:30).

Tart or sour cherries promote healthy blood sugar levels. They have the same natural sugar content as sweet cherries but contain more bitter and sour tasting phytochemicals which are the same compounds which give them their enormous antioxidant excellence, according to science. Tart cherries are also effective at suppressing the pain induced by inflammation, as are citrus fruits. They also contain significant quantities of the sleep-inducing hormone melatonin, which influences, regulates and controls the sleep cycle. Melatonin is a potent and unique antioxidant and hormone that can not only cross the blood-brain barrier, but also the cell membranes. One of its roles is to help maintain a healthy immune system. Melatonin is effective at raising glutathione levels in many tissues such as the liver, brain, muscles, and blood serum. Melatonin also plays a role in stimulating other antioxidants, which makes it a truly unique antioxidant. It is produced at night in the pineal gland in the centre of the brain to help regulate the circadian rhythm. Melatonin is not only produced in the pineal gland but is also naturally present in edible plants such as cherries. When these are digested their melatonin can transfer into the blood from the gut to the brain as it is easily capable of crossing the blood-brain barrier. It has soothing effects on the brain neurons and thereby it can help to relieve insomnia, headaches, and neurosis while also calming the nervous system. Melatonin is considered more powerful than vitamins A, C, and E because it is both water and fat-soluble and can enter cells that vitamins cannot.

"When thou liest down, thou shalt not be afraid: yea, thou shalt lie down, and thy sleep shall be sweet" (Proverbs 3:24).

Delectable cherries are abundant in the flavonoids isoquercitrin and quercitrin, which researchers have found to be potent antioxidant and anti-cancer agents. These two flavonoids eliminate the by-products of the oxidation process by aiding in removing damaged cells and allowing healthier ones to regenerate. These flavonoids are released when cherries are consumed, which helps to attack and destroy cancerous cells in the body.

"The LORD shall reign for ever and ever" (Exodus 15:18).

Perillyl alcohol (POH) is a phytonutrient contained in cherries, which is extremely powerful at reducing the development, progression and occurrence of all types of cancer. It targets cancer stem cells and has been found to be successful with every type of cancer that it has been tested on. Researchers have discovered that POH stops the growth of cancer cells by depriving them of the proteins that they need to grow.

"Ye are blessed of the LORD which made heaven and earth"
(Psalm 115:15).

GRAPES

Grapes are a member of the berry family and belong to the Vitaceae family group of dicotyledonous flowering plants. Their botanical name is derived from the Vitis genus.

Gorgeous grapes are said to be the oldest cultivated fruit and have a very long and abundant history. They are depicted in hieroglyphics in ancient Egyptian burial tombs. Evidence also suggests that they were cultivated in Asia thousands of years ago. In the second century AD, over ninety varieties of grapes were already known and are now grown in multitudinous varieties, and with the exception of Antarctica, grapes are cultivated on all the continents of the Earth. Depending on the varieties that are grown, grapes can be round or elongated and can contain seeds or be seedless. Grapes come in a variety of sizes and colours

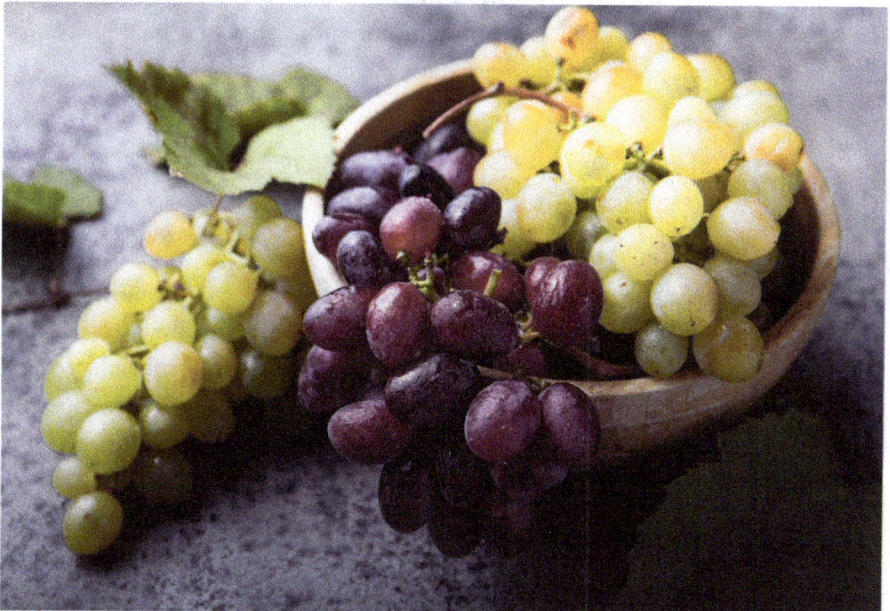

and can be black, purple, dark blue, crimson, pink, pale yellow, or green, with the darker coloured grapes generally being the most nutritious. Grapes are also mentioned in Biblical texts.

"But I say unto you, I will not drink henceforth of this fruit of the vine, until that day when I drink it new with you in my Father's kingdom" (Matthew 26:29).

Sumptuous grapes have hundreds of different antioxidant nutrients, and as a group, have the following nutrients for health support: anthocyanins, beta-carotene, caffeic acid, carotenoids, catechins, coumaric acid, epicatechins, ferulic acid, fibre, fisetin, folate, flavanols, gallic acid, isorhamnetin, kaempferol, lutein, myricetin, phenolic acids, piceatannol, pterostilbene, proanthocyanidins, procyanidins, quercetin (natural anti-inflammatory), resveratrol, stilbenes, viniferones, and zeaxanthin.

Grapes contain many nutrients which include vitamin A, vitamin B-complex, vitamin C, vitamin K, carotenes, copper, fibre, folate, iron, manganese, Omega-3, and potassium. Manganese and copper are essential co-factors of the antioxidant enzyme superoxide dismutase.

Consuming grapes can improve many health issues including cancer, cardiovascular disease, Alzheimer's disease, asthma, diabetes and diabetic neuropathy, constipation, allergies, weight loss, immune function, skin and hair problems, migraines, eye health, macular degeneration, cataracts, and kidney disorders.

"He will swallow up death in victory; and the Lord GOD will wipe away tears from off all faces; and the rebuke of His people shall he take away from off all the earth: for the LORD hath spoken it" (Isaiah 25:8).

Juicy and flavourful grapes are abundant in the powerful polyphenolic antioxidant compound resveratrol, which has been found to have a protective role against cancers, Alzheimer's disease, coronary heart disease, stroke, degenerative nerve disease, and fungal and viral infections. Resveratrol is a fat-soluble compound and a stilbene phytonutrient that is present not only in grape flesh but also in the grape seeds and grape skins, with the skin and seeds containing the richest concentration of antioxidants. It has been shown to have the ability to target cancer stem cells and to increase blood flow to the brain. Resveratrol reduces the risk of strokes by altering the molecular mechanisms inside the blood vessels. It does so by reducing the blood vessels' susceptibility to clotting through the decreased activity of angiotensin, which is a systemic hormone that causes blood vessel constriction. Resveratrol increases the production of the vasodilator nitric oxide, which helps with the reduction of blood vessel constriction, thereby grapes can help to combat many diseases. Resveratrol is also capable of killing dozens of lethal cancers, including the cancer stem cells within them.

"Peace I leave with you, my peace I give unto you: not as the world giveth, give I unto you. Let not your heart be troubled, neither let it be afraid" (John 14:27).

Luscious grapes contain powerful antioxidant polyphenols, which may prevent many types of cancers, and their high potassium content helps to prevent death from all causes. Anthocyanins are polyphenolic antioxidants that are abundant in red grapes and these phytochemicals engage in anti-cancer, anti-allergic, anti-microbial, and anti-inflammatory activity. The antioxidant flavonoids quercetin and myricetin contained in grapes help the body to counteract harmful free radical formations, while catechins, a type of disease-fighting flavonoid antioxidant found in the green varieties of grapes, have also been shown to possess health-protective functions. Chronic inflammation and chronic oxidative stress are key factors in the development of cancer and the anti-inflammatory and antioxidant properties of grapes offer natural protection against cancers. Grapes are also high in the antioxidants zeaxanthin and lutein, which are important for eye health.

Chronic inflammation and chronic oxidative stress are key factors in the development of cancer and the anti-inflammatory and antioxidant properties of grapes offer natural protection against cancers.

"This was the Lord's doing, and it is marvellous in our eyes?" (Mark 12:11).

The wisdom of the *doctrine of signatures* is revealed in grapes, which hang in a cluster that has a similar shape to that of the heart. Each grape has the appearance of a blood cell and they are also a profound heart and blood-vitalizing food. They also prevent decreased blood flow to the brain. The resveratrol which they contain prevents platelet aggregation. Thrombocytes (platelets) are cell-like blood particles that perform an important role in the blood clotting process. They form in the bone marrow from megakaryocyte cells (large polyploid nuclei, or cells containing at least two homologous sets of chromosomes) which break up into fragments and become platelets, which are tiny, colourless, disc-shaped particles that circulate in the blood. They do not reproduce or have a nucleus, yet they are produced when needed and last for about ten days. Platelets help the blood clotting process by forming a plug and sticking to the lining of blood vessels, which helps to repair and prevent blood vessel leakage and blood loss by initiating the first phases of the clotting process. Evidence illustrates that the highly active compounds in grapes and their seeds protect cardiovascular health by helping with chronic inflammation.

"For this is my blood of the new testament, which is shed for many for the remission of sins" (Matthew 26:28).

The name currant originated in the ancient city of Corinth. Currants often come from the dried black Corinth grape or dark red seedless grapes.

Sultanas are dried white grapes from seedless varieties which turn golden when dried and are juicy, sweet and plump, which distinguished them from dark-coloured raisins. Sultanas are mostly produced in Turkey.

Raisins are dried white Muscatel grapes that are grown in hot climates and produce dark-coloured dried fruit which results in their being especially concentrated in iron. Some golden raisins are chemically treated with sulphur dioxide prior to drying to preserve their golden colour.

Grape seeds contain higher concentrations of many of the beneficial compounds found in grapes. There is evidence that high antioxidant grape seed extract is beneficial for a number of cardiovascular conditions and a study has found that it provides superior antioxidant efficacy as compared to vitamins C, E, and beta-carotene. The main flavonoids in grape seeds and skins are gallic acid, catechin, epicatechin, ellagic acid, quercetin, kaempferol, myricetin, and trans-resveratrol. Studies also suggest that grape seed extract reduces swelling and helps with eye diseases related to diabetes. Polyphenol extracts from grape seeds have the ability to inhibit the production of neurofibrillary tangles, which is a primary marker for Alzheimer's disease.

"But let all those that put their trust in thee rejoice: let them ever shout for joy, because thou defendest them: let them also that love thy name be joyful in thee" (Psalm 5:11).

RASPBERRIES

Raspberries belong to the flowering rose family (Rosaceae) of the diverse Rubus genus, which is the main species of both the cultivated and the wild raspberry. There are over 200 species of raspberries, all belonging to the same large botanical genus. Raspberries are classified as aggregate drupes and there are three basic groups: red raspberries, black raspberries, and golden raspberries. Although naturally golden in colour, yellow raspberries are special forms of black or red raspberries. Purple raspberries are a hybrid of black and red. Raspberries can also be any colour from white through to orange and pink shades and the difference is in the structure. Raspberries also have two hybrids—boysenberries and loganberries.

These glorious and flavourful berries are thought to have originated in Asia Minor. The ancient Greeks were the first known to have cultivated raspberries and the first recorded raspberry harvest was from Mount Ida in AD 45. They were grown by the Romans and records concerning them have been found from the fourth century in the writings of the Roman agriculturist Rutilius Taurus Aemilianus Palladius. Seeds have been discovered at ancient Roman forts in Britain and it seems likely that the Romans could have spread raspberry cultivation throughout Europe. There is evidence of raspberries dating back about 2,000 years in Europe, and it was the English who popularized, hybridized, cultivated, and improved them throughout the Middle Ages and onwards. They were also used as a medicine as well as a food. Raspberries have been one of the important bush fruits of Europe for many years. Raspberry plants were exported to New York by 1771, and New York State began cultivating raspberries in the late 1800s. By 1925, there were 415 varieties available.

Wild raspberries grow on at least five continents and have enormous species diversity. When wild raspberries are compared with the cultivated variety they are similar in total anthocyanin and total phenol content.

Exquisite raspberries contain outstanding phytonutrients that include anthocyanins, caffeic acid, catechins, chlorogenic acid, coumaric acid, cyanidins, delphinidins, ellagic acid (an excellent source), ellagitannins, epicatechins, ferulic acid, flavonoid gallotannins, flavonols, gallic acid, glycosides, hydroxybenzoic acids, hydroxycinnamic acids, kaempferol, lambertianin, lignans, lutein, malvidins, pelargonidins, phenolic acids, proanthocyanidins, quercetin, resveratrol, sanguiin, stilbenoids, tannins, tiliroside, vanillic acid, and zeaxanthin.

Tangy and tasty raspberries are good sources of vitamin B2, vitamin B3, vitamin B5, vitamin C, vitamin E, vitamin K, biotin, copper, fibre, folate, iron, magnesium, manganese, Omega-3 fatty acids, and potassium. Black raspberries contain preventative compounds that include vitamin A, vitamin C, vitamin E, ellagic acid, and quercetin, which can help to prevent strokes.

Consuming raspberries can improve many health issues. Among these are cancer, cardiovascular disease, diabetes, arthritis, stroke, gout, macular degeneration, cataracts, inflammation, digestion, immune problems, eye diseases, memory loss, and fertility in both men and women.

"Peace I leave with you, my peace I give unto you: not as the world giveth, give I unto you. Let not your heart be troubled, neither let it be afraid" (John 14:27).

The great diversity of anti-inflammatory and antioxidant phytonutrients in raspberries is quite outstanding and provides significant amounts of nutrients which protect against the dangers of excessive inflammation and oxidative stress. These compounds help to scavenge free radical molecules which lower the risk of chronic diseases. Raspberries are high in anti-inflammatory Omega-3 fatty acids. Raspberries are also anticoagulants (which prevent clot formation) and fibrinolytic (which has clot-dissolving abilities).

"But the meek shall inherit the earth; and shall delight themselves in the abundance of peace" (Psalm 37:11).

Scientists have discovered that the nutrients in raspberries can boost the metabolism, which makes them valuable for combating obesity. Research demonstrates the potential of raspberries in improving the management of obesity, as the metabolism of fat cells can be increased by the phytonutrients contained in them, especially rheosmin, a raspberry ketone.

"And the LORD shall guide thee continually, and satisfy thy soul in drought, and make fat thy bones: and thou shalt be like a watered garden, and like a spring of water, whose waters fail not"
(Isaiah 58:11).

The anti-cancer benefits of raspberries are attributed to their powerful anti-inflammatories, antioxidants, and phytonutrients. Their properties also target cancer stem cells. Phytonutrients such as ellagitannins, which are present in both the red and black varieties, have the ability to change the signals that are sent to existing cancer cells, thereby decreasing the number of cancer cells by sending signals that encourage them to execute apoptosis. Ellagitannins are converted in the body to ellagic acid, the well-recognized cancer-fighting antioxidant. These phytonutrients can also trigger signals that encourage non-cancerous cells to remain non-cancerous.

"He giveth power to the faint; and to them that have no might He increaseth strength" (Isaiah 40:29).

Raspberries contain measurable amounts of oxalates, and in peer-reviewed research studies, the ability of oxalates to lower calcium absorption is comparatively small.

"Pleasant words are as an honeycomb, sweet to the soul, and health to the bones" (Proverbs 16:24).

Raspberry leaf has a long history of use in botanical medicine and has been used to support functions in various body systems. Its most well-known use has been in conjunction with helping menstrual issues, pregnancy, and childbirth. Raspberry leaf tea can also be a caffeine-free replacement for unhealthy black tea as it is said that the flavour and aroma are similar.

"Behold, I am the LORD, the God of all flesh: is there any thing too hard for me?" (Jeremiah 32:27).

The Black raspberry (Rubus occidentalis) is only indigenous to North America and has been called the *king of berries* for its superior health benefits. The difference between black raspberries and blackberries is the core, where the stem attaches to the berry. Blackberries always have a white core, whereas black raspberries have a hollow centre, the same as red raspberries do. Black raspberries are less tart, they can withstand colder temperatures and are harvested earlier than blackberries. They are a small, black-coloured raspberry, covered with very small hairs similar to a red raspberry, whereas blackberries are sometimes described as shinier than black raspberries and are usually larger. A study demonstrated that black raspberries have astonishingly high antioxidant levels. They are anti-inflammatory, vaso-protective, antioxidative, and anti-neurodegenerative. Research also indicates that they are anti-cancer and are highly effective at preventing oesophageal cancer and colorectal tumours. Black raspberries also significantly improve vascular function and cardiovascular disease with the bioactives of anthocyanins, ellagitannin, flavonols, resveratrol, and tannins. They are amongst the foods that are highest in anthocyanins and show approximately 1000% greater health benefits than blackberries and red raspberries. Anthocyanins not only impart deep dark colours to berries but have also been shown to improve vision and memory.

"And sow the fields, and plant vineyards, which may yield fruits of increase." (Psalm 107:37).

STRAWBERRIES

Strawberries are the fruits of the flowering rose family (Rosaceae) and belong to the Fragaria genus. Apples and plums, as well as blackberries, cherries, and raspberries, also belong to the rose family. Botanically, strawberries are not categorized as berries but instead, are classed as fleshy receptacles; with the dry seeds that speckle the outside of the strawberry being classed as fruits. The actual edible ripe fleshy part of the strawberry plant is classified as the achenes. Strawberries are the only fruit that have their seeds on the outside. There are well over 600 known varieties of strawberries which differ in texture, size, and flavour.

Delightful and delectable strawberries have grown wild throughout the world for many centuries. They were utilized in Roman times and evidence shows that they grew wild in Italy well before 200 years BC. Their history not only goes as far back as the Romans but possibly also to the Greeks. Strawberries were first recorded as a medicinal herb around AD 1300 when France began to cultivate them as a medicine. They were thought to be good for curing gout and digestive upsets and by the 1500s the cultivation of this delicious berry was being developed. During the sixteenth and seventeenth centuries, wild strawberries appeared in gardens where they were carefully cultivated. The beautiful berry of today was originally grown in Northern Europe, and the development of the big-fruited commercial strawberry occurred during the first half of the seventeenth century. However, it was not until the late eighteenth century, when its cultivation began to be pursued in earnest, that the first garden strawberry was grown in France. The first American strawberries were cultivated in 1835.

Bioflavonoids (vitamin P) are responsible for the flavour and colour of spectacular tasting strawberries and provide an important and outstanding variety of powerful antioxidant and anti-inflammatory phytonutrients. These bioflavonoids are found in the ripe, fresh berries and include anthocyanins (principally cyanindins and pelargonidins), caffeic acid, catechins, cinnamic acid, coumaric acid, cyanidins, ellagic acid, ellagitannins, epicatechins, ferulic acid, flavonols (principally catechins, epicatechins, epigallocatechins, fisetin, gallocatechins, kaempferol, procyanidins and quercetin), gallic acid, gallocatechins, gallotannins, hydroxy-cinnamic acids, (including caffeic, cinnamic, coumaric and ferulic acids), hydroxy-benzoic acids (principally ellagic acid), kaempferol, lutein, pelargonidins, phenolic acids, procyanidins, quercetin, salicylic acid, stilbenes, tannins, terpenoids, resveratrol, and zeaxanthin.

Succulent strawberries are an excellent source of many B vitamins, immunity-boosting vitamin C, vitamin K, manganese and potassium. They are also a very good source of fibre, folate and iodine, and a good source of ascorbic acid, biotin, copper, iron, magnesium, Omega-3 fatty acids, phosphorus, and potassium with its co-factoring enzyme superoxide dismutase.

In addition to anti-cancer abilities, strawberries also contain potential neurological disease-fighting substances. Their health benefits also include proper brain function, relief from gout, arthritis, and various cardiovascular diseases. Several research studies have shown that strawberry phytonutrients work together synergistically to provide cardiovascular benefits. Furthermore, the blood glucose-levelling abilities and free radical eliminating antioxidant activities of strawberries are outstanding.

"But seek ye first the kingdom of God, and His righteousness; and all these things shall be added unto you" (Matthew 6:33).

There are compounds in strawberries that have demonstrated anti-cancer activity and the ability to block the initiation of carcinogenesis. They also suppress the progression and proliferation of tumours. The impressive polyphenolic and antioxidant content of strawberries improves the immune system as well as protecting against various types of cancers.

"Great is the LORD, and greatly to be praised; and His greatness is unsearchable" (Psalm 145:3).

The healthful fibrous elements in strawberries help to entrap heavy metals in the digestive system and escort them out of the body. When slicing a strawberry in half from the top to the bottom, small fibres are visible on the inside edge of the strawberry and these connect to the outer seeds. Because inorganic fruit juice is often heavily laden with pesticides, which are water-soluble, these juices are often a toxic cocktail. It is more beneficial to eat whole, organic fruit as nature intended so that the ingested fibre can help to eliminate unwanted substances and also feed the gut microbes.

"O give thanks unto the LORD; for He is good; for His mercy endureth for ever" (1 Chronicles 16:34).

Triterpenes from the phytosterol family are found specifically in strawberries. Lupeol, a triterpene in strawberries, has been found to have immense anti-inflammatory potential. Strawberries also lower blood levels of C-reactive protein, which is a signal of inflammation in the body. Strawberries contain the important bone health nutrients—vitamin K, magnesium, and potassium.

"For length of days, and long life, and peace, shall they add to thee" (Proverbs 3:2).

A recent study showed that the abundant flavonoid fisetin in strawberries can kill breast cancer cells without harming normal breast cells. Fisetin is also found in apples, cucumbers, grapes, onions, and persimmons and it has been proven to cause apoptosis in prostate cancer, cervical cancer, breast cancer, and colon cancer cells.

"Verily, verily, I say unto you, The hour is coming, and now is, when the dead shall hear the voice of the Son of God: and they that hear shall live" (John 5:25).

Beautiful and luscious strawberries have an abundance of biotin (vitamin B7) which helps to beautify the skin and build strong nails and hair. Biotin is also contained in mushrooms, avocados, cauliflower, and legumes. The content of the antioxidant ellagic acid and vitamin C in strawberries protects the elastic fibres in the skin and thereby helps to prevent a loss of skin elasticity.

> *The powerful life-promoting properties of God's beautiful berries are not only delicious but also life-enhancing and life-sustaining and can be enjoyed as part of a healthy whole plant-food diet.*

"But if a woman have long hair, it is a glory to her: for her hair is given her for a covering" (1 Corinthians 11:15).

The primary reasons for nearly all health problems related to the eyes are a deficiency of antioxidant nutrients and free radical damage. Amidst a lack of protective nutrients, free radicals can cause substantial damage to the eyes such as the degeneration of the optic nerves, ocular pressure, vision defects, macular degeneration, cataracts, and excessively dry eyes. Strawberries contain powerful antioxidant potential which can reduce macular degeneration, help to prevent cataracts, and associated eye problems and also assist in protecting the brain.

"And Jesus said unto him, Receive thy sight: thy faith hath saved thee" (Luke 18:42).

The powerful life-promoting properties of God's beautiful berries are not only delicious but also life-enhancing and life-sustaining and can be enjoyed as part of a healthy whole plant-food diet.

"Trust in the LORD with all thine heart; and lean not unto thine own understanding. In all thy ways acknowledge Him, and He shall direct thy paths" (Proverbs 3:5, 6).

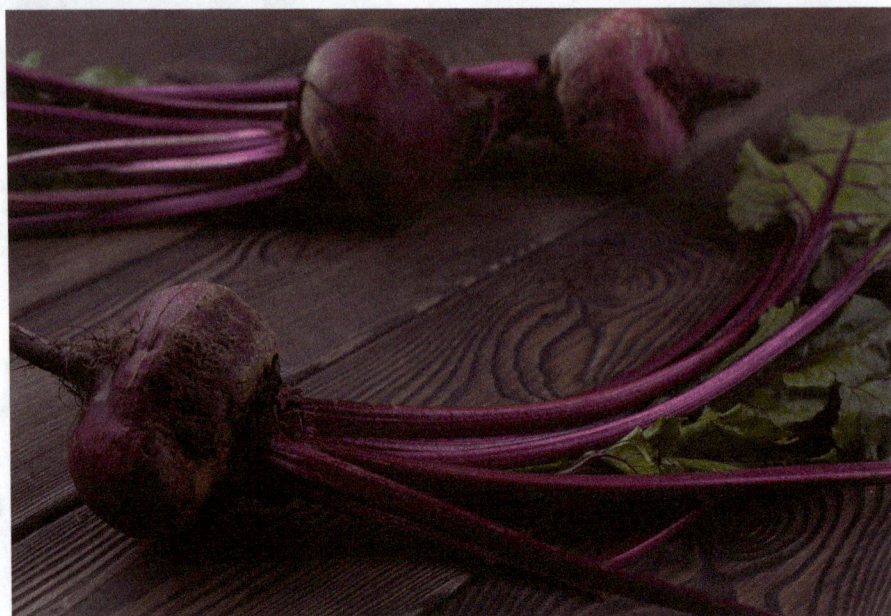

Chapter 9

Beetroot

"THE GREATEST MEDICINE OF ALL IS TO TEACH OTHERS HOW NOT TO NEED IT."

Beetroot is a member of the flowering plant species scientifically known as Beta vulgaris. The Beta genus is a member of the flowering plant family Amaranthaceae. Other well-known species of this family include spinach, amaranth, sugar beet, and quinoa. Both beetroot and Swiss chard are different varieties of this same plant family and their edible leaves share a resemblance in both taste and texture. The earliest known written mention of beetroot was in an Assyrian text that mentioned it was growing in the Hanging Gardens of Babylon. The remains of beetroot have been excavated in the third dynasty Saqqara pyramid at Thebes, Egypt. The wild beetroot is the ancestor of the beetroot which is a familiar vegetable today, and in earlier times the beetroot greens and not the roots were exclusively consumed. Beta vulgaris was initially prized for its leaves and for the fleshy elongated leaf midribs that characterize Swiss chard. Chard is a beetroot which has been bred for its leaves instead of its roots, to be used as a leafy vegetable. Hippocrates, *the father of medicine*, advocated beetroot leaves to bind wounds, while other Greeks offered it to the sun god Apollo in the temple of Delphi. The ancient Romans were one of the first civilizations to cultivate beetroot and use its roots for food. They described early varieties as being black and white, and their texts discuss more uses for the root of the beet than its leaves. Beetroot was so well regarded in ancient Rome and Greece that methods were developed for producing them during the hot summer months. In the first century BC, sources of Jewish and Roman literature indicate that domestic beetroot was grown in the Mediterranean basin. The Greek physician, botanist, pharmacologist ,and author Pedanius Dioscorides records two types of beetroot in the first century AD. Archaeologists also discovered depictions of beetroots painted on walls in the ancient towns that were preserved in ash from the eruption of Mount Vesuvius in AD 79. Beetroot was used by the ancients and consumed generally for its medicinal properties but mainly to relieve fever and as a laxative. It was also used for the treatment of anaemia, ulcers, malignant growths, liver problems, and low blood sugar.

"Our help is in the name of the LORD, who made heaven and earth" (Psalm 124:8).

From Eastern Europe and the Middle East, cultivated Beta vulgaris was carried on trade routes to East Asia. In ancient times it was consumed in Asia Minor and later in India. It was also recorded in writings in China from the seventh century AD. The tribes that invaded Rome were responsible for spreading beetroot throughout northern Europe, where the plant adapted very easily to the cooler climates and was first used as animal fodder and later for human consumption. It was first recorded in 1542 that the root of the beet was cultivated for consumption in Italy and Germany where new varieties were developed, particularly the common red variety of today. The beetroot of the Middle Ages looked quite different from the beetroot of today and was used to aid digestion. Its earliest shape had long thin roots and more closely resembled the shape of a parsnip rather than the plump, round shape of more recent times, which began appearing near the end of the 1500s. Soon the round shape became the most popular but it was not until about two centuries later that it became a worldwide culinary success.

The Italians developed different types of beetroot during the fifteenth and sixteenth centuries and some of these early varieties were introduced from Italy into northern Europe by the sixteenth century. Northeastern Europe was the first area to embrace the beetroot as a dietary staple and it was valued as one of the only vegetables that grew well throughout the winter. The sixteenth-century saw the creation of delicious Borscht, and from this century forward populations mainly consumed beetroot as a vegetable. During the sixteenth and seventeenth centuries uncontrolled hybridization between chards, leaf beets, and long-rooted beetroot produced a wide variety of forms. By the nineteenth century, beetroot was widely consumed across Europe where it has been used as a treatment for cancer for centuries.

"For they are life unto those that find them, and health to all their flesh" (Proverbs 4:22).

Creativity has resulted in various cultivars of Beta vulgaris. There are four main cultivar groups: the beetroot, with its roots and leaves consumed as a vegetable, though it was originally prized for its leaves and not for its roots; the sugar-producing sugar beet, from which approximately 30% of the world's sugar production is derived; the mangel-wurzel, which can easily be stored and used for livestock feed; and Swiss chard, which is cultivated for its edible leaves. The sugar content in the garden beetroot is no more than 10%, while the sugar content in the sugar beet is typically 15%–20%. Beetroot has the highest sugar content of all vegetables, containing more sugar than sweet corn or carrots. Although beetroot is a vegetable that comes from the same family as sugar beets, these two vegetables are very different. Sugar beets are white in colour and are commonly used to produce sugar. It was grown as a garden vegetable long before it was prized for its sugar content. Unlike sugar beets, beetroot cannot produce sugar. In 1747, German chemist Andreas Marggraf established that sugar beets contain sucrose. His student Franz Karl Achard built a sugar beet processing factory at Cunern in Silesia, which was destroyed during the Napoleonic Wars of 1802–1815. Napoleon banned cane sugar imports in 1833, the consequence of which ensured that the emerging sugar beet industry thrived. Sugar beet production requires four times less water than sugar cane production. Betaine is a nutrient which was named after its discovery in sugar beet juice in the nineteenth century, and this nutrient is valuable for the health of the cardiovascular system.

"Pleasant words are as an honeycomb, sweet to the soul, and health to the bones" (Proverbs 3:24).

This powerful red root is potent, time-tested, accessible, and affordable. It is a rich source of outstanding antioxidants and nutrients. It is a very good source of vitamin C, calcium, copper, farnesol, folate, manganese, potassium (which helps to enhance cerebrum capacity and avert strokes and cancers), and rutin. It is also a good source of vitamin A, vitamin B1, vitamin B2, vitamin B3, vitamin B5, vitamin B6 (needed to make melatonin, dopamine and serotonin), iron, magnesium (for stress and muscle tension), phosphorus and insoluble and soluble fibre. It also contains boron, glycine, iodine, Omega-3, selenium, silicon (for stronger and healthier hair), sodium, sulphur, and zinc. It also contains traces of rare caesium and rubidium, which are critical for cancer protection. Zeaxanthin and lutein are two carotenoid phytonutrients contained in beetroot that play an important role in health. Science reports them to be extremely beneficial for eye health and especially the retina. The combination of special elements created only in specific concentrations and combinations within beetroot afford its disease preventing and cancer-fighting powers.

"But seek ye first the kingdom of God, and His righteousness; and all these things shall be added unto you" (Matthew 6:33).

Beetroot greens are not only delicious but also boost bone strength. They can be prepared in the same way as spinach or Swiss chard and contain even more iron than spinach, which is another leafy green in the same botanical family. Including the stems when preparing them makes more nutrients available as the largest majority of nutrients are in the fibre. They are also incredibly abundant in valuable nutrients such as the antioxidant carotenoids: beta-carotene, lutein, and zeaxanthin (which are protective against eye disease). They also contain vitamin A, vitamin B5, vitamin B6, vitamin C, vitamin E, vitamin K, calcium, copper, fibre, folate, iron, magnesium, manganese, phosphorus, potassium, and zinc.

"The LORD will give strength unto His people; the LORD will bless His people with peace" (Psalm 29:11).

Some of the many benefits of beetroot include its ability as the following: adaptogenic, analgesic, anti-ageing, anti-allergenic, anti-anaemic, anti-anxiety, anti-arthritic, anti-asthmatic, anti-atherogenic, antibacterial, antibiotic, anti-carcinogenic, anti-diabetic, anti-depressant, anti-fungal, anti-inflammatory, anti-ischaemic, anti-malarial, anti-mitotic, antioxidant, antiparasitic, antiphlogistic (prevents or relieves inflammation), antipyretic, antisclerotic, antiseptic, anti-tumour, anti-ulcer, anti-viral, anxiolytic, apoptotic, cytotoxic (to cancer stem cells), detoxicant, digestive, diuretic, epigenetic, hepatoprotective, immune-protective, immunomodulatory, laxative, neuroprotective, neurorestorative, radio-protective, remineralizing, tonic, vasodilator, vasoprotective, and vulnerary.

"It shall be health to thy navel, and marrow to thy bones"
(Proverbs 3:8).

The following health issues are included in the many health-protecting benefits afforded by beetroot: cancer (including leukaemia), epilepsy, anaemia, influenza, inflammation, multiple sclerosis, cirrhosis, cardiovascular disease, epithelial and endothelial dysfunction, asthenia, jaundice, hepatitis, gallbladder and liver disease, diarrhoea, nausea, Alzheimer's disease and dementia, constipation, strokes, rabies, tetanus, kidney disorders, macular degeneration, cataracts, and hemorrhoids. It also inhibits the Epstein-Barr virus. Beetroot pectin inhibits the synthesis of types A and B staphylococcal enterotoxins.

"Behold, I will bring it health and cure, and I will cure them,
and will reveal unto them the abundance of peace and truth"
(Jeremiah 33:6).

The humble beetroot is considered to be one of the most rejuvenating of all vegetables, with numerous proven health benefits for virtually every system of the body. It contains trace amounts of various amino acids, which help to build proteins for the body, including alpha-amino acids and D-amino acids. Some of the many known capabilities of beetroot include: faster formation of red blood corpuscles, thereby improving cellular oxygenation; liver function support; relief of constipation; improving digestive disorders; detoxification properties; assisting with fatigue elimination and convalescence; benefits for nails, skin, hair and bronchial ailments; boosting stamina, mood, metabolism, energy, vitality, endurance and strength; promoting cognitive health; stimulating lymphatic circulation and the immune system; accelerating bile secretion; anti-fungal Candida-fighting properties; strengthening of skin and vein walls; revitalization of blood, thereby obstructing cancer cell development; assisting capillary fragility; improving blood circulation; helping to prevent macular degeneration, cataracts and respiratory problems. Thereby, beetroot promotes health in addition to fighting disease.

"Praise ye the LORD. O give thanks unto the LORD; for He is
good: for His mercy endureth for ever" (Psalm 106:1).

Potent beetroot is not only a superfood but also a powerful cleanser of the body and a treasure-trove of health-affirming nourishment. It is also a gift from God to the colon. There are numerous different types of beetroots, many of which are distinguished by their colour and which, although typically a beautiful reddish-purple hue, also come in varieties that feature white, crimson, golden yellow, pink, orange, dark purple, and even alternate red and white coloured concentric whorls. It contains the substance geosmin, which is responsible for its earthy taste and which some people are quite sensitive to, even at very low amounts.

"For He satisfieth the longing soul, and filleth the hungry soul with goodness" (Psalm 107:9).

Beetroot is a very powerful source of anti-cancer nutrients, created, and combined together to fight against disease. Chemotherapy and other highly lethal regimens harm normal cells and often lead to the demise of the whole system. However, this delicious crimson bulb does no harm to the body, but rather strengthens, detoxifies and speeds it on its way to health. Genotoxic chemotherapy causes mutations by interacting with DNA and is a well-known risk factor for developing primary and also secondary cancers. This destructive pernicious carcinogen not only causes cancer but also destroys the erythrocytes (red blood cells) and vital organs. It also devastates the immune system, which is designed to protect the body. If every oncologist were asked to test lethal chemotherapy on themselves in an attempt to demonstrate its safety in the sight of those that they recommend it to, then the incidences of destructive chemotherapy-induced deaths would be significantly diminished. Chemotherapy vehemently and adversely affects the whole body, and especially the blood, the digestive system, the skin, nails, and hair, and can cause permanent damage to various parts of the body including the brain, the liver, the ears, and reproductive organs. The presence of a growing cancer indicates a very strong possibility that the immune system is not functioning at optimal levels or is suppressed. If this is the case, deadly chemotherapy will further weaken the immune system, which, when it is already striving to deal with a toxic load, any remaining cancerous cells will rapidly overrun the already weakened body as there will be hardly any defences left available to prevent the reproduction of the remaining cancer cells.

"For the eyes of the Lord are over the righteous, and His ears are open unto their prayers: but the face of the Lord is against them that do evil" (1 Peter 3:12).

Radiation destroys haemoglobin, but beetroot helps the body to build it as compounds contained in the betalain phytonutrients in beetroot reduce toxicity associated with gamma radiation exposure. Using radiation for cancer is damaging to the body as there are multiple harmful effects of this dangerous protocol. The types of radiation used on cancer patients are gamma rays, high-energy radiation, X-rays, and charged particles. Systemic radiation uses radioactive substances such as radioactive iodine. Even low levels of exposure to radiation can lead to the alteration of the blood, headaches, fatigue, itchy and dry skin, scalp discolouration and scalp tenderness, brain damage, mood changes, memory problems, reproductive issues, nausea, reduced listening and psychomotor capabilities, an increase in information processing times, major digestive imbalances, and the destruction of many cellular structures in key tissue and organ systems. It also reduces lymphocytes (white blood cells that are one of the main types of immune cells) which can cause infections and increase the likelihood of developing leukaemia. The lignin-containing dietary fibres in beetroot are very effective at protecting against radiation poisoning. Self-education of sound knowledge is a powerful tool for combating diseases through natural means, but fear of disease weakens the whole body. Hippocrates said: "Let food be thy medicine and medicine be thy food". He also said: "Whenever a doctor cannot do good, he must be kept from doing harm."

> *Beetroot is a very powerful source of anti-cancer nutrients, created, and combined together to fight against disease.*

"That the wicked is reserved to the day of destruction? they shall be brought forth to the day of wrath" (Job 21:30).

Betacyanins, from the betalain group of phytonutrients, have a very important function and contain pigments that are reddish crimson in colour and are the dominant pigments in red beetroot. A study of these phytonutrients demonstrated that they help to slow the growth of tumours and are also efficacious for the liver, kidneys, and gallbladder. Betacyanins and betaxanthins absorb light differently because of their different structures, and each type donates a different spectrum of colour to a plant.

"And God made two great lights; the greater light to rule the day, and the lesser light to rule the night: He made the stars also" (Genesis 1:16).

The amino acid betaine in beetroot has significant anti-cancer properties due to its natural red colouring agent. This red pigment has shown strong growth inhibition against colon cancer, central nervous system cancer, breast cancer, and lung cancer cells. When the betaine pigment is absorbed into the blood it can increase the oxygen-carrying ability of the blood by up to 400%. Betaine is an important nutrient for cardiovascular health and fights acidic conditions that can lead to strokes, heart disease and other cardiovascular diseases. It also provides anti-inflammatory, antioxidant, and detoxification support. Betaine is made from the B-complex vitamin choline, which is a key vitamin for assisting in the regulation of inflammation in the cardiovascular system as sufficient choline is important for preventing the unwanted accumulation of homocysteine. It is known that inflammation in the body not only increases the risk of cardiovascular disease and cancer but also countless other diseases. A study has shown that those who consume the most choline have significantly reduced levels of inflammation. Betaine normalizes stomach acid secretion by increasing the acid levels in the stomach if there is an insufficiency and acts as an antacid if there is an overabundance. Betaine hydrochloride (betaine and hydrochloride) is a compound that is naturally found in beetroot and is frequently used to aid digestive issues as it contains digestive enzymes to properly break down food. Betaine is one of the most abundant sources of the amino acid glutamine, which is essential to the health and maintenance of the intestinal tract. Betaine supports the liver and encourages the liver cells to eliminate toxins. It also triggers the gallbladder to release bile, thins the bile, and aids in the prevention of gallstones. It acts to protect the liver and bile ducts which are important for optimum liver function. Artichokes are also a liver protector and bile producer.

The betaine and methionine in beetroot support liver healing and detoxification. Without this function toxins can accumulate both in the liver and fatty tissues of the body, thwarting weight loss and contributing to sluggishness, mood swings, and more serious illnesses. The important betaine compound in beetroot donates a methyl group of one carbon and three hydrogen atoms that subsequently reduces high levels of homocysteine, which damage the DNA. B vitamins also assist in this process. Not only is beetroot a powerful food for detoxifying and supporting liver function whilst also protecting it from chemical toxicity, but it also detoxifies the kidneys and lymph system while promoting the regeneration of healthy new cells. It also stimulates the production of new liver cells. Beetroot also contains a myriad of important substances which cause a marked improvement in both liver health and overall wellbeing. Beetroot and carrots are extremely high in plant-flavonoids and beta-carotene, and consuming these two vegetables can help to stimulate and improve overall liver function. DNA is constantly being damaged and attempting to repair itself. Beetroot supports this repair by improving the process of methylation. Beetroot is considered to be one of the best cleansing foods and has long been used for medicinal purposes.

"Then shall thy light break forth as the morning, and thine health shall spring forth speedily: and thy righteousness shall go before thee; the glory of the LORD shall be thy rereward"
(Isaiah 58:8).

Betalains are phytonutrients and plant pigments that are somewhat rare in the plant world because they are only found in the order of Caryophyllales (an order of dicotyledonous shrubs and herbs) and only in some of the plants of this order. Beetroots are a unique source of these highly water-soluble betalains, of which the most studied is betanin, followed by vulgaxanthin. The combination of these provides anti-inflammatory, antioxidant, and detoxification support. Such abilities make beetroot a highly likely candidate for reducing the risk of many types of cancer. This support includes some especially important Phase II detoxification measures, which involve glutathione, the master detoxifier of all the antioxidants that the body produces. Unfortunately, an unhealthy lifestyle depletes this vital antioxidant. The glutathione molecule is one of the most important places to find sulphur in the body. It is formed from the amino acids glutamine, cysteine, and glycine. Glutathione performs many functions, including operating as an anti-inflammatory, an antioxidant, and a detoxifier that binds metals and toxins, thereby rendering them water-soluble and able to be easily excreted from the body. When detoxifying, specific enzymes in betalains stimulate glutathione production and connect toxins to glutathione molecules, which are then neutralized and excreted harmlessly from the body. All betalains derive from the same original molecule, which is betalamic acid. The addition of amino acids or amino acid derivatives to betalamic acid determines the specific type of pigment that is produced. Betalain pigments in beetroot have frequently been shown to help neutralize toxins by rendering them sufficiently water-soluble for excretion in the urine. These same pigments contain nitrogen and are stored within the plant cell vacuoles (microscopic water sacs within each cell). They are also contained in chard, amaranth, rhubarb, and in the flower petals, leaves, stems, fruits, and roots of various plants.

Each betalain component supplies a specific structure and function to every cell and also provides a reward system for cells that have internal deficiencies and are distressed by toxins. This helps to strengthen the cell wall, which results in the cell being rehydrated. These components also provide a mineral balancing function with the correct ratio of minerals inside and outside of the cells, thereby maintaining the integrity of the cells. Betalains are concentrated in the leaves, flesh, and peel of beetroot and are an incredibly powerful, natural anti-inflammatory. Beetroot is not only high in betalains but also polyphenols, which have excellent antioxidant properties. Betalain antioxidants play an important role in the prevention of most chronic diseases, due to their ability to neutralize and counteract the effects of oxidative substances in the body. Many betalains function both as antioxidants and anti-inflammatory molecules. Their properties significantly aid the ability of the body to fight many inflammation-related diseases. Inflammation and the immune response are guided by the gut bacteria, which directs approximately 80% of the immune response. Commensal bacteria can manufacture powerful anti-inflammatory substances, but ingesting even small amounts of animal products can generate higher levels of inflammatory compounds in the gut. Hundreds of scientific studies have shown the incredible health benefits available through the antioxidant power of betalains. There are two basic categories of betalains whose protein structure is extremely beneficial and vital to life, and these are the betacyanins and the betaxanthins. Included among the betacyanins that are present in plants are betanin, isobetanin, probetanin, and neobetanin. Included among the betaxanthins that are present in plants are vulgaxanthin, miraxanthin, portulaxanthin, and indicaxanthin. Research indicates that the betalains in beetroots provide special antioxidant support for eye and nerve tissue better than other antioxidant-rich vegetables, as betalains work in conjunction with the manganese and vitamin C in beetroot. Betalains are attached to a glucose molecule and have nitrogen in their structure. They help the body to make carnitine, which is a nutrient that helps the body to turn fat into energy. Betalains also replace anthocyanins in the plants where they are found, as plants will only have one or the other of these two substances.

Taking betalains into the body system helps to restore vitality on a cellular level. They help the body to reduce the toxins surrounding the cells and enable essential nutrients to reach each cell whilst reducing the inflammation in the body that leads to disease. Betalains protect many types of cells from toxins that are known to trigger tumours—especially brain cells. Scientific research shows that betalains not only help to reduce inflammation but also help to protect the endothelial cells, which constitute a monolayer of the inner lining of blood vessels and also the blood-brain barrier, which is formed by highly specialized high-density brain microvascular endothelial cells. They also provide significant protection from toxins that directly affect the liver and are incredibly effective at preventing chronic health problems as well as helping the body to maintain wellness. Betalains neutralize toxins, reduce the enzymes responsible for causing inflammation, and support the natural detoxification process of the cell. By preserving the integrity of the cell and preventing the accumulation of toxins, chronic inflammation can be avoided.

"O give thanks unto the LORD; call upon His name: make known His deeds among the people" (Psalm 105:1).

The betalin pigments in beetroot have repeatedly been demonstrated to support activity in the body's Phase II detoxification process. Phase II detoxification is the metabolic step that cells use to combine activated, unwanted toxic substances with small nutrient groups, which effectively neutralizes the toxins and causes them to be sufficiently water-soluble for excretion from the body. Betalins not only have detoxification effects but are also antioxidant and anti-inflammatory. The liver is the first line of defence against cancer and needs to function at optimal levels to prevent and help reverse any cancerous condition. Betalins allow toxins in the body to be bound to other molecules, which are then transported out of the body, thereby assisting to cleanse the system and support the liver. Studies have shown that coarse vegetables release their nutrients from the fibre when they are cooked, and a new study reveals that betalins are lost from beetroot if they are overcooked, unlike some other food pigments.

"Create in me a clean heart, O God; and renew a right spirit within me" (Psalm 51:10).

Betanin, the most common pigment in beetroot, is responsible for its strong red colour, which is also used commercially as a natural food dye. It assists in protecting the liver by encouraging bile stimulation, preventing the accumulation of fatty deposits, and acting as a powerful anti-oxidant. Betanin also helps the liver to eliminate toxins by supporting its natural function as an organ of detoxification while assisting in the elimination of harmful substances from the body. Studies on tumour cells show that the antioxidant properties of the betanin pigment can reduce tumour growth in breast, colon, nerve, stomach, and testicular tissues. It is believed that it does this by inhibiting pro-inflammatory enzymes.

The phytonutrients betanin, isobetanin, and vulgaxanthin reduce inflammation and possess the ability to inhibit the activity of cyclo-oxygenase enzymes (including both COX-1 and COX-2). COX enzymes are extensively used by cells to produce messaging molecules that provoke inflammation. In most circumstances, when inflammation is required, this production of pro-inflammatory messaging molecules is of benefit. However, under different circumstances when the body has unwanted and chronic inflammation, the production of these inflammatory messengers can worsen the outcome. Many of the unique phytonutrients contained in beetroot have been shown to function as anti-inflammatory compounds, especially in their ability to inhibit unwanted and chronic inflammation.

*"O LORD my God, I cried unto thee, and thou hast healed me"
(Psalm 30:2).*

Betaxanthins are any of the betalain pigments which appears yellow to orange, but generally in lesser amounts than betacyanins, which means that the red colour of the betacyanins dominates the vegetable. Betaxanthins dominate in a variety of yellow beetroot and particularly the betaxanthin called vulgaxanthin. This phytonutrient is also found in some varieties of Swiss chard. Indicaxanthin, a type of betaxanthin, has a yellow or orange pigment and is also a powerful antioxidant.

"To the only wise God our Saviour, be glory and majesty, dominion and power, both now and ever. Amen" (Jude 1:25).

Crimson-coloured root vegetables contain powerful nutrient compounds that help to protect against birth defects, heart disease, and cancers. Scientific evidence continues to support beetroot as a natural healer for cancer, and research reveals astounding cases of cancer remission in those with cancer who consumed high concentrations of beetroot. The powerful alkaloid allantoin in beetroot has anti-tumour effects, which researchers demonstrated in the 1960s. Beetroot is extraordinarily rich in unique disease-fighting and anti-cancer chemicals. It improves the function of many body systems and enables the body to prevent and reverse many health conditions, including cancer. Beetroot also strengthens the immune system by stimulating the production of white blood cells and antibodies which are responsible for detecting and eliminating abnormal cells. Consuming beetroot assists with the boosting of immune function and prevents chronic diseases because of the antioxidants, vitamins, and minerals that it contains. The anti-cancer fighting properties of beetroot are known to kill cancer cells in pancreatic, prostate, and breast cell lines and have also been responsible for apoptosis in lung tumours. It also contains phytosterols, which have been proven to reduce joint inflammation and the symptoms of an enlarged prostate in addition to inhibiting the growth of cancer cells. Beetroot has a healing and blood-building effect, which is what is needed to combat leukaemia, as it increases the red blood corpuscles. Its high iron content acts as a regenerator and activator of red blood corpuscles, thereby supplying cancer cells with more oxygen, which thwarts cancer because it cannot survive in an oxygen-rich environment. When leukaemia is present, the white blood cells increase and the erythrocytes decrease and break down. There are also decreased amounts of the oxygen-carrying haemoglobin, which is caused by the disappearance of the red blood corpuscles, and as a result the body gradually dies.

"Whoso sheddeth man's blood, by man shall his blood be shed: for in the image of God made He man" (Genesis 9:6).

Consuming foods rich in nitrates, such as beetroot, can increase blood flow to the brain and carry oxygen to areas where it is lacking. Because of this one factor, it can stop the decline in cognition, assist with the proper functioning of the brain, and protect against the progression of dementia. When nitrate is converted into nitrite it assists with better transmission of neural impulses and brain functioning. Beetroot's favourable influence on the brain and nerves is due to its high content of the amino acids asparagine, betaine, and glutamine. It removes toxins and heavy metals from the brain and is also a source of melatonin.

"For, behold, I create new heavens and a new earth: and the former shall not be remembered, nor come into mind" (Isaiah 65:17).

The ancient wisdom of the *doctrine of signatures* reveals itself in the colour of the heart-shaped red beetroot, of which even the leaves are heart-shaped. This *heart beet* not only nourishes the blood and circulatory system but is also one of nature's finest cardiovascular tonics, with its long rootlets having a similar shape to arteries. Beetroot not only contains betaine but also folate, which lowers homocysteine levels. Homocysteine is an amino acid that increases the formation of blood clots. Beetroot has an exceptionally high concentration of folate (vitamin B9), which helps to prevent birth defects and is important for healthy tissue growth and cell function. Folate aids in the generation and upkeep of cells and beetroot is one of its richest sources. Beetroot also contains potassium and produces nitric oxide, which both normalise heart rhythm and heart rate.

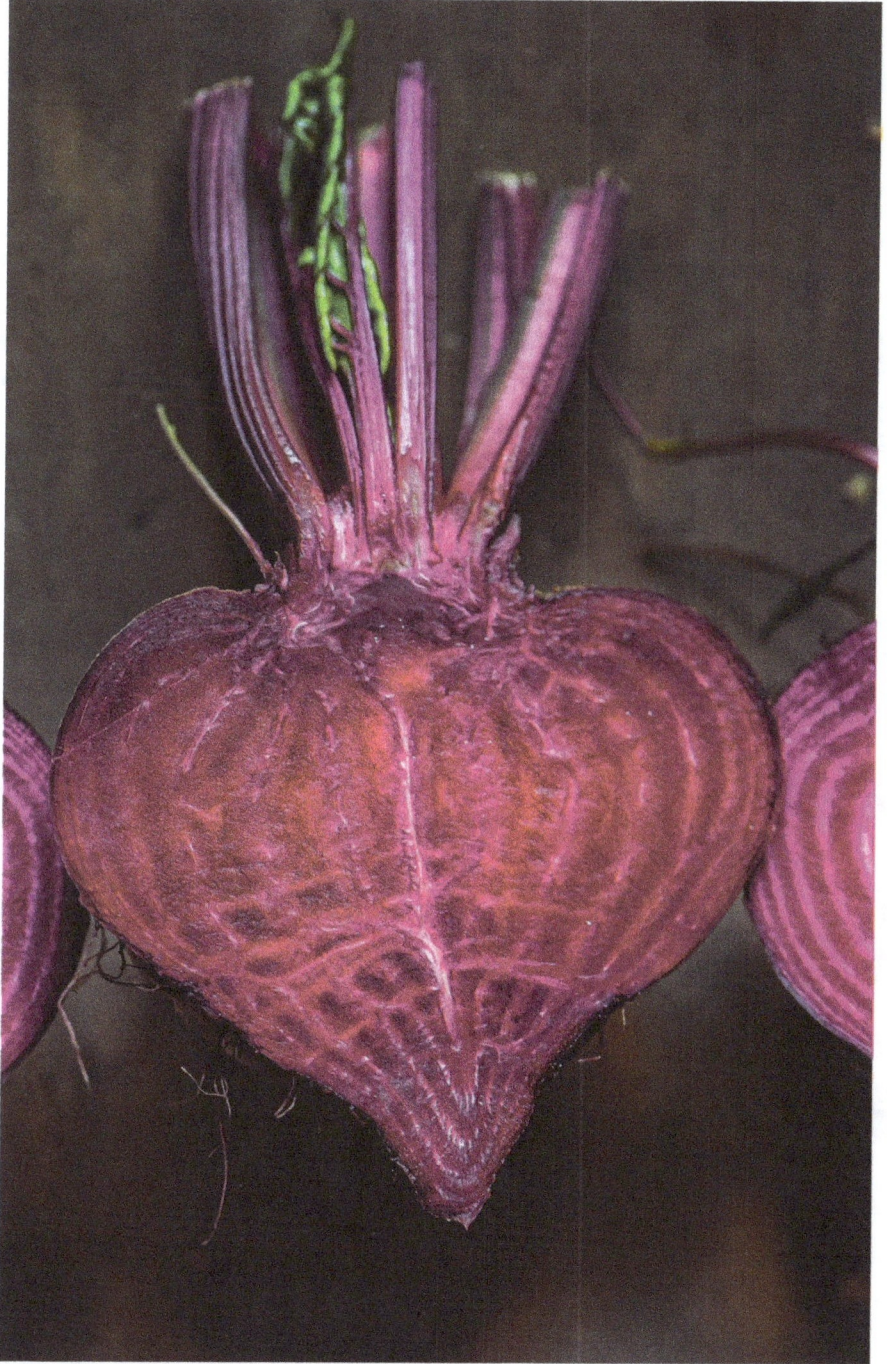

"Delight thyself also in the LORD; and He shall give thee the desires of thine heart" (Psalm 37:4).

This beautiful crimson root aids in the absorption of iron, which is one of its many nutrients. It improves the blood circulation and increases the blood count and oxygen capacity of the erythrocytes. Iron is not only essential for the production of red blood cells but it also helps with low haemoglobin and anaemic conditions. The large amount of iron that beetroot contains assists in the formation of haemagglutinin, which is a part of the blood that helps to transport nutrients and oxygen to various parts of the body. Iron not only helps to battle against disease and conveys oxygen to the cells but is also critical for muscle proteins. The high iron content of beetroot not only has anti-tumour effects but is also designed to regenerate red blood corpuscles that supply more oxygen to cancer cells. This higher oxygen content improves cellular respiration, which helps to kill cancer cells. Other iron-rich foods do not have the same effect as beetroot as its copper content makes the iron more available to the body. Although other foods contain iron, the human body is able to assimilate iron from beetroot more readily than almost any other known food, and researchers suspect that a catalyst in beetroot helps the body to more easily assimilate the available iron.

> *This heart beet not only nourishes the blood and circulatory system but is also one of nature's finest cardiovascular tonics, with its long rootlets having a similar shape to arteries.*

"But if we walk in the light, as He is in the light, we have fellowship one with another, and the blood of Jesus Christ His Son cleanseth us from all sin" (1 John 1:7).

Beetroot contains both soluble and insoluble fibre and there is evidence to suggest that not all dietary fibre is the same. Beetroot and carrot fibre are two specific types of plant fibre that may contribute special health benefits, particularly with respect to the health of the cardiovascular system and digestive tract. The high volume of soluble fibre found in beetroot also feeds the beneficial bacteria in the gut while exerting favourable effects on bowel function, which assists in preventing constipation due to its powerful digestive effects. Beetroot fibre is a nutrient of interest in health research, and some beetroot fibre benefits may be due to the pectin polysaccharides that significantly contribute to the total fibre content. Research provides evidence that some types of beneficial anti-inflammatory gut bacteria may be able to inhibit the development of cancer by slowing or completely halting the progression of some cancer types by reducing not only inflammation but also DNA damage, which are significant factors for causing cancer. The pectin fibre in beetroot can help to flush out toxins that have been removed from the liver and eliminate them from the system instead of their being reabsorbed by the body. It has also been shown to increase the level of anti-oxidant enzymes in the body, specifically glutathione peroxidase.

"O give thanks unto the LORD; for He is good: for His mercy endureth for ever" (Psalm 118:29).

The high concentration of nitrates in beetroot (and largely in other leafy vegetables) is converted to nitric acid within the body, which relaxes and dilates the blood vessels and affects how efficiently the cells use oxygen. This increases a proficient uptake of oxygen during exercise. The vasodilator gas nitric oxide, which is the master signalling molecule of the entire cardiovascular system, travels through the artery walls sending signals to relax to the tiny muscle cells around the arteries. When these tiny muscle cells relax the blood vessels dilate. Sunlight also charges blood vessels, thereby increasing blood flow. When the rays of the sun penetrate the skin it causes an enormous increase of nitric oxide. As much as 60% of the blood can be redirected to the skin's surface through the action of nitric oxide, which assists with the absorption of solar radiation. Nitric oxide is manufactured in the endothelium and diffuses out of the endothelium and into the underlying layer of smooth artery muscle. There it signals the muscles to relax and expand and undergoes a vasodilation process. Beetroot has approximately twenty times more nitrates than most other vegetables, and not only are high concentrations of nitrates found in beetroot but also cabbage, celery, and other leafy green vegetables such as spinach.

"Be of good courage, and He shall strengthen your heart, all ye that hope in the LORD" (Psalm 31:24).

This awesome vegetable is safe for those with diabetes as it contains the antioxidant alpha-lipoic acid, which may help to lower glucose levels, reduce peripheral and autonomic neuropathy, increase insulin sensitivity, and prevent the oxidative stress caused in those with diabetes.

"I will be glad and rejoice in thee: I will sing praise to thy name, O thou most High" (Psalm 9:2).

Beetroot, and especially beetroot greens, are among the small number of foods that contain measurable amounts of oxalates, which are naturally occurring substances found in plants. When oxalates become too concentrated in the fluids of the body they can crystallize and cause stones. Beetroot greens contain levels of oxalates that are about ten times higher in the leaves of the beetroot plant than in the root. The oxalic acid content becomes higher when cooked but enjoying them with fresh lemon juice helps to counteract stone formations.

"Oh that men would praise the LORD for His goodness, and for His wonderful works to the children of men!" (Psalm 107:15).

The consumption of beetroot can cause urine to become pink or red. This condition is known as beeturia and is not considered harmful but may be a potential concern if it involves problems with iron metabolism. Those with iron excess, iron deficiency, or known problems with iron metabolism are more likely to experience beeturia. It can also be a sign of insufficient stomach acid which beetroot can help to correct.

"Iron sharpeneth iron; so a man sharpeneth the countenance of his friend" (Proverbs 27:17).

Beetroot has a high antioxidant and polyphenol content which protects the body from free radical damage. Polyphenols operate as antioxidants which block the action of enzymes that cancer cells need for growth. Beetroot has also been found to increase the production of glutathione, the master antioxidant and detoxifier, which is naturally produced in the body. It is used by virtually every cell of the body to neutralize toxins. The body needs glutathione to protect the liver, eyes, kidneys, skin, and many other organs from toxic by-products that are produced by the body through normal metabolism, and beetroot improves the metabolism. If the body is rich in glutathione from the consumption of beetroot it can perform its essential function of drawing harmful toxins into the colon where they can be eliminated. Without adequate levels of glutathione, many environmental toxins can remain inside the body and possibly cause unwanted health problems. The antioxidants betalain, betanin, and vulgaxanthin in beetroot promote the production of glutathione. Red beetroot has been demonstrated to be an important therapy against X-ray, radioactive damage, and digestive problems. Studies have shown that it inhibits the formation of cancer-causing compounds and is also protective against stomach and colon cancer. In addition to being renowned for being a powerful liver cleanser, it is also excellent for alkalizing the system. Hypochlorhydria is a condition of abnormally low levels of stomach acid and beetroot increases stomach acidity, which is essential for the proper digestion of food and the assimilation of nutrients. Beetroot also contains methionine, which is the only essential amino acid containing sulphur. It is the precursor of the other sulphur-containing amino acids and is essential for the synthesis of proteins and many other biomolecules which are required for optimal health. Research indicates that the daily consumption of beetroot is excellent at breaking down and eliminating cancer-causing poisons. Beetroot has an incredibly strong ability to break up cancer in the body.

"For I am persuaded, that neither death, nor life, nor angels, nor principalities, nor powers, nor things present, nor things to come, Nor height, nor depth, nor any other creature, shall be able to separate us from the love of God, which is in Christ Jesus our Lord" (Romans 8:38, 39).

To fully heal from cancer or other health issues, regaining healthy function of the digestive system and waste elimination is of the utmost importance. Unwanted toxins should be removed from the body and stressful and emotional issues need to be resolved as well as any underlying health conditions.

"If ye abide in me, and my words abide in you, ye shall ask what ye will, and it shall be done unto you" (John 15:7).

Beetroot is a very powerful gift from God to help the body heal itself by supplying nutrients, eliminating toxins, and building up the body naturally.

"For the Lord Himself shall descend from heaven with a shout, with the voice of the archangel, and with the trump of God: and the dead in Christ shall rise first: Then we which are alive and remain shall be caught up together with them in the clouds, to meet the Lord in the air: and so shall we ever be with the Lord. Wherefore comfort one another with these words" (1 Thessalonians 4:16–18).

Summary

"NATURAL FORCES WITHIN US ARE THE TRUE HEALERS OF DISEASE." —HIPPOCRATES

Disease emanates from inflammation, which is not the root cause of disease but is merely a symptom of underlying causes of disease. Inflammation can be a natural, healthy immune response to a perceived threat or a natural, healthy response to cellular damage. Tissue damage cannot heal without an inflammatory response. It can also be a natural response of the body to an infection, which can be caused by organisms such as parasites, viruses, fungi, or bacterium. Inflammation can be acute or chronic and is an attempt of the body to protect itself by signalling the immune system to instigate a healing response and repair and heal damaged tissue. Without the physiological response of inflammation, infections could become deadly. Harmful stimuli can include pathogens, damaged cells, irritants, or anything else that negatively affects the body and elicits a biological acute response in an attempt to remove them. Cells malfunction because of either trauma from an external force or from an internal trauma caused by toxicity or nutritional deficiencies. When a damaged body part is inflamed it is either deteriorating or healing. Inflammatory signs, such as swelling and redness, affirm that the body is attempting to heal itself. Without inflammation, the body cannot heal as it brings nutrition and disease-fighting cells to heal the damaged area. However, chronic inflammation can eventually cause many severe conditions and diseases if it is not kept in check and is simply a failure to eliminate the cause of acute inflammation.

Inflammation has a reason for existing and can be quenched by removing its cause and utilizing anti-inflammatory foods as part of a healthy whole plant-food diet and lifestyle. Candida is typically a root cause of disease. ALL animal products are acid-forming and cause inflammation. In addition to animal products, other causes of inflammation not only include pathogens such as fungi, viruses, parasites, and bacteria but also infections, stress from any cause, various environmental toxins, pollutants, pesticides, heavy metals, root canals, amalgam fillings, an insufficiency or overabundance of sleep, GMOs, artificial sweeteners, drugs, including vaccines, refined grains, smoking, electro-magnetic radiation, intemperance from any cause, artificial colours, flavours and preservatives, alcohol, de-mineralized white salt, excess weight, excitotoxins such as MSG, unhealthy beverages, and any needed chiropractic adjustments. Inflammatory insufficiencies include pure water, healthy salt, exercise, sunshine, fresh air, and adequate nutrients, including adequate healthy fats and antioxidants. Maintaining a high level of vital antioxidants such as vitamins A, C, and E plus Omega-3 fatty acids, the B vitamins (particularly B12) and vitamin D3 will help to ensure a high level of health which will assist with facilitating the prevention and elimination of disease. Symptoms are not a disease but an expression of the innate God-given self-healing design of the body, as the body is constantly striving to be disease-free. If the body receives what it needs to function efficiently and is not subjected to that which is harmful, symptoms should dissipate. Detoxifying is also extremely beneficial for the body and can be undertaken with the help of the foods contained in this book.

"Now therefore stand and see this great thing, which the LORD will do before your eyes" (1 Samuel 12:16).

This is a very simplified explanation of the function of vitamin C when inflammation is present in some vital areas of the body. Inflammation causes pain and adequate vitamin C can extinguish pain. The reason why adequate vitamin C is so effective for many diseases is because of its very powerful antioxidant and anti-inflammatory properties. The protein zonulin is the glue that bonds the epithelial and endothelial cells together to form tight junctions for critical barriers. These barriers line various vital structures in the body including the brain, heart, arteries, veins, capillaries, skin, and the gut. These cells form the extremely important blood-brain barrier, which can become unstuck due to inflammation. Adequate vitamin C together with other antioxidant nutrients and a nutritious whole plant-food diet and healthy lifestyle halts this inflammation, thereby preventing and reversing inflammatory diseases in their tracks. These diseases include mental disorders, where the endothelial cells of the blood-brain barrier become leaky because the zonulin has given way due to inflammation; immune diseases, where the epithelial cells of the gut lining become leaky because the zonulin has given way due to inflammation; And heart disease, hemorrhagic strokes, and aneurysms, where the endothelial cells of the blood vessel lining become leaky because the zonulin has given way due to inflammation. These blood vessel health issues can also be caused by a copper deficiency, which manifests itself in grey, white, or silver hair (unless the hair colour is genetic), as copper is required as a co-factor to manufacture hair pigment. Vitamin C needs to be taken throughout the day in adequate amounts as the human body cannot store it. If the body is inundated with a high amount of toxins, then much higher doses of vitamin C need to be taken much more frequently throughout the day as additional antioxidant molecules will be required to quench higher amounts of free radicals.

The key is to keep inflammation under control with a healthful diet and lifestyle to prevent diseases, including cancer. The body will heal itself if the appropriate conditions are created and the cause of the problem is discontinued. Vitamin C is a life-saving nutrient. Irrespective of what health issue is manifest, the outcome will be favourable if the principles contained in this book are implemented. The preservation of health is much easier than curing disease. Finally, to have spiritual healing with Jesus Christ is more important than anything else, and being at peace with Him is the only true healing.

"And God said, Let the earth bring forth grass, the herb yielding seed, and the fruit tree yielding fruit after his kind, whose seed is in itself, upon the earth: and it was so" (Genesis 1:11).

"Behold, I show you a mystery; We shall not all sleep, but we shall all be changed, In a moment, in the twinkling of an eye, at the last trump: for the trumpet shall sound, and the dead shall be raised incorruptible, and we shall be changed. For this corruptible must put on incorruption, and this mortal must put on immortality. So when this corruptible shall have put on incorruption, and this mortal shall have put on immortality, then shall be brought to pass the saying that is written, Death is swallowed up in victory. O death, where is thy sting? O grave, where is thy victory?" (1 Corinthians 15:51–55).

The Price of Love

In the garden of Gethsemane our Saviour bade us watch and pray.
"Watch and pray dear friends:" He pleads: "It's for your soul Satan intercedes."
But His friend betrayed Him with a kiss, for silver he could not resist.

An angry mob took Him away, when Him His good friend did betray.
Christ could have saved Himself, but no; for Satan is a defeated foe.
Much sport of Him they all did make: not once did He retaliate.

They spat on Him and smote Him too; rejecting One who was so true.
They pulled His hair and knocked Him down, our Saviour, who'll soon wear His crown.
But the angry mob called for His blood, His precious name they'd turned to mud.

They tied Him up and beat Him raw, the whip into His flesh it tore.
Great chunks of flesh came from His back, His bones laid bare when the whip did crack.
Much blood was lost, it made Him weak, but words of love was all He'd speak.

Huge thorns into His brow they sank, it was our cup from which He drank.
Our cup of sin, our cup of woe, our Saviour drank it long ago.
They stripped Him bare, they killed out Lord, because He brought a two edged sword.

They put on Him a gorgeous robe, then mocked Him staggering down the road.
When cross upon His back they laid, His way along the road He made.
He stumbled, fell, and was so weak, our Saviour, who was kind and meek.

They drove huge nails into His hands, that pled with us, making no demands.
Into His feet they drove nails too, the feet that led to paths so true.
What kind of love is this He sends? The kind of love that has no end.

They hung Him there on Calvarys' tree, the One who came to set us free.
Such love for us we'll never know. He reaped the price which we do sow.
Betrayed by friends whom He so loved, while trusting in His Father above.

His mangled form was all they left, so bruised and battered and bereft.
Unrecognized as One who came to take away their guilt and shame.
The prince of love who paid the price, our Saviour, we did sacrifice.

The price of death for us He paid, when in that tomb so dark He laid.
But Gods' dear Son rose from that tomb to take away our sin and doom.
He died that He might set us free. He died for you; He died for me.

Author – THE HOLY SPIRIT through Pauline White.

Resources

Cowan, Thomas. "The Heart Is Not a Pump!" YouTube Video. Accessed June 6, 2021. https://1ref.us/1ou.

_____. "Heart May Not Be a Pump: Thomas Cowan on Cardiovascular Disease." YouTube Video. Accessed June 6, 2021. https://1ref.us/1ov.

Curtis, Ernest. *The Cholesterol Delusion.* Indianapolis: Dog Ear Publishing, LLC, 2010.

Dastani, Mostafa, et al. "The Effects of Curcumin on the Prevention of Atrial and Ventricular Arrhythmias and Heart Failure in Patients with Unstable Angina: A Randomized Clinical Trial." *Avicenna Journal of Phytomedicine 9*, no. 1 (Jan-Feb 2019). Accessed June 6, 2021. https://1ref.us/1p4.

Goldacre, Ben. *Bad Pharma: How Drug Companies Mislead Doctors and Harm Patients.* New York: Farrar, Straus, and Giroux, 2014.

Hazum, E., et al. "Morphine in Cow and Human Milk: Could Dietary Morphine Constitute a Ligand for Specific Morphine (mu) Receptors?" *Science,* August 28, 1981. PubMed. Accessed February 28, 2021. https://1ref.us/1ni.

Informed Consent Action Network (ICAN). News Release July 13, 2018. Accessed June 6, 2021. https://1ref.us/1or.

Lindqvist, P.G., et al. "Avoidance of Sun Exposure as a Risk Factor for Major Causes of Death: A Competing Risk Analysis of the Melanoma in Southern Sweden Cohort." *Journal of Internal Medicine* 280, no. 4 (October 2016). Accessed June 6, 2021. https://1ref.us/1oz.

Llamas, Michelle. "Big Pharma's Role in Clinical Trials." Accessed February 28, 2021. https://1ref.us/1nj.

Marinelli, Ralph, et al. "The Heart Is Not a Pump: A Refutation of the Pressure Propulsion Premise of Heart Function." *Frontier Perspectives* 5, no. 1 (Fall-Winter 1995). Accessed June 6, 2021. https://1ref.us/1ot.

McEwen, B.S. "Stress: Homeostasis, Rheostasis, Reactive Scope, Allostasis and Allostatic Load" in *Reference Module in Neuroscience and Biobehavioral Psychology, 2017.* Accessed June 6, 2021. https://1ref.us/1os.

McKenna, Kyle Christopher. "Use of Aborted Fetal Tissue in Vaccines and Medical Research Obscures the Value of All Human Life." *The Linacre Quarterly* 85, no. 1. Accessed August 4, 2021. https://1ref.us/1pp.

Mercola, Joseph. "How Cells from an Aborted Fetus Are Used to Create Novel Flavor Enhancers." Organic Consumers Association, from Mercola.com, March 17, 2013. Accessed August 4, 2021. https://1ref.us/1pn.

Michaëlsson, Karl, et al. "Milk Intake and Risk of Mortality and Fractures in Women and Men." *BMJ* 2014. Accessed February 28, 2021. https://1ref.us/1nh.

Myer, Stassi. "13 Studies on Coconut Oil and Its Health Effects." Healthline. Accessed June 6, 2021. https://1ref.us/1ox.

"Otto Warburg Biographical." The Nobel Prize. Accessed August 4, 2021. https://1ref.us/1oy.

Peck, Peggy. "FDA Documents Say Drugs Increase Rish of Asthma-Related Death." *MedPage Today* (December 5, 2008). Accessed June 6, 2021. https://1ref.us/1p5.

People for the Ethical Treatment of Animals (PETA). Accessed September 8, 2021. https://1ref.us/1q5.

Perry, Susan, and Jim Dawson. *The Secrets Our Body Clocks Reveal*. United States: Rawson Associates, 1988.

"Prostate Specific Antigen (PSA) Test." National Cancer Institute. Accessed June 6, 2021. https://1ref.us/1p6.

Richardson, Valerie. "Aborted Fetus Cells Used in Beauty Creams." *The Washington Times*, November 3, 2009. Accessed August 4, 2021. https://1ref.us/1po.

Schmidt, Morten, et al. "Non-steroidal Anti-inflammatory Drug Use and Risk of Atrial Fibrillation or Flutter: Population Based Case-control Study." *BMJ* (July 4, 2011). Accessed June 6, 2021. https://1ref.us/1p3.

Scully, Jackie Leach. "What Is a Disease?" EMBO Reports, July 2004. Accessed February 28, 2021. https://1ref.us/1ne.

Stokel, Kirk. "Curcumin Starves Cancer Cells to Death." Urology of Virginia. Accessed June 6, 2021. https://1ref.us/1p0.

Wallace, Alfred Russel. "A Summary of the Proofs that Vaccination Does Not Prevent Small-pox but Really Increases It." National Anti-Vaccination League, 1904. Accessed June 6, 2021. https://1ref.us/1p1.

Zhu, Caroline, et al. "A Review of Traumatic Brain Injury and the Gut Microbiome: Insights into Novel Mechanisms of Secondary Brain Injury and Promising Targets for Neuroprotection." *Brain Sciences* 8, no. 6 (June 2018). Accessed June 6, 2021. https://1ref.us/1p2.

Zong, Geng, et al. "Monounsaturated Fats from Plant and Animal Sources in Relation to Risk of Coronary Heart Disease Among US Men and Women." *The American Journal of Clinical Nutrition* 107, no. 3. Accessed June 6, 2021. https://1ref.us/1ow.

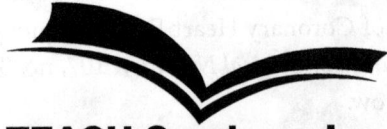

TEACH Services, Inc.

P U B L I S H I N G

We invite you to view the complete
selection of titles we publish at:
www.TEACHServices.com

We encourage you to write us
with your thoughts about this,
or any other book we publish at:
info@TEACHServices.com

TEACH Services' titles may be purchased in
bulk quantities for educational, fund-raising,
business, or promotional use.
bulksales@TEACHServices.com

Finally, if you are interested in seeing
your own book in print, please contact us at:
publishing@TEACHServices.com

We are happy to review your manuscript at no charge.